The Post-Traumatic Stress Disorder Sourcebook

ALSO BY GLENN R. SCHIRALDI:

Conquer Anxiety, Worry and Nervous Fatigue: A Guide to Greater Peace

Building Self-Esteem: A 125-Day Program

Facts to Relax By: A Guide to Relaxation and Stress Reduction

Hope and Help for Depression: A Practical Guide

Stress Management Strategies

The Post-Traumatic Stress Disorder Sourcebook

A Guide to Healing, Recovery, and Growth

Glenn R. Schiraldi, Ph.D.

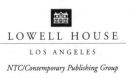

LOWELL HOUSE

LOS ANGELES

NTC/Contemporary Publishing Group

The Post-Traumatic Stress Disorder Sourcebook is intended solely for educational and informational purposes and not as medical advice. Please consult a medical or mental health professional if you have any questions about your health.

Library of Congress Cataloging-in-Publication Data
Schiraldi, Glenn R. 1947–
    The post-traumatic stress disorder sourcebook: a guide to healing, recovery, and growth / Glenn R. Schiraldi
      p. cm.
    Includes bibliographical references and index.
    ISBN: 0-7373-0265-8 (alk. paper)
    1. Post-traumatic stress disorder. I. Title.
RC552.P67 S3226 1999
616.85'21—dc21   99-047837

"River of Feelings" from *Peace Is Every Step* by Thich Nhat Hanh. Copyright © 1991 by Thich Nhat
    Hanh. Used by permission of Bantam Books, a division of Random House, Inc.
"Principles of Recovery" from *More Help For Your Nerves* by Claire Weekes. Copyright © 1986 by
    Claire Weekes. Used by permission of Bantam Books, a division of Random House, Inc.
Excerpts from *Trauma and Dreams* edited by Deirdre Barrett. Copyright © 1996 by the President and
    Fellows of Harvard College. Reprinted by permission of Harvard University Press.
"The Elderly Child Remembers" and "Normalizing the Genital Area" reprinted with permission of The
    Free Press, a Division of Simon & Schuster, Inc. from *Treating Traumatized Children, New Insights
    and Creative Interventions* by Beverly James. Copyright © 1989 by Lexington Books.

Published by Lowell House
A division of NTC/Contemporary Publishing Group, Inc.
4255 West Touhy Avenue, Lincolnwood, Illinois 60712-1975 U.S.A.

Printed in the United States of America

International Standard Book Number: 0-7373-0265-8

03 04 RRD 18 17 16 15 14 13 12 11 10 9 8 7 6

Contents

APPENDICES

Acknowledgments

In recent years, so much has been learned about post-traumatic stress disorder (PTSD). No one compiles a synthesis such as this one without relying on the cumulative efforts of many brilliant theorists, researchers, and clinicians who have advanced our understanding of PTSD and its treatment. I am grateful to dissociation pioneers Drs. Pierre Janet, Richard P. Kluft, Frank W. Putnam, and Richard J. Loewenstein. I am thankful to Drs. Bessel van der Kolk for his insights regarding the brain and trauma, George S. Everly, Jr., Charles R. Figley, Edna B. Foa, Judith L. Herman, Mardi Horowitz, Donald Meichenbaum, James W. Pennebaker, Beverly Raphael, Francine Shapiro, John P. Wilson, and many others who have so diligently labored to further our knowledge.

I am most grateful for those who gave so generously of their time to review this book and suggest helpful improvements. These include Drs. Bethany Brand, Charles R. Figley, George S. Everly, Jr., Donald Meichenbaum, Raymond M. Scurfield, Francine Shapiro, Mary Beth Williams, John P. Wilson; and Robert L. Bunnell, John W. Downs, Esther Giller, and Mary Beth Quist.

Finally, I am exceedingly grateful to the survivors of trauma—in all walks of life—who have battled to overcome their symptoms, and by their courage inspired us all.

Portions of this book have been adapted from some of my previous works: *Conquer Anxiety, Worry and Nervous Fatigue: A Guide to Greater Peace; Building Self-Esteem: A 125-Day Program; Facts to Relax By: A Guide to Relaxation and Stress Reduction; Hope and Help for Depression: A Practical Guide;* and *Stress Management Strategies.*

The book provides information on the most promising treatment approaches for post-traumatic stress disorder. It will likely inform you and help you make wise decisions regarding your healing, recovery, and growth. However, this book is not a substitute for treatment by a qualified mental health professional, when such help is needed.

Pace yourself when reading this book so as not to become overwhelmed. The treatment approaches described herein can be very effective if properly timed, paced, and applied within the context of a sound working relationship with a skilled mental health professional. Conversely, some approaches (sometimes even certain symptom management approaches), when applied too early, too fast, or alone, might actually increase symptoms. A skilled therapist can help ensure that issues of pacing and safety are attended to, while helping to provide perspective amidst the complexities of recovery. If in doubt, discuss any questions you have with a mental health professional specializing in post-traumatic stress disorder before attempting any approach described herein.

Finally, research regarding the treatment of PTSD is in its early stages. As yet no one treatment approach has been shown to be superior to any other for all people. Thus, it is important that survivors and clinicians be informed about the range of treatment options so that they can make the best decisions possible about the treatment or combination of treatment approaches.

Introduction

We are never prepared for what we expect.
—James A. Michener, Caravans

A firefighter cradles a lifeless little girl. Seven months later he leaves his beloved profession because of post-traumatic stress disorder (PTSD). In a dimly-lit campus parking lot, a bright coed is assaulted. Three weeks later she drops out of college. PTSD has claimed yet another victim.

Life doesn't prepare us for trauma. Following exposure to traumatic events, millions of people develop PTSD, or lesser forms of this condition—with symptoms ranging from nightmares to headaches, flashbacks, withdrawing from people, profound sadness, anxiety, anger, guilt, fatigue, pessimism, sexual problems, and emotional numbing. Unless proper treatment is found, many, perhaps most, of these people will secretly and needlessly battle distressing symptoms for life. The good news, however, is that PTSD can be treated successfully. With the right treatment, victims can begin to heal and return to the journey of joyful living.

This book is written for all victims of trauma. You will find it useful if you are a survivor of rape, abuse of any kind, domestic violence, war, crime, natural disasters, industrial disasters, accidents, terrorism, and other traumatic events. It will also be helpful to those whose work exposes them to trauma. Such professions include police officers, fire fighters, rescue and disaster workers, military service personnel, emergency medical service workers, paramedics, physicians, and nurses. The book will help you understand the changes that traumatic events cause in people, the process of recovery, and the full range of treatment options. In addition, this book will be of great use to concerned friends, family, and health professionals who associate with survivors of traumatic events.

If you are a survivor, the book will involve you in your own healing and help you to take control of your recovery process. It will also help you to recognize your limitations, determine if help is needed, and find the right help. Once you understand the promising range of treatment options available, you will be better able to choose the best ones for you and benefit from their use. Should you decide to seek the services of a mental health professional, this book will be a valuable resource to you both.

In one sense, PTSD is described by great emotional upheaval and the shattering of the soul. From another view, however, PTSD is also the story of courage, determination, resilience, and the ultimate triumph of the human spirit. Today there is much cause for hope. People with PTSD *can* be helped. We now know many ways to lessen the great suffering caused by traumatic events, to help victims deal more comfortably with lingering or recurrent symptoms, and to help them move beyond the trauma. It seems that these words apply especially to this book:

> Pain is a great teacher. Yet the greatest teacher imparts little wisdom if the student has not eyes to see and ears to hear. I write this so that we may benefit from our suffering and triumph over our pain . . . and in the process become better, stronger, warmer, more compassionate, deeper, happier human beings—realizing that the ultimate value of pain reduction is not comfort, but growth.[1]

The goal of this book, then, is to help you move beyond survival, toward the realm of living well. Because you are certainly more than a survivor . . . and much more than just a victim.

The book is organized as follows: Part I explains all about PTSD. You'll understand that the symptoms you are experiencing make sense, and that you are not going crazy. You'll understand anxiety, dissociation, memory networks, and triggers. And you'll get answers to commonly asked questions.

Part II explains that healing, recovery, and growth are possible. You'll understand the principles of treatment and healing, and the broad types of treatment approaches that are available.

Part III prepares you for healing and recovery. You'll be guided to establish physical and emotional safety, and to take care of important needs.

In Part IV you will learn how to manage troubling symptoms of PTSD so that you can be more comfortable and progress more successfully and confidently in treatment.

Part V explains the broad range of treatment options that are available to you. Chapters 19 to 22 explain important basic principles and skills for neutralizing traumatic memories, including changing commonly held negative and guilt-promoting thoughts. You'll learn how confiding traumatic wounds begins the healing process. Promising newer therapeutic approaches are described in chapters 23 to 27. These are applied under the direction of a therapist; however, you'll know what to ask for and will tend to be more comfortable with these approaches once you've read about them. Chapters 28 to 39 describe other important approaches to healing. Some approaches, such as those in chapters 29, 33, and 38 are applied under the direction of a therapist. Other chapters will be useful to discuss in a therapeutic setting and/or to try as homework under a therapist's direction. The reminder is constant: read for understanding—there is power in being informed. If there is any doubt about what to apply or when, discuss your questions with a trauma specialist before attempting anything in this book.

Part VI will help you move beyond PTSD and grow despite your experience with trauma. We'll explore positive aspects of living including intimacy, sexuality, meaning and purpose, spiritual and religious satisfaction, happiness, pleasure, and humor. And finally, you'll be shown how to plan for setbacks and cope with them confidently.

Finally, a range of appendices will direct you to additional important information, including a very comprehensive resource list.

Read this book with hope, for indeed there is good reason to hope. Remain committed to your well-being and to the enjoyment of life, and you will become a more valuable resource to others and to yourself.

PART I

About PTSD

CHAPTER 1

PTSD Basics

Humpty Dumpty sat on a wall

Humpty Dumpty had a great fall

All the king's horses and all the king's men

Couldn't put Humpty Dumpty together again

WHAT IS PTSD?

Post-traumatic stress disorder (PTSD) results from exposure to an overwhelmingly stressful event or series of events, such as war, rape, or abuse. It is a normal response by normal people to an abnormal situation.

The traumatic events that lead to PTSD are typically so extraordinary or severe that they would distress almost anyone. These events are usually sudden. They are perceived as dangerous to self or others, and they overwhelm our ability to respond adequately.[2]

We say that PTSD is a normal response to an abnormal event because the condition is completely understandable and predictable. The symptoms make perfect sense because what happened has overwhelmed normal coping responses.

THE HUMAN FACE

In another sense, however, the mental and physical suffering in PTSD is beyond the range of normalcy and indicates a need for assistance.[3] People with PTSD call to mind the Humpty Dumpty nursery rhyme. They often report feeling:

- shattered, broken, wounded, ripped, or torn apart
- like they'll never get put back together
- bruised to the soul, devastated, fallen apart, crushed

- shut down, beaten down, beaten up
- changed: I used to be happy-go-lucky, now I'm serious and quiet; My life seems to be divided into two periods: before the trauma and after; It really threw me; my life was derailed; nothing seems sacred or special anymore.
- as though they are in a deep black hole, damaged, ruined, different from everybody else, losing their mind, going crazy, doomed, dead inside, "on the sidelines of life's games"[4]

WHAT CAUSES PTSD?

As Table 1.1 indicates, PTSD could be caused by a wide range of events, grouped into three categories. As a general rule, Intentional Human causes are the most difficult to recover from,[5] followed by Unintentional Human causes. Acts of Nature are the least complex and typically resolve more quickly than the other categories.

WHAT SPECIFICALLY IS PTSD?

A trauma is a wound. PTSD refers to deep emotional wounds. In 1980, following the Vietnam experience, the American Psychiatric Association formally defined PTSD, categorizing it as one of the anxiety disorders. Table 1.2 lists the diagnostic criteria, or requirements for determining if one has PTSD, as described in the *Diagnostic and Statistical Manual* (DSM) of the American Psychiatric Association. A discussion of these criteria will follow.

DSM CRITERIA EXPLAINED

At first, PTSD might seem quite confusing. However, you'll soon realize that the symptoms are very understandable. They make sense, and seeing this is, in itself, somewhat curative. The explanations that follow will help to clarify these criteria.

Exposure to Stressor

PTSD is the only DSM condition where the occurrence of a stressor is part of the diagnosis. Unlike other anxiety disorders that are simply described by their symptoms, PTSD requires the occurrence of a catastrophic event. You might wish to refer again to Table 1.1 for a listing of such events. PTSD can result from any severe stressor, and the symptoms are similar if the stressors are severe enough.

Table 1.1
POTENTIALLY TRAUMATIC EVENTS/STRESSORS

I. **Intentional Human (man-made, deliberate, malicious)**
  - Combat, civil war, resistance fighting
  - Abuse
    - sexual—incest; rape; forced nudity, exhibitionism, or pornography; inappropriate touching/fondling or kissing
    - physical—beating, kicking, battering, choking, tying up, stalking, forcing to eat/drink, threatening with weapon, elder abuse by own children
    - emotional—isolation, threats to leave or have affair, intimidation, degrading names, economic neglect, minimizing or denying abuse, taking away power/control, destroying property, torturing pets, neglect (leaving alone, not feeding or bathing)[6]
  - Torture (the worst form is sexual because it combines physical, emotional, and spiritual cruelty)
  - Criminal assault, violent crime, robbery, mugging, family violence/battery
  - Hostage, POW, concentration camp, hijacking
  - Cult abuse
  - Terrorism
  - Bombing (e.g., Hiroshima, Oklahoma City)
  - Witnessing a homicide, sexual assault, battering, torture, etc.
  - Sniper attack
  - Kidnapping
  - Riots
  - Participating in violence/atrocities (e.g., Nazi doctors, soldiers, identifying with the aggressor)
  - Witnessing parents' fear reactions
  - Alcoholism (due to its effects on family members)
  - Suicide or other form of sudden death
  - Death threats
  - Damage to or loss of body part

II. **Unintentional Human (accidents, technological disasters)**
  - Industrial (e.g., a crane crashes down)
  - Fires, burns (e.g., oil rig fire)
  - Explosion
  - Motor vehicle accidents, plane crash, train wreck, boating accidents, shipwreck
  - Nuclear disaster (e.g., Chernobyl, Three Mile Island)
  - Collapse of sports stadium, building, dam, or sky walk
  - Surgical damage to body or loss of body part

III. **Acts of Nature/Natural Disasters**
  - Hurricane
  - Typhoons
  - Tornado
  - Flood
  - Earthquake
  - Avalanche
  - Volcanic eruption
  - Fire
  - Drought, famine
  - Attack by animal (such as a pit bull)
  - Sudden life-threatening illness (e.g., heart attack, severe burns)
  - Sudden death (e.g., loss of unborn child)

Table 1.2
PTSD DIAGNOSTIC CRITERIA*

A. **Exposure to Stressor.** The person must be exposed to a traumatic event involving both of the following:

(1) person experienced, saw, or learned of event(s) that involved actual or threatened death, serious injury, or violation of the body of self or others

(2) person's response involved intense fear, helplessness, or horror (in children, the response may involve disorganized or agitated behavior)

B. **Event Re-experienced.** The trauma is persistently re-experienced in at least one of the following ways:

(1) recurrent, intrusive recollections of event (images, thoughts, or perceptions—in children repetitive play may express themes or aspects of the event)

(2) recurrent, distressing dreams of event (children may have no recognizable content in dreams)

(3) acting or feeling as if the trauma were recurring (sense of reliving, illusions, hallucinations, and dissociative flashback episodes, including those on awakening or when intoxicated—children may reenact the trauma)

(4) intense psychological distress upon exposure to internal or external cues that symbolize or resemble an aspect of the trauma

(5) physiological reactivity upon exposure to such cues

C. **Avoidance.** Persistent avoidance of stimuli associated with the trauma and numbing of general responsiveness that was not present before the trauma, as indicated by at least three of the following:

(1) efforts to avoid thoughts, feelings, or conversations that remind one of the trauma

(2) efforts to avoid activities, places, or people that arouse recollections

(3) inability to recall an important aspect of the trauma

(4) markedly diminished interest or participation in significant activities that used to be pleasurable

(5) feeling of detachment/estrangement from others

(6) restricted range of affect (e.g., can't have loving feelings, especially those associated with intimacy, tenderness, or sexuality)

(7) sense of foreshortened future (e.g., does not expect to have career, marriage, children, or normal life span)

D. **Arousal.** Persistent symptoms of increased arousal that were not present before the trauma. At least two of the following occur:

(1) difficulty falling or staying asleep

(2) irritability or outbursts of anger

(3) difficulty concentrating

(4) hypervigilance

(5) exaggerated startle response

E. **Duration of symptoms in Criteria B, C, and D is more than one month.**

F. **Life Disrupted.** The disturbance causes clinically significant distress or impairment in social, occupational, or other important areas of functioning.

Reprinted with permission (with slight adaptation) from the Diagnostic and Statistical Manual of Mental Disorders. 4th ed. Copyright © 1994 American Psychiatric Association.

Thus, the PTSD resulting from rape or violent crime is quite similar in appearance to the PTSD resulting from combat.

Of the three categories of stressors in Table 1.1, Intentional Human traumas are usually the worst. PTSD symptoms resulting from such stressors are usually more complex, are of longer duration, and are more difficult to treat for a number of reasons. Such traumas are typically the most degrading and cause the most shame. They often involve feelings of being stigmatized, marked, different, or an outcast (as in rape). Man-made traumas also are most likely to cause people to lose faith and trust in humanity, in love, and in themselves. By contrast, natural disasters are, typically, less difficult to recover from. Survivors often bond. Often heroism and community support is evident. Survivors often feel a reverence or awe for nature that leaves faith in humanity intact.

Categories may be combined in traumatic stress. For example, a hurricane (a natural disaster) might cause the collapse of improperly built homes (unintentional or intentional trauma).

We shall discuss the next three symptom groups in the sequence in which they logically occur (B, D, C). That is, people re-experience the trauma in distressing ways, and become very aroused as a result. They then make various attempts to avoid the PTSD symptoms.

Event Re-experienced

In one sense, PTSD can be viewed as a fear of the unpleasant memories of the traumatic event that repeatedly intrude into one's awareness. Intrusive recollections can occur in the form of thoughts, images, or perceptions. These intrusions are unwelcome, uninvited, and painful, and the person wishes that they could put a stop to them. They often elicit feelings of fear and vulnerability, rage at the cause, sadness, disgust, or guilt. Sometimes they break through when one is trying to relax and one's guard is down. Sometimes a trigger that reminds one of the trauma will start the intrusions. For example, a survivor of a Russian prisoner-of-war camp often daydreams, absorbed in unpleasant memories and out of touch with his surroundings. A number of cues can trigger this re-experience, including thin soup, walking in the woods, Russian music, a harsh rebuke by a supervisor, or any unpleasant confrontation.[7] Sometimes there is no apparent connection to the thoughts or feelings that are replayed.

Nightmares are a common form of re-experiencing the trauma. The nightmares might be fairly accurate replays of the traumatic event, or they might symbolically depict the trauma with themes of threats, rescuing self or others, being trapped or chased by monsters, or dying.

Flashbacks are a particularly upsetting form of re-experiencing the traumatic event. In flashbacks, we feel that we are going back in time and reliving the trauma. Typically, flashbacks are visual re-experiences. However, they can also involve sensations, behavior, or emotions. For example, a war veteran hits the ground when a car backfires, sees a battle recurring, begins to hear sounds of battle, and feels hot, sweaty, and terrified. Later, he does not remember the incident. Flashbacks can last from seconds to hours, and even days. They are usually believed to be real, then forgotten, but sometimes the person will realize that the flashback was not reality. Flashbacks are often triggered by insomnia, fatigue, stress, or drugs.[8]

Experiencing the intrusive memories is very distressful, both psychologically and physically. Although one might not realize that a cue triggers the distress that accompanies intrusive thoughts, some searching can usually find a trigger. The trigger might be either a cue in the environment, such as the backfiring car that reminded the veteran of gunfire, or an internal trigger, such as a nauseous feeling that is similar to one experienced after a rape.

Arousal

Like other anxiety disorders, PTSD is characterized by extreme general physical arousal, and/or arousal following exposure to internal or external triggers. The nervous system has become *sensitized* by an overwhelming trauma. Thus, two things happen. General arousal becomes elevated, while the nervous system overreacts to even smaller stressors. Signs of arousal include:

- Troubled sleep includes difficulty falling or staying asleep, twitching, moving and/or awakening unrested. Awakenings may be due to nightmares. Fear of nightmares might then lead to fear of going to sleep, especially if one was violated in bed.[9]
- Irritability or outbursts of anger might be displayed as smashing things, heated arguing, flying off the handle, screaming, intense criticizing, or impatience. Unresolved anger is fatiguing. It might be mixed with shame, frustration, betrayal, or other uncomfortable emotions that lead to moodiness and explosions of pent-up anger. One might then feel embarrassed or guilty.
- Difficulty concentrating or remembering. It is difficult to concentrate and remember when one is still battling for control of intrusive memories.

- Hypervigilance. People who have endured a trauma will be on guard against intrusive memories. They are also likely to be unusually cautious to ensure that further injury does not occur. Hypervigilance might be demonstrated as:
  - feeling vulnerable, fearful of lots of things, unable to feel calm in safe places
  - fear of repetition
  - anticipating disaster: needing to sit in the corner of a room with back to the wall—looking for exits, places to hide (one fireman carried around a fire extinguisher for a year after being burned by a petroleum ball)[10]
  - rapid scanning, looking over one's shoulder
  - keeping a weapon or several weapons
  - being overprotective or overcontrolling of loved ones
- Exaggerated startle response means you are easily frightened. A sensitized nervous system will overreact to frightening or even unusual stressors. Thus, one might jump, flinch, or tense when someone appears suddenly or from behind, when a sudden noise occurs, when someone wakes you up when sleeping, or when someone touches you. Eye blinking may become more rapid. One who was struck in a head-on car accident will now jerk the steering wheel when she sees another car approaching.[11]

In addition to the above symptoms, symptoms of a sensitized nervous system might include:

- elevation of certain stress hormones in the blood[12]
- elevated heart rate (either resting or in response to stress)
- elevated blood pressure
- hyperventilation (i.e., expelling CO_2 too fast, usually caused by rapid, shallow "chest breathing," but can also result from deep breathing); tight chest or stomach
- lightheadedness
- sweating
- tingling, cold, or sweaty hands

These might occur generally, or in response to a trigger.

Avoidance (Numbing)

Because the intrusive thoughts and accompanying arousal are so unpleasant, people with PTSD desperately try to avoid all reminders of the trauma. They might refuse to talk about it. They might block from their mind thoughts, images, or feelings about the event. They might avoid activities, places, people, or keepsakes that arouse recollections. Some might become housebound in attempts to avoid fearful encounters. Some turn to drugs or overwork to avoid their painful feelings, while others simply shut down all feelings in order to avoid their pain. Some live in a fantasy world, trying to pretend that nothing bad happened.[13]

Some shut out memories of painful periods in their lives (amnesia). Thus, one cannot remember when their spouse died in a car accident. Another who was abused has gaps in her memory of childhood.

When memories are so painful, it makes sense that one would try to numb them. However, one cannot numb painful memories without also numbing joyful memories. One must suppress *all* feelings in order to numb painful feelings. So people with PTSD often avoid even pleasant activities, including those that were pleasurable before the trauma—such as travel, babies, hobbies, or relaxation. You might hear people say, "I don't know how to have fun or play anymore." Without feelings, these people naturally feel uninvolved with life.

Not surprisingly, people with PTSD commonly feel detached or estranged from others. People who have endured combat, rape, disaster work, and other forms of trauma often assume that they are now different and that no one could possibly relate to their experiences. They might feel that they can't tell others about what happened or what they did for fear of judgment, and the secrets and fear of being shunned leads to their feeling disconnected from others. Because they no longer feel comfortable in social situations, they might avoid gatherings—or they might go but find no pleasure in them. Of course, to connect with others, people need to be emotionally open. This is difficult when one is still struggling to contain memories of the past.

Restricted range of affect refers to the "psychic numbing" or "emotional anesthesia" that one does to try to escape from the painful memories. As we mentioned, anything that numbs pain acts as a general anesthesia. Thus, one with PTSD might have trouble laughing, crying, or loving. Feeling numb and closed down, this person might wrongly assume they have lost their capacity to feel or be compassionate, intimate, tender, or sexual. Certain family or work environments such as the military or emergency service work might encourage the suppression of feelings. However, at some point the healthy experience and expression of grief and pain must occur if one is to become a healthy emotional person.

As trauma can lead one to feel disconnected from others, it can also lead one to feel disconnected from his or her future. This is called *a sense of foreshortened future*, which means that trauma victims can't envision or look forward to a normal, happy life. They might not expect to have a career, marriage, children, community connections, or a normal life span—so it is difficult to make plans for the future. Instead, their pessimistic expectations for the future might include disasters, repetition of the trauma, dying young, or simply finding no joy. This outlook has been called the "doomsday orientation"—no matter how good life seems, trouble is coming.[14] Said one with PTSD, "I can't get past the past, so how can I think about the future?" If people are stuck in the past—preoccupied with unresolved pain, guilt, anger, grief, or fear and desperately trying to block these feelings out—they will often lack the energy or interest to plan for the future. If they worry that intrusive memories can spoil their moods at will, they will hardly make plans for a joyful future. Said another with PTSD, "I placed my memories behind prison doors and stand guard. I realized, however, that it is I who is the prisoner. I am so tired of standing guard that I no longer seem to care." It is a sad irony that when one tries to block out the past, one blocks out both the present and future as well.

Duration

The symptom picture described in B, C, and D must persist for at least one month for a diagnosis of PTSD. PTSD is specified as *acute* if the diagnosis resolves within three months, *chronic* if the diagnosis persists beyond three months, and *delayed* if the onset of PTSD occurs at least six months after exposure to the stressor. It has been observed that a large percentage of PTSD cases improve considerably within three months.

Impaired Social and Occupational Functioning

The diagnosis of PTSD means that symptoms are significantly interfering with your relationships or work. Communication is disrupted by numbing, pulling inward, avoiding people and social situations, or by hostility and anger. Work suffers due to absenteeism, fatigue, or impaired concentration.

CHAPTER 2

Making Sense of the Bewildering Symptoms
Understanding Anxiety and Dissociation

This chapter describes two of the major symptoms of PTSD—anxiety and dissociation, to include the role of memory networks and the triggering of trauma-related memories.

ANXIETY

PTSD is considered an anxiety disorder. Many of PTSD's arousal symptoms are common to anxiety. There is no mystery about this condition. Anxiety is comprised of worrisome thoughts plus excessive emotional and physical arousal.

Normally, when the brain perceives a threat, it sets off a chain of physical changes that prepare the body for fight or flight. Messages are sent via nerves and blood-borne hormones to the body's various organs. Muscles tense, the heart beats faster and more strongly, and the rate of breathing increases. The brain becomes sharper and able to react more quickly. This is called the *stress response,* or just stress. Stress is very adaptive in the short-term. It prepares the body for emergencies. The energy of the stress response is designed to be worked off physically; the body then returns to the resting state.

In anxiety, the mind stays vigilant, ever on alert. This, in turn, keeps emotions and the body aroused. Chronic or severe arousal changes the nervous system. We say that the nervous system becomes *sensitized* from overstimulation. The brain's alarm centers stay on alert and sound the alarm for smaller threats than usual, while the body takes longer to return to the resting state. A traumatic event (or even an overload of smaller stressors) can change the structure and function of nerve cells. The amounts of neurotransmitters (chemical messengers) in the brain can change, as can the number of receptor sites for these chemicals on the nerves. A vicious cycle is set off whereby worry maintains physical and emotional arousal and arousal maintains worry. It feels like worry and arousal cannot be shut off. Anxiety seems to take on a life of its own, and is not always proportional to what is going on in your life. Anxiety accounts for a bewildering array of symptoms:

- *physical*: tension, fatigue, trembling, tingling, nausea, digestive tract problems, hyperventilation (rapid breathing), pounding heart, suffocating feelings, even panic attacks
- *emotional fatigue*: irritation, moodiness, fear, exaggerated emotions, loss of confidence
- *mental fatigue*: confusion, inability to concentrate, remember, or make decisions
- *spiritual fatigue*: discouragement, hopelessness, despair

The symptoms of anxiety are merely an exaggerated stress response. They lessen as we retrain our nervous system to be calmer. They increase as we tell ourselves that they are unbearable and must stop.

Avoidance is a hallmark of anxiety. We try to flee the things that trigger it. This brings temporary relief, but at quite a cost. First, we maintain the fear of the triggers. We don't allow ourselves to let the fear in and watch it subside as we relax. So we don't learn to master our fears. Each time avoidance is rewarded with short-term anxiety reduction, we will tend to use it again in the future. The distractions that we use to escape the fear, such as work, will become associated with the fear through conditioning. Soon the distractions become triggers by association. The antidote to avoidance is to face the things we fear and flow with the symptoms until the stress response runs its course and we retrain our nervous system to be less reactive. This is learned in a gradual fashion.

Although PTSD is considered an anxiety disorder, also viewing it as a dissociative disorder helps us to better understand the symptoms. In order to understand dissociation, let's first understand normal "associated" consciousness.

NORMAL "ASSOCIATED" CONSCIOUSNESS

In normal consciousness or awareness, people are fully engaged in life's experiences. They are mindful of their surroundings, are tuned in to people, and feel all their feelings. Despite feeling various emotions or being in different situations, they always feel like the same person. When normal memories are triggered or intentionally retrieved, they can examine them and then put them away at will. Distractions from present awareness are either pleasant or at least controllable. For example, if you are paying your bills and your mind drifts off to Bermuda, you can bring your mind back to the task at hand if you choose to. If adding numbers brings back an unpleasant memory of failing math, you might think about it for a moment and then bring your focus back quickly to the bills.[15] In other words, your mind functions in a smooth, integrated way. Memories are filed away in an organized way. They can be retrieved and smoothly put away again.

DISSOCIATION

Have you ever observed an antelope clamped in a lion's jaws? It seems to stop struggling as its consciousness shifts. Where does its consciousness go?[16] There seems to be an innate mechanism—called *dissociation*—that allows mammals to temporarily escape distressing experiences. Thus, we can mentally escape a present distressing experience, as the antelope did, by mentally "going away." Or, we can temporarily escape a traumatic memory by separating and walling off the memory. Instead of being smoothly connected to all other memories, the highly charged traumatic memories become dissociated or isolated. While the memory may be walled off for awhile, it is not filed in long-term memory. Instead of taking its place alongside other memories on file, the traumatic memory remains "on the desktop" where it repeatedly intrudes upon awareness and cannot, it seems, be put away for long. Dissociated traumatic memory material is said to be walled off, split off, fragmented, separated off, or compartmentalized such that the information does not become integrated with the rest of one's memory material, nor is it fully connected to present awareness.

Traumatic memories contain many aspects: thoughts, images, feelings, behaviors, and physical sensations. Wrapped up in the trauma material may be a unique sense of identity, or who you are, since people often feel very different during the trauma. So you might feel like a different person since the trauma or when traumatic memories intrude into your awareness.

MEMORY NETWORKS

A simplified picture helps to show how associated and dissociated memories are stored in the brain (see Figure 2.1).

Figure 2.1
AWARENESS AND MEMORY

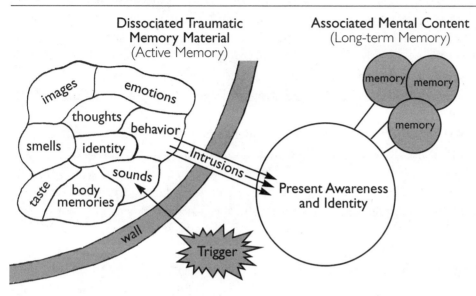

Associated Mental Content

On the right of the wall is normal *associated* mental material. Normal memories are smoothly connected or integrated. Lessons learned and useful ideas from previous life experiences can be blended into present awareness and coping efforts. So a person who has had a very safe and secure childhood might approach a new challenge with the thought, "I'm safe; I'll probably be alright." Across all memories is the sense that you are the same person. Scientists have learned that under normal conditions various parts of the brain are activated to process memories in an organized way (see Appendix 3). That is, the brain connects diverse aspects of a single memory to form an integrated whole. That memory is also filed alongside other memories in a way that a person can place it in time and space. Normal memories are processed logically and verbally. They are understood and make sense, and are then filed away. Although the memories contain appropriate emotions, they can be recalled without overwhelming emotion.

Dissociated Traumatic Memory Material

On the left is *dissociated* trauma material. Notice several aspects of this material.

The "walled off" material is highly unstable. The parts of the brain that would normally file traumatic memories in long-term storage were overwhelmed during the trauma. So traumatic memories remain near the forefront of awareness, easily triggered by reminders of the trauma—or even things associated with the *trigger*. For example, a woman who was raped on an elevator two years ago now re-experiences terror when she approaches any elevator. Since she got into the elevator after parking her car, parking garages have also become frightening. In fact, she feels frightened almost any time she parks her car, even when outside. A new association has been formed between the elevator and the act of parking. Now either can trigger intrusive memories. Sometimes traumatic memories can be triggered by stressful emotions that might seem unrelated to the trauma. For example, a firefighter "trapped" in traffic remembers being helpless to rescue a child in a burning building; one who was abused as a child experiences intrusive memories when his boss criticizes him. These are called *state-dependent memories*, and the process called *mood-dependent retrieval*. A trigger may or may not be obvious as it passes through our awareness.

The "wall" is highly permeable. It is like a leaky dam. We expend much energy trying to maintain the wall, but memories keep seeping through, into awareness.

The dissociated material is highly emotional and relatively nonverbal. Unlike normal memories which are rather logically and verbally processed before storage, trauma material is walled off prior to complete processing. If verbal processing is done at all it is usually quite incomplete, and thoughts related to the trauma will usually be automatic, unspoken, unchallenged, and disorganized. During a trauma a person might have thought, "I am completely vulnerable." Now any stressful situation automatically triggers the same thought. The person may not even be aware of the unspoken thought. Instead, she just feels the intense emotions resulting from the thought. In this case, the very ideas that would help the person cope with traumatic memories are already stored in the associated memories. Normally, for example, she knows that all situations are not unsafe, especially when proper precautions are taken. However, the intrusive traumatic material, separated from this adaptive thinking, dominates her experience.

Trauma material is not only walled off from associated adaptive material, but the traumatic memory itself might be fragmented into various aspects. The aspects of memory include thoughts, images, emotions, behavior, identity, and physical sensations. Physical sensations include sounds, smells, tastes, and "body memories" (tactile or touch sensations, pain, and kinesthetic—the sensation of movement, tension, or position). Because of this fragmentation, a trigger does not usually set off all aspects of a memory. For instance, emotions from a traumatic memory might flood awareness without images or other memory aspects. Sheila was enjoying dinner with a group of friends. She became unaccountably anxious and sick to her stomach. She didn't realize that a man in the group was wearing the same cologne as the man who raped her. In this case, only fragments of the unprocessed memory (i.e., the emotions and physical sensations) were triggered by the fragrance.

Trauma material is like a screaming, emotional two-year-old trying to escape from a playpen in the middle of the living room while you try to watch a television program. You wish for a few moments of peace but the more you ignore the child, the more the child demands attention, and the more effort it takes to concentrate on the show. Seeing a child on television reminds you of your own child. Eventually you give the child attention and the intrusions stop. This suggests how recovery will occur in PTSD.

Triggers

Many triggers in the present environment can activate traumatic memory material and stimulate intrusions. *Triggers* are cues—often harmless—that have become associated with the original trauma. In some way, they remind us of the trauma or recall traumatic memories. The association may be obvious or subtle. They may trigger most of the memory or just certain fragments of it. Often, they trigger intrusions against our will. Recognizing triggers, and realizing that their power to elicit intrusions is understandable, are steps toward controlling PTSD symptoms. Table 2.1 lists a range of triggers and the traumatic memories they can stir up.

Some people find it helpful to understand triggers by their twelve categories.

1. *Visual*: seeing blood or road kill reminds one of wounded bodies; black garbage bags reminds a veteran of body bags; a secretary sees her boss standing over her and is reminded of her abusive father.
2. *Sound* (auditory): a backfiring car sounds like gunshot to combat veteran; sounds during lovemaking with spouse remind one of sexual abuse.
3. *Smell* (olfactory): the smell of semen or another's body during intercourse, or the smell of aftershave reminds one of sexual assault.[17]
4. *Taste* (gustatory): eating a hamburger reminds one of an automobile accident that occurred as one drove away from a fast food restaurant.
5. *Physical or Body*
   - *Kinesthetic* means the sensation of movement, tension, or body position.

Table 2.1
TRAUMATIC EVENTS AND TRIGGERS

Trigger	Original Traumatic Event
dark clouds; strong winds	tornado
entering subway tunnel	trench warfare or tunnel rats in Vietnam
lasagna or milk cartons	firemen recovering bodies of eighty children buried in school cafeteria by tornado
firecracker	combat, gun shots
popcorn popping	helicopter in Vietnam, small arms fire
campfire, cooking, barbecue grill	burn victim or fireman who rescued burn victim
rumbling truck	earthquake
aging, hospitalization	POW camp—loss of freedom, family, and purpose; helplessness
warm damp day	Vietnam
rain, clouds in sky	flood
bedroom, lying down, closing eyes	rape
asthmatic breathing	hand held over mouth of rape victim
nausea from illness or something eaten	date rape (which led to nausea)
neighbors	child dies in neighborhood auto accident, neighbors at scene
fuel at gas station	airplane crash rescue worker
perpetrator on television	violent robbery
pretzels	eaten at frat party before being raped
boss criticizes	abuse by father
depression, guilt, anniversary month, becoming a parent	miscarriage
throat swab during medical exam leads to nausea and shakiness[18]	oral rape
physical intimacy (emotional expressiveness elicits fear of losing control)	sexually abusive, raging father
cold snowy weather, uniformed security guards, hunger, watery soup, walking along roads in winter, German vehicles, any unpleasant confrontation or rebuke by supervisors	POW in Germany
fire fighting, police, other paramilitary jobs	soldiering
elevator	sexual assault
SCUBA diving, beach	rescue workers searching for bodies following airliner crash in ocean
injection, vaginal exam	torture
seeing a crime on television	policeman seriously wounded
rushing, overload, stress	a disastrous decision made under pressure, without time to think

Thus, running when tense might be reminiscent of trying to flee a beating; trying to do progressive muscle relaxation (tensing muscles, lying on one's back with eyes closed) might trigger memories of sexual abuse.

- *Tactile* or touch: pressure around wrists or waist, being gripped, held, or otherwise restrained (perhaps even a hug) reminds one of torture or rape; feeling someone on top of you; a man accidentally kicked in bed by his wife while sleeping recalls torture; being touched during sexual relations with a spouse in the same place or in the same way as occurred during abuse will likely trigger traumatic memories.
- *Pain* or other internal sensations: surgical pain, nausea, headaches, or back pain might trigger memories of torture or rape. Elevated heartbeat from exercising might remind one of a similar sensation during a bombing.

6. *Significant dates or seasons*
   - anniversary dates of the trauma
   - seasons of the year with their accompanying stimuli (temperature, lighting, colors, sounds)
   - other dates (e.g., a mother becomes distressed on the date when her murdered son would have graduated)

7. *Stressful events/arousal*: sometimes changes in the brain due to trauma cause it to interpret any stress signals as recurrence of the original trauma.[19] At other times, seemingly unrelated events are actually triggers. Examples include:
   - A woman visits her spouse in the hospital which triggers a flashback of abuse. As a little girl she was treated in the same hospital, following the abuse.
   - An argument with a spouse triggers memories of parents arguing violently.
   - Criticism from a boss reminds a person of being abused by his father.
   - A frightening dream with no apparent related theme activates the fear of a traumatic memory. (Of course, a nightmare of the trauma would understandably elicit strong feelings of distress.)
   - Athletic competition reminds an athlete of being abused when she performed poorly.

8. *Strong emotions*: feeling lonely reminds one of abandonment; feeling happy reminds a woman of a rape that occurred after having dinner with

her best friends; anything that makes one anxious, out of control, or generally stressed, such as PMS. Some memories are state-dependent, meaning that the brain activates them only when the emotional state is the same as the original memory.[20] Thus, if one was drunk when raped, she may feel symptoms only when drinking; if raped when sober, then drinking might provide an escape from the symptoms.[21]

9. *Thoughts*: rejection by a lover leads to the thought "I am worthless," which triggers the same thought that occurred when one was abused as a child.

10. *Behaviors*: driving reminds a person of a serious accident.

11. *Out of the blue*: Sometimes intrusions occur when you are tired, relaxing, or your defenses are down. Often a thought or something you're not aware of will elicit symptoms; so might the habitual act of dissociating during stressful times.

12. *Combinations*: often triggers contain several memory aspects at once. For example:
    - walking to the parking lot on a dark summer's night (visual + kinesthetic + season) triggers a memory of violent crime.
    - fireworks (sounds plus flarelike sight) triggers combat memories.
    - intercourse (weight, touch, sounds, relaxing, the smell of aftershave or semen, the pressure of a hug or a squeezing sensation on the wrists) triggers memory of rape.

WHY DOES DISSOCIATION OCCUR?

Dissociation is a defense against extremely distressful, painful experience. The mind walls off trauma material to try to contain it in much the same way as the body walls off infection. Dissociation is most likely to occur if the trauma was severe, repeated, or occurred at a very young age. We might regard dissociation as a very understandable coping mechanism.

As long as we wall off painful material, we gain some protection. However, the protection is temporary. Without exploration and processing, the material remains negatively and emotionally charged and will intrude in distressing ways. Intrusions are the mind's way of telling us that painful material needs processing. If we can view intrusions as such, then we will likely experience less distress when they occur.

WHEN DOES DISSOCIATION OCCUR?

Dissociation might occur during traumatic events that seem too painful to cope with. For example, a teenager who was raped reported that she felt as if she were on the ceiling during the rape, looking down and feeling sorry for the person being raped. In this way, called *depersonalization,* she could "separate" herself from the trauma. Her usual self was watching the event from afar, while another part of her was walled off in the trauma memories. This defense is entirely understandable. It protects for awhile. Yet notice what has happened. Walled off material has been created. This material will eventually intrude in a distressing way until it has been processed enough to take its place among other memories on file. The sense of self has been split as well. Another way to dissociate during the traumatic event is called *derealization.* Here the person looks at the event as if it is not really happening—a dream, far away or covered by fog. Dissociation at the time of the trauma will make healing more difficult.

Dissociation can also occur later in life as an escape from stress. We might simply be trying to escape an everyday stressful situation or we may be reacting to intrusions or triggers. We are more likely to dissociate in the present if dissociation happened at the time of the trauma. Dissociation at the time of trauma is more likely when the victim is very young or if the offense was repeated or horrific. One seems to learn to use dissociation as a defense. We are also more prone to dissociate in the present if we are tired, drunk, sleepy, anxious, or depressed.[22]

THE VARIETIES OF DISSOCIATION

People dissociate in many ways that do no harm. For example, immersing yourself in a book, movie, or play and "tuning out" your surroundings is generally a harmless escape. Daydreaming is another way to escape from reality. Usually, these are harmless because they are pleasant and under our control. We become concerned when dissociation occurs often, is not under our control, becomes distressing, or makes us feel detached from life. Let's take a look at the more distressing forms of dissociation. All signal that the person is elsewhere, not focused in the present, and is using energy to contain troubling material. All signal that the person is trying to distance himself from the unacceptable.

In *depersonalization,* one feels as if they are an outside observer of self (e.g., on ceiling looking down, across the room watching a movie of self).

Amnesia means forgetting all or parts of the trauma. Some forget the entire trauma. Some forget only the most stressful aspects of the trauma, such as the moment when one was thrown from a car. Some experience gaps in their life story, for example, an entire year of school during which abuse occurred, or for all the years before it occurred. Others simply have a poor general memory, as if remembering anything might invite more intrusions. Amnesia is not explained by normal forgetfulness, but is more severe and distressing.

Dissociative Flashbacks

After people try for so long to wall off traumatic memories, they eventually break through into awareness. *Dissociative flashbacks* pull us away from the present and into the memory. We suddenly and vividly experience the memories as if they are happening in the present. For instance, Bob was a combat veteran of the Vietnam war. While at a Fourth of July celebration, a teenager carelessly threw a fire-cracker near his young daughters. Bob immediately flashed back to the war, pounced on the teenager and was choking him when bystanders pulled him off. He later had no recollection of the flashback.[23] As people explain what happened he begins to think he is going crazy. He is not. It is simply the result of walled-off material that has never been processed. As with other intrusive memories, one might re-experience many aspects of a traumatic memory or just certain aspects. One may or may not act as if they are back in the situation. Some still retain some awareness of present reality during flashbacks, as though they were watching a movie of the trauma. Some remember having the flashback.

Fugue

Fugue is a form of amnesia where a person suddenly travels to another town with no recollection of how they got there. They may start a new life and forget their old identity.

Dissociative Identity Disorder (DID)

DID is the most severe dissociative state. Here people form at least two different personality states, or identities, in order to cope with unacceptable material. Ellen was a happy little girl until her father began to sexually abuse her. She could not figure out how a father who was often loving to her could also mistreat her. Her young mind could not make sense of this, nor was she old enough to seek help or talk about it. It seemed that part of her must be bad to deserve this. As she developed, Ellen formed two identities. Ellen was the good and outwardly happy girl that most people knew. At other times, particularly when trauma-related triggers occurred, she switched to an identity known as Trixy—a seductive, promiscuous woman who frequented bars to be picked up. Trixy is a way to contain the unacceptable trauma material. To Ellen, it seems that the trauma "didn't happen to me—it happened to someone else," in this case, Trixy. In DID, there may be many more personality states (sometimes called *alter egos* or *alters*). Each feels like a different person and may have a different self-image. This is why DID used to be called multiple personality disorder. However, there is only one person and one personality—but the aspects of the personality have not yet been integrated. There may be a host identity that knows the other identities, and may be influenced by the alters' voices. The host is often compulsively good, logical, depressed, and overwhelmed. There may be an angry identity who blows up at people. Alternate identities might differ in age, may conflict with or deny knowing each other, or may hold different fragments of memories. The identities might have names (like Barbara) or symbolic names (The Tramp, The Crazyman, etc.). Identities might sound or speak differently. DID almost always results from a history of horrific childhood trauma. If, for example, a close relative repeatedly abuses a child before her personality integrates and parents are not there to help the child integrate the experience, then DID could occur. In treatment, the individual learns to challenge the distortions (e.g., "I must have deserved this") and to accept and integrate all aspects of the personality.

The above forms of dissociation are rather dramatic. However, dissociation is not always so. Some may just seem to "go away" or "space out" when triggers or intrusive thoughts occur or when present situations are stressful. If the skill was learned during the trauma as a protective defense, it makes sense that one would use the device in the present.

HOW DO WE KNOW WHEN ONE IS DISSOCIATING?

While it may not always be apparent which form dissociation takes, a number of signs suggest that one is trying to avoid the unacceptable. Page 24 provides a listing of such signs, which are likely to continue until the trauma material is processed.

IS DISSOCIATING BAD?

It depends. Dissociation is something most people do. At times it can be helpful. You might "escape" from work for a few moments to daydream about a romantic evening. The famous concentration camp survivor, Viktor Frankl, mentally escaped the prison at times to consider a brighter future.

INDICATIONS OF DISSOCIATION

- body becomes still or stiff
- person is slow to respond to others
- things seem to move in slow motion or fast-forward
- emotions become flat, numb; no feelings
- not feeling expected pain
- out of touch with surroundings
- drifts off, goes away, spaces out (gets spacey), blanks out, loses track of what's happening
- stares off into space, blank stare
- downward stare
- eyes darting anxiously from side to side, or rolling upward
- eyes blink rapidly or flutter
- far away or dazed look
- tunes out
- not involved in present
- feels like an observer of the present situation, rather than a participant
- inattention
- memory lapses
- fantasies, excessive daydreaming
- overactivity or withdrawal
- being on autopilot (automatism behavior), feeling like a robot
- falling asleep
- disoriented

- misses conversation
- derealization (people or world don't seem real; feel like a stranger in a familiar place; don't recognize yourself in the mirror; world seems like a dream, veiled, like you're not really there)
- feels like one is watching things from outside his/her body
- life split before and after (I'm a different person since the trauma)
- twitching or grimacing
- clouding of alertness; foggy feeling (if you're suppressing traumas, you can't focus your thoughts; your mind goes blank)
- unusual, inexplicable behavior (hitting the ground when a car backfires; a dependable woman suddenly leaves the house for two days)
- attempts to remain grounded in the present (stroking side of chair, tapping, jiggling leg)
- self-soothing (rocking back and forth)
- things look or sound different: colors are faded or brighter, tunnel vision, "wide-angle view," sounds are louder or more muffled than expected, things seem far away or unclear/fogged

Dissociation provides some relief, and some protection from overwhelming pain. In that sense, dissociation serves a useful purpose. On the other hand, continually blocking out memories requires enormous energy that can leave one fatigued and irritable. In numbing out the painful memories we also lose pleasant memories and feelings. Inevitably, distressing intrusions will occur. Dissociation also delays or prevents healing because it keeps us from coming to terms with the walled-off material and prevents us from associating it with mastery and control experiences. Dissociation might be likened, then, to a baby's bottle or security blanket. Both served a useful function at one time.

WHAT CAN I EXPECT IF DISSOCIATION IS NOT MANAGED?

As a rule, unprocessed trauma material will continue to intrude until it makes sense, until you have processed it to the point where it can settle into long-term memory. We shall learn shortly how this is done.

CHAPTER 3

Associated Features

To complete our understanding of PTSD, we must understand a variety of symptoms that commonly occur following a traumatic event. In this chapter, we'll discuss thirteen associated features.

1. SELF-RECRIMINATION

Time and again we see traumatized people feel shame and guilt, whether they are responsible for the event or not. Although shame and guilt are similarly defined in the dictionary, guilt usually implies a feeling of responsibility, and shame has come to mean a feeling of badness, of worthlessness to the core. Soldiers who return from war often experience survivor's guilt. Upon examination, we often see questions of worth arise ("Why did I survive when John was a much finer human being?"). Victims of sexual abuse or rape often feel responsible ("I must have done something to cause it—if I had been more careful it would not have happened."). Often shame and guilt are experienced as a result of what the survivor sees as inappropriate behavior. For example, a child in the Oklahoma City bombing stepped on an electrical cord, and assumed that she set off the explosion. A firefighter reflexively runs from an exploding building. Five seconds later he returns to try to find his buddy. Years later he reproaches himself for being a coward. The question often arises, "What kind of person would do that?" The answer, fair or not, is often, "One who is worthless, useless, unlovable, bad to the core." That is a difficult—and very erroneous—belief to live with.

Often people feel shame and guilt for what they did not do. Children who are victims of repeated sexual abuse self-recriminate, thinking, "Why didn't I do something to stop it?" Or the sibling thinks, "Why didn't I do something to rescue her, when I knew it was going on?" A police officer freezes for an instant as criminals open fire. His buddy is shot and he later thinks, "If I had returned fire immediately, he might still be alive."

Sometimes people with PTSD feel guilty for being unable to control their symptoms ("I must be a wimp to be depressed") or behaviors ("I can't believe I blew up at my wife like that—what's wrong with me?").

Guilt can be adaptive if it is realistic and if it leads to improvements in our behavior or character. Self-condemnation is never helpful. Unprocessed guilt and shame will make recovery very difficult. Fortunately, a number of very effective approaches can help to neutralize these emotions. We'll discuss them in chapter 22.

2. SHATTERED ASSUMPTIONS

Each of us holds basic assumptions that give order to our chaotic world and make stress bearable. A number of researchers have indicated that PTSD is due to the shattering of views of self, the world, and other people. In the now famous musical *Les Miserables,* Fantine is left by the man she loves with a newborn. In a stunned and socially isolated state she is accused of being a whore at work and thrown out on the streets, where she later takes up prostitution to feed her child. In poignant song she recalls a time when men were kind, when God was loving and forgiving, when the future was bright. Then all went wrong. Life killed her dreams, shredded her hope, and filled her with shame. Such are the changes often experienced by trauma victims. Table 3.1 lists several ways that people typically think before and after traumatic events. These assumptions summarize the work of Janoff-Bulman, Epstein, and others.[24] The shattered, post-trauma assumptions are often imbedded in the walled-off material, so they are not well challenged or integrated.

3. MOOD DISTURBANCES

Mood disturbances are common among those with PTSD, including:

- *Depression.* This follows logically from lowered self-esteem, hopelessness, shame, loss, feeling permanently damaged, and pessimism. Thus, victims of trauma might be at risk for suicide until such negative thoughts and feelings have been resolved.

Table 3.1
SHATTERED ASSUMPTIONS

Pre-Trauma Assumptions	Post-Trauma Assumptions
Views of Self	
Invulnerability (It can't happen to me; I'm not vulnerable, I'm safe and secure, I know what to expect, I can control things.)	Recurrence preoccupation (It will happen again; I'm vulnerable and helpless, fragile, threatened, endangered, insecure; I'm no longer safe.) I can't succeed in relationships. I can't control my behavior, symptoms, or sanity.
I see myself in a positive light (decent, worthwhile, good, competent, guiltless).	I'm bad, unworthy, shameful ("tramp mentality"), incompetent, weak, different from others, permanently damaged. Self-questioning. I can't count on myself anymore. Abused people conclude, "I'm an object existing for the needs of others—my needs are irrelevant." Self-denigration, shattered identity (don't know who I am anymore; identity split into before and after trauma).
I will have a happy future.	My life-long goal of protecting others feels shattered. I am unworthy of a good life. I can't conceive of a happy future anymore or of finding love. I am not good enough.
Views of the World	
The world is meaningful, fair, good, predictable, orderly, comprehensible, pleasurable, rewarding, kind, and safe. It makes sense and follows accepted social laws.	It just doesn't make sense. The world is confusing ("Why did this happen to me? What's the meaning of life?"). I can't believe in a God who permits this. God hates me.
People get what they deserve—if I'm cautious I can prevent disaster. Bad things won't happen to me.	What I do just doesn't matter. I have no control.
Views of Others	
People are good, trustworthy, comprehensible, worth relating to.	I can't trust people anymore—they're bad, exploitive, hurtful, etc. I can't relate to others; I feel alienated and isolated. Nobody understands.

- *Anxiety*
- *Hostility.* This is an attitude of dislike and distrust of others. It might show up as irritability, rage, or angry outbursts at:
  - those who didn't go through the trauma and can't understand
  - a perpetrator
  - those who did not protect the victim (such as parents)
  - secondary victimizers (those who are supposed to protect you but hurt you instead, such as police or insensitive doctors)
  - family members who happen to be nearby
- *Grief for losses.* This may not always be obvious for reasons we'll discuss later.

4. ADDICTIONS

Substances such as alcohol, cocaine, barbiturates, opiates, amphetamines, or other drugs are frequently abused in attempts to relieve the pain. Such self-medication provides only temporary relief from symptoms and interferes with healing.

5. IMPULSIVE BEHAVIORS

In further attempts to escape the pain, people with PTSD might take impulsive trips, suddenly be absent from work, or make sudden changes in lifestyle (compulsive shopping, eating, or sudden changes in sexual behavior).[25]

6. SOMATIC (BODILY) COMPLAINTS

When trauma material cannot be processed and verbally expressed, the pain is often expressed physically, frequently around body areas that were physically traumatized. Often the physical pain serves as a distraction from emotional pain. Physical complaints can include:[26]

- chronic pain—headaches, heart pains, painful joints, back pain, pelvic pain
- hypertension
- allergies, asthma, rheumatoid arthritis, skin problems
- heavy limbs, lump in throat, fainting, numb or tingling body parts, hypochondriasis

- exhaustion—trying to contain the symptoms of PTSD is fatiguing, making one vulnerable to more physical (and psychological) symptoms[27]
- gastrointestinal disturbances include ulcers, irritable bowel/spastic colon (the term "gut-wrenching" is apt to describe traumatic events[28])

It is often observed that physical complaints are more likely to occur in people who were traumatized in preverbal childhood. The physically painful part of dissociated memory might then intrude as present pain. Other physical complaints are simply the common symptoms of anxiety and a sensitized nervous system.

7. OVERCOMPENSATIONS

In an effort to regain lost control, some people with PTSD become driven for success, achievement, or fitness.[29] This can be a positive outcome of trauma, although it might also distract from healing.

8. DEATH ANXIETY

A brush with death or serious injury will understandably lead to fear of recurrence until that fear is processed and completed.

9. REPETITION COMPULSION

Freud observed that people will often reenact traumas in attempts to master and complete them. (We hope this time to make things right.) This might take several forms:

- Many combat vets go into police, fire protection, emergency medical services, or crisis intervention, perhaps in an attempt to transfer their experience in a meaningful way.
- High-risk behaviors might include skydiving, rock climbing, scuba diving, or reckless speeding. As with high-risk professions, living on the edge creates an adrenaline rush that might ward off depression and the feeling of helplessness experienced during trauma. At the same time, stress-triggered opiates in the brain act like a natural pain killer.
- A woman abused as a child marries an abuser and stays with him.
- A man who was abused as a child enlists in the military, seeking to do violence against the enemy.[30]

- Someone who was forced to go without food as a child might develop problems with eating such as bingeing and purging.

Repeating the trauma gives an oddly comforting feeling of familiarity, predictability, and control. However, the original trauma is rarely resolved by such acts.[31] In fact, these acts might help one continue to avoid the original trauma.

10. SELF-MUTILATION (self-injury or self-injurious behavior)

One of the ironies of PTSD is that victims might further harm themselves. As Matsakis observes, self-mutilation includes "burning, hitting, cutting, excessive scratching, using harsh abrasives on skin or scalp, poking sharp objects into flesh, head banging, pulling out hair or eyebrows for noncosmetic purposes, inserting objects into body orifices," excessive fasting, self-surgery, excessive tattooing, or refusing needed medication.[32] This seems like such a paradox. Why in the world would those who are already in intense pain further injure themselves? It seems to make no sense, yet it does. Most often, it follows a history of protracted childhood trauma (such as physical and/or sexual abuse), not a single exposure.[33] The person harms himself in response to overwhelming, dissociated pain. At least sixteen reasons account for this complex behavior. Self-mutilation:

1. *Expresses pain that can't be verbalized.* It can be expected when the abused child was told to keep the offense a secret, or when the abuse happened before the child learned to talk. The nonverbal outcry says, "Something terrible has happened." It may be a plea for help.

2. *Attempts to convert emotional pain to physical pain.* Physical pain can be localized, displaced, and released, providing a temporary distraction from psychic pain.

3. *Paradoxically relieves pain.* Stress triggers natural painkillers in the brain, temporarily easing psychic and physical pain. This so-called stress-induced analgesia might also help explain why trauma victims become addicted to trauma-related stimuli.[34]

4. *Is a way to feel alive.* Numbing and dissociation feel dead. Perhaps feeling pain is better than feeling nothing. Physical pain grounds one in reality and counters dissociation. It returns focus to the present, providing relief from intrusions. Some people report that blood provides a soothing, warm sensation that relieves stress and reminds them they are still alive.

5. *Provides an illusory sense of power, a sense of mastery and control of pain.* Reversing roles and assuming the role of the offender, the person might think, "This time when I am hurt, I am on the controlling end. I can determine when the pain begins and ends."[35]

6. *Attempts to complete the incompleted.* The idea of repetition compulsion states that we repeat what we've experienced until we've completed old business—processing it and learning a better way. Unfortunately, simply reenacting the abuse doesn't change the trauma material. Complete processing of the material does.

7. *Is a way to contain aggressive tendencies and pain.* The person thinks, "If I discharge my anger and hurt on myself, then I won't hurt anybody else." Maybe it is the only way to stop anger, at least for a time. Learning constructive ways to express emotions is the antidote for this approach.

8. *Vents powerful emotions that cannot be vented directly* (e.g., I can't rage at the powerful perpetrator, so I vent on myself instead).

9. *Makes the body unattractive to spare further abuse.* This harmful defense makes sense to a child who was powerless to stop sexual abuse. Excessive thinness or weight might accomplish a similar purpose.

10. *Might become associated with pleasant moments.* Following abuse, some abusers become remorseful, attentive, and loving for a time. Thus, victims might be conditioned to think that pain signals the beginning of good times.

11. *Imitates what the child has seen.* Children naturally imitate behavior that is modeled by adults. They learn to abuse if their parents are abusive, just as they will learn kindness if the parents model that.

12. *Can be an attempt to attach to parents.* Children have a deep need to attach to parents, even if they are rejecting. In order to gain the abusive parent's approval, the child might internalize his punishing attitudes. The child's thinking might be, "I'll show I'm good and devoted to Mom by doing what she does to me." This makes more sense when we realize that abusers often isolate the victims, making them more dependent on them for approval. Need for approval causes the victim to identify with the aggressor. A child might confuse abuse with emotional closeness, especially if abuse was the only form of attention the parent showed. The child might think, "If I keep hurting myself, eventually they will love me."

13. *Can mark a return to the familiar, understandable past.* The child thinks, "I don't understand loving, soothing behavior, but I do understand pain. It does not always feel good, but at least it is predictable."

14. *Is consistent with one's view of self.* People treat themselves consistent with their self image. Abuse teaches the victim, "I'm worthless, bad, no good, an object—so it makes sense to treat myself like an object." Self-punishment consistently follows from feeling blameworthy, bad, or inadequate.

15. *Is consistent with one's view of a maimed world and a nonexistent future.*[36]

16. *May ensure safety if it results in hospitalization.*

The fact that you hurt yourself does not mean you are insane. You are simply repeating what you learned to cope with intolerable pain. As you learn productive ways to meet your needs you'll no longer need to do this. The antidote is learning to honor yourself and soothe yourself in healthy ways.

11. OTHER ADDICTIONS AND SELF-DESTRUCTIVE BEHAVIORS

Other self-destructive behaviors include eating disorders, accident proneness, compulsive exercise, gambling, sex/prostitution, and shopping. Of course, suicidal tendencies could be included here. Although these behaviors can be complex, understanding them in light of PTSD can help make them less confusing. Much of our discussion of self-mutilation sheds light on these as well.

Flannery estimates that 80 percent of prostitutes come from homes with abuse and/or alcoholism.[37] In alcoholic or abusive homes, children often learn that sex is separate from love, and is useful for purposes other than love. Thus, a prostitute might use sex as the only means of survival she knows. Or she might use it to control men and relationships, a form of repetition compulsion. Prostitution is also consistent with one's core beliefs about self:

- "Sex is not only the only thing I'm good *at,* it's the only thing I'm good *for.*"
- "What am I worth? Nothing, except for the morale of the troops."

Flannery adds that sex addiction is not really an attempt to appease the sex appetite, but is an attempt to rework and master trauma. The victim hopes that this time sex will provide self-esteem, a sense of being lovable, and relief from the pain of rejection, abandonment, and loneliness. Of course, isolated from love, sex provides none of these. Nor does the addiction resolve the problems of dissociated material.

Much like self-mutilation, compulsive gambling can provide an adrenaline rush, a sense of control, and distraction from the pain of dissociation. The vet who starts barroom brawls does so for similar reasons. The abused child who becomes an abusive spouse might wish to stop. Yet following the abuse, they feel a sense of control, a calmness attributable to the release of endorphins in the brain. Food becomes another way to soothe pain for overeaters.[38]

A final form of self-destruction that we'll discuss is revictimization. Repetition compulsion only partially explains why a woman would stay in an abusive relationship. Abuse tends to leave one feeling stunned, numbed, and unable to protect oneself.[39] The adult who was abused as a child will often seek a powerful authority figure to rescue her. Too often this is another abuser who can spot defenseless prey. Abusers typically isolate their victims, making them feel helpless, dependent upon them, and grateful for "any shred of affection." The victim increasingly views the abuser as powerful and respected. It becomes harder and harder to leave the relationship,[40] as the cycle of victimization continues.

12. ALEXITHYMIA

Alexithymia is another name referring to the general shutting down of feelings. One becomes like a robot, capable of functioning but expressing little feeling. One might describe bodily symptoms to the doctor but be unable to connect them to emotional pain. Recall that traumatic memories are highly emotional. To permit any feelings will also invite negative emotions into awareness. So we dread and bottle up all feelings, even love, joy, and relaxation. People make us feel, so people might be avoided. Since empathy requires feelings, giving or receiving love will be challenging. People with alexithymia may appear overly intellectual or businesslike. They will deny that anything is wrong ("Nothing bad happened; I didn't do anything wrong; It didn't bother me; It bothered me then, but not now because I don't think about it"). When resulting from trauma, alexithymia is a defense against painful dissociated material.[41] Some hold the view that showing feelings is a sign of weakness rather than a normal aspect of being human and a necessary step in healing. This view tends to promote alexithymia.

13. CHANGES IN PERSONALITY

Changes in personality may result from traumatic events. These changes may be substantial, especially if the events are severe, repeated, or happen early in life. As already suggested, an individual might become chronically distrustful, cynical, angry, irritable, aggressive, destructive, socially withdrawn, perfectionistic, dependent, anxious, moody, or depressed. Self-esteem often drops. Three common personality disorders—antisocial, borderline, narcissistic—and dissociative Identity disorder are described in Appendix 4.

CHAPTER 4

Frequently Asked Questions

We'll complete our overview of PTSD by answering some commonly asked questions.

WHO GETS PTSD?

Anyone can get PTSD. The best predictor is the stressful event. PTSD is most likely if you are close to a severe event. A longer duration of the event, or events, increases the chances of PTSD, although a single exposure to an extreme event could also lead to PTSD.[42]

It is estimated that at least 40 percent of Americans have experienced at least one major trauma,[43] and that 8–12 percent of U.S. adults will experience PTSD at some point in their lives. These figures might increase with certain changes in society such as rising crime rates and the weakening of the family unit. Certain populations are at risk including children and people whose work exposes them to trauma. The latter group includes the armed forces, police, firefighters, rescue workers, emergency medical service workers, dispatchers, and disaster workers. However, anyone can be exposed to potentially traumatic events.

ARE THERE FACTORS THAT MAKE US MORE VULNERABLE TO PTSD?

The primary cause of PTSD is the stressful event. The risk for PTSD increases if the events

- are sudden and unpredictable[44]

- last a long time

- recur or are thought likely to recur—especially if there is insufficient time or resources to recover

- contain real or threatened violence (e.g., sexual abuse combined with violence is generally more traumatizing than sexual abuse alone)

- involve multiple forms (e.g., after an earthquake, a plane with relief supplies crashes into a village)

- occur in early years before the personality is fully integrated. Abuse from family members is generally more destructive than abuse from strangers because a child's most significant relationships are involved.

Consensus is emerging, however, that a variety of secondary factors can increase the risk of developing PTSD following exposure to traumatic events. These factors become more influential as the severity of the traumatic event decreases.[45] They include pre- and post-trauma vulnerabilities and initial distress following the trauma.

Pre-Trauma Vulnerabilities

Individual differences. People are different; we meet traumatic events at varying degrees of preparedness. There is no shame in this. Some of the risk factors include:

- A history of prior traumatization (e.g., Vietnam veterans with PTSD were more likely to have experienced childhood abuse than those without PTSD. This is understandable since present traumas are likely to reactivate unresolved traumas from the past.)

- Underdeveloped protective skills, problem-solving skills, self-esteem, resilience, creativity, humor, discipline, ability to express emotion to others, ability to tolerate distress. (All are learnable. PTSD can stimulate us to develop these skills.)[46]

- Personality and habitually negative thought patterns (e.g., pessimism, depression, introversion). These also are modifiable.

- Biology. Some people appear to have overreactive nervous systems. Heredity and a history of drug abuse appear to influence this factor.

Family characteristics. For optimal mental health, children need to bond to warm, loving adults in a secure, predictable setting. Here they can learn to trust others and themselves. They learn to experience and express emotions appropriately and safely. Given reasonable demands, they discover that the world is predictable and that they can cope. They learn that in difficult times they can share their burden with others who will support them. Yet a variety of family environments can predispose the child to insecurity, shame, guilt, secrecy, distrust, alienation, or bottling of emotions—all of which increase vulnerability to PTSD. Consider a few of the possibilities:

- Watching parents divorce, children might conclude: The world is not safe; people don't stand by you, so don't trust.

- By watching parents cope with stress, a child might learn to blame others, take out anger on others, use illegal drugs to self-medicate, or avoid emotions.

- Parents with PTSD can indirectly transmit their wounds.[47]
  - A combat vet may parent according to the following rules of war, thereby teaching his children the same rules:
    - destroy your enemies lest they destroy you
    - don't show feelings such as grief or tenderness
    - do whatever it takes to protect yourself
    - it's safer to disguise your intentions

    Fearing angry outbursts, the children of such vets learn to keep quiet. Since the outbursts are unpredictable, they learn to feel unsafe and out of control. They have no way of knowing the cause of their father's pain, but self-esteem will be disrupted if they do not realize that they are not causing the problem.
  - A police officer protects his family but is emotionally disengaged. He takes the children to the park but is worried about danger instead of enjoying the experience with them. Another enmeshes the family ("We must always stick together for protection; avoid outsiders; don't leave home; never argue"). In both situations, the children learn to be anxious and distrustful.

- An abusive, alcoholic father threatens to harm a child if she tells. The child learns to be secretive and ashamed. The child learns to "look normal" rather than heal.

Recent life stressors. These can weaken resistance. Accumulated stressors might include recent divorce, illness, financial pressures, natural death of a friend or relative, or losing a job.

Pre-trauma vulnerabilities might have limited you in the past, and probably have limited your growth since the trauma. Sometimes the trauma highlights the opportunity to grow in these areas, which is why trauma can present certain positive aspects.

Initial Distress at the Time of Trauma

PTSD is more likely to develop if one:

- dissociates[48]
- has the perception that they were responsible or acted inappropriately—how one thinks about the traumatic event is crucial, a point we shall repeatedly return to
- perceives that they are alone or isolated (e.g., a batterer threatens to kill his wife if she tells anyone; an abused child feels different from her friends and is too ashamed to talk with anyone)

Post-Trauma Factors

Recovery environment. Lack of support from family, friends, and community can make the victim feel more alone, helpless, or worthless. Ideally, support systems will be believing, uncritical, and supportive. They will encourage you to take care of yourself and express your feelings—they can feel and accept your pain, even if they don't understand it. Risk factors include:

- *Emotional unavailability.* Some adults feel threatened by pain. They don't know how to talk about it. Perhaps they too were victims and feel their unresolved memory material will be triggered by your trauma.

- *The victim's being disbelieved, stigmatized, shamed, or shunned.* Think of a rape victim who is blamed or rejected by her husband, or our troops returning from Vietnam.[49] The rejection adds to the wound, while the victim is denied the healing balm of sharing one's burdens. In contrast, consider cultural homecoming or decompression rituals such as the Native American sweat lodge or homecoming parades for soldiers which help integrate individuals into society.

- *Secondary victimization.* This occurs when those who are supposed to help instead inflict further harm.
  - The police or lawyers treat a victim of rape as if she asked for it or could have prevented it had she been more careful.

- A physician minimizes the symptoms, belittles one seeking assistance, or even refuses to render treatment ("There's nothing wrong with you, it's all in your head.").
- *Conspiracy of silence.* Perhaps the wife tells the child to keep silent about the father's incest for fear that he will be thrown in jail.

Lack of treatment. This reinforces the victim's belief that she is alone and different from others. By contrast, some organizations provide group meetings and education to help prevent the development of PTSD, and provide follow-up individual counseling.

Ineffective coping. Some people keep the pain inside—unexpressed and unprocessed. They might then turn to drugs or alcohol to kill the pain, or to self-destructive behaviors. None of these solve the root problem—painful dissociated material. Effective copers take care of themselves and seek necessary help.

WHAT COURSE WILL PTSD TAKE?

Horowitz has described the normal sequence of the traumatic stress reaction and recovery:[50]

1. *Outcry.* This stage involves strong, distressing emotions. One freezes or feels stunned, overwhelmed, or frightened. Perhaps one begins to feel strong emotions after having coped with an emergency, maybe when home relaxing. Strong anger might have helped them to cope.
2. *Avoidance and denial.* One thinks, "Oh, no! It can't be true." One feels numb/blunted. They withdraw, avoid potential supporters, constrict emotionally, and stare blankly into space. In a frantic attempt to keep life as usual, they compulsively return to pre-trauma tasks that were important then (perhaps work, sports, sex, or cleaning). But the world looks gray. Feeling physically and emotionally numb, unable to talk about it, they might turn to drugs for relief.
3. *Intrusions.* Intense emotions and thoughts related to the stressful event begin to break into awareness, accompanied by signs of arousal. The strong waves of thoughts and emotions might wane for a time, giving one hope of coping. But they return. Arousal is signaled by startle reactions, hypervigilance (excessive alertness, looking around for threats), and com-

pulsive repetition of actions that are linked to the event (constant search-ing for lost persons or situations, reenacting the event, and rehearsing ideal responses to regain control).

4. *Working through until completion.* Eventually, one faces the reality of the event, experiences all thoughts and feelings, talks it through with oth-ers, corrects erroneous thoughts, comes to terms with the experience, grieves, and restores equilibrium. New commitments are made to live, ac-cept self, accept losses, find the silver lining in the trauma (e.g., find re-siliency, wisdom, or compassion), grow beyond the pre-trauma condition, and move on.

If one gets stuck at a step before completion, then the symptoms of PTSD will continue, including swinging between stages. If stuck, Horowitz recommends early treatment so that maladaptive coping does not get fixed. Treatment involves going through the four stages to find out where one is stuck, and then progress-ing through to completion.

Most people will experience at least some symptoms of PTSD following a se-verely stressful event. As a general rule, about half of all adults diagnosed with PTSD will recover within three months.[51] Others will continue to experience PTSD for months to years if not treated. Without treatment, many people who do not meet the full criteria for PTSD will continue to experience symptoms for decades; people might indeed manage their symptoms for decades only to find them multiplying during retirement years. Perhaps one finally becomes exhausted from a lifetime of battling. Perhaps a hospital stay or failing health triggers old memories of helplessness and loss of control.[52]

PTSD usually begins within three months of the trauma, although there might be a delay of months to years. However, so-called delayed PTSD is rare. Careful examination will usually detect PTSD early on, although the symptom profile and associated features might change over the course of the disorder.[53] Some people experience periods of remission followed by recurrence.

IS IT A SIGN OF BEING CRAZY OR WEAK THAT I AM STILL BOTHERED BY THE TRAUMA AFTER ALL THESE YEARS?

PTSD symptoms are simply a sign that the trauma overwhelmed your coping abil-ities at the time and that you have not yet learned effective ways to cope or re-duce the symptoms. As you learn new skills, you will likely feel much better.

WHAT ARE THE COSTS AND CONSEQUENCES OF PTSD?

Wilson summarizes that PTSD impacts one's psychology, self-concept, development, and attachment capacities (including the capacities for intimacy, love, bonding, and sexuality).[54] Untreated, PTSD is associated with greater rates of the following:

- depression
- anxiety disorders (e.g., panic disorders, phobias)
- suicide
- low self-esteem
- guilt
- personality disorders
- dissociative disorders
- cynicism
- revictimization
- family disruption (e.g., conflict, divorce, secondary wounding)
- impaired relationships
- social isolation
- sexual dysfunction or sexual acting out
- unemployment
- drug addictions
- eating disorders (e.g., anorexia, bulimia)
- medical illness
- homelessness
- loss of religious faith
- child and spousal abuse
- difficulty handling stress
- violence

Just a few notes will suffice for explanation.

Suicide

Suicide may be viewed as an attempt to escape overwhelming pain. The rate for incest victims is two to three times higher than rates for the depressed; the latter comprise the majority of suicides. Suicide attempts among rape victims occur ten times more frequently than the population average.[55] It is apparent that sexual abuse violates not only the body but the mind and soul as well. It sends the message that a victim is but an object. The lasting danger is that the victim accepts that message and fails to realize that things can get better. Battered women also attempt suicide at alarming rates, consistent with findings that women are on average more distressed by troubled relationships than are men.

Revictimization

Incest victims are more likely to be sexually victimized in later years and to marry abusive spouses. Here is a complex irony. There is a great need to protect oneself.

Yet experience might have taught the victim that self-protection is futile. One who dissociates is not in contact with lessons of the past. Vulnerable and in need of assurance, one becomes a "sitting duck" for an abuser.[56]

Intergenerational Secondary Wounding

PTSD victims can infect their families. For example, children of Vietnam vets can feel neglected by emotionally absent fathers who transmit the expectation of silence. Children of Holocaust survivors might also bear scars of their parents' wounds. Through their parents they might learn to fear separation, avoid intimacy, or overachieve. They might experience Holocaust-related nightmares, anxiety, concentration difficulties, aggression, and psychosomatic disorders. Frequently children of victims wish to empathize and understand their parents but the parents remain emotionally closed. The children might then take on the symptoms themselves as a way to feel close. In short, any parental difficulties can be passed on to the family. The difficulties are compounded by the family's frustration at being unable to help the victim.[57]

Sexual Dissatisfaction[58]

Many symptoms common to PTSD interfere with the enjoyment of wholesome sexual intimacy: difficulty trusting, guilt, depression, self-loathing, emotional numbness, preoccupation with emotional survival, disgust, drug abuse, and anger, to name several. The challenge is even greater when inappropriate sexuality was part of the traumatic experience. For example, home is no longer safe to incest survivors, who are most often females. Unhelped survivors are more likely to enter sexualized relationships to replace deeper intimacy, and often become pregnant during teen years. They are more likely to experience sexual dysfunction and report that they do not like being a woman. They will often experience flashbacks during sexual closeness.[59] In relationships they might experience great ambivalence about sex. They often find sex aversive and wish to avoid it. At other times they need and seek closeness. So they might flip-flop between avoidance and excessive sexuality. Partners might interpret the flashbacks or the wish to avoid sex as rejection.[60]

WILL TIME HEAL THE WOUNDS?

Perhaps. Some people seem to recover without treatment within a few months. For others, however, "work hard and forget" does not necessarily work.[61] Often effects can be prolonged and may worsen without treatment. The good news is that research has taught us much about PTSD, including many strategies that help people to heal, recover, and grow.[62]

WHAT ABOUT TRAUMATIC BRAIN INJURY?

Sometimes injuries to the brain can cause PTSD symptoms. Head injury can occur if someone is knocked out or whipped around, or if someone experienced a coma or concussion. Such conditions might be a result of violence, a car accident, or other traumatic events. The victim might look the same but act differently.

Many of the symptoms of head injury are similar to PTSD including concentration difficulties, aggression, depression, anxiety, irritability, mood swings (being demanding or verbally abusive), amnesia (usually loss of recent memory), fatigue, disrupted sleep, headache, decreased sexual interest (although 5 to 10 percent will exhibit increased interest), and shame.

However, additional signs might suggest brain injury. Look for:

- slowed processing (slowed memory storing or retrieval)
- difficulty with abstract or complex thinking (e.g., a person can't explain what "people who live in glass houses shouldn't throw stones" means)
- decreased muscle strength
- seizures (sometimes looks like a fainting spell)
- loss of coordination
- difficulty with vision, speech, hearing, smell, or taste

Brain injury is best treated by a neuropsychologist, who is trained to detect abnormalities that might not be obvious on normal medical tests. State head injury foundations can assist in care of the victim and support of the family.

WHAT ABOUT FALSE MEMORIES?

The accuracy of trauma memories is one of the most controversial aspects of PTSD. Perhaps no one has summarized the research on this topic better than Dr. Jon G. Allen of the Menninger Clinic. He relates that a full range of recall is possible. Some people remember the gist of the trauma reasonably accurately and consistently. Some remember parts of the trauma consistently with varying degrees of precision. Some totally forget the trauma, and some of these later have varying degrees of recall. Sometimes the recall occurs spontaneously. Sometimes recall is prompted by a psychotherapist or hypnotist. Sometimes this recall can be relatively accurate, and sometimes totally false. Allen points to the need for caution in evaluating the accuracy of traumatic memories. We recall that traumatic memories are often stored in fragmented, dissociated bits, which are not filed in memory in proper perspective with respect to time. Trying to reconstruct them might lead to interpretation and the changing of details over time. Spontaneously recalled memories tend to be more reliable than those suggested by a therapist or gained through hypnotism because some people are somewhat prone to suggestion.[63] Thus it is generally considered unethical for a therapist to try to persuade a client that abuse has occurred, or to even suggest it.

PART II

About Healing, Recovery, Growth

CHAPTER 5

Principles of Healing, Recovery, and Growth

The story of PTSD is the tale of the indomitable and indefatigable human spirit to survive and adapt.

—*Dr. Donald Meichenbaum*[64]

You might, like many other people, find it somewhat healing just to understand your PTSD symptoms and realize that they make sense. You are not crazy, although your symptoms might indicate the need for assistance. This book is to help you heal, recover, and grow. "Healing" and "recovery" are often used interchangeably, although we will use them to mean slightly different things. *Healing* means "to make whole." It, in fact, derives from the same root as "health" and "whole." We'll use the word to refer to the process of becoming whole again. *Recovery* means a return to your former state of functioning. Although we are never the same following any new experience, we can again feel strong, whole, and functional—ready to move beyond the suffering and turn the negative experience of PTSD into growth.

When you recover you will notice that your symptoms will be fewer, less severe, and less troubling when they occur. You'll notice that:[65]

1. You can recall or dismiss the traumatic event at will, instead of suffering from intrusive memories, frightening dreams, troubling flashbacks, and distressing associations (i.e., triggers).

2. You can remember the event with appropriately intense feeling—not false detachment.

3. Feelings about the traumatic event can be named and endured without overwhelming arousal, dissociation, or numbing.

4. Symptoms of anxiety, depression, and sexual dysfunction, if not absent, are at least reasonably tolerated and predictable.

5. You are not isolated from other people but have restored your capacity for affinity, trust, and attachment.

6. You have assigned meaning to the trauma and discarded a damaged sense of self, replacing it with a belief in your own strength. Losses have been named and mourned; self-blame has been replaced by self-acceptance and self-worth; obsessive rumination about the past has been replaced by realistic evaluation.

7. You will be more comfortable with all feelings—positive, negative, and neutral.

8. You will again commit to your future and take responsibility for your life, no matter how badly you were treated or defeated.

The road to recovery and growth is different for each person. In some cases, symptoms will resolve fairly quickly. In many cases, recovery will be a marathon, not a sprint. We might picture the process as shown in Figure 5.1.

PTSD puts one in the dark valley. This is a detour, a temporary derailment, not an endpoint. Steps to healing begin the upward climb, sometimes two steps forward and one step back. Often the course is not smooth and you might feel like you are getting worse before you get better. Over time you will reach the recovery point and be ready to pick up where you left off.

THE SEVEN PRINCIPLES OF HEALING

1. *Healing starts by applying skills to manage PTSD symptoms.* These include skills to reduce distressing arousal, manage anger, and manage intrusions. These skills are not curative but they do help to reduce troubling symptoms to the point where life becomes more manageable. They enable us to begin the steps of healing.

2. *Healing occurs when traumatic memory is processed or integrated.* Recall that a dissociated traumatic memory is walled off, or separated, from adaptive memories that are associated and stored in long-term memory. Fragments of the memory are also separated from one another. Highly charged

Figure 5.1
HEALING, RECOVERY, AND GROWTH

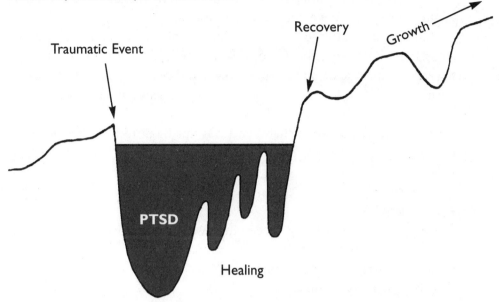

and stored in active memory, the traumatic memory intrudes into awareness as a call for processing and integration. In integration, memory fragments are recalled and explored so that they can be connected to each other—making the memory whole. The memory is connected to adaptive material, including adaptive thoughts and emotions. Inaccurate or unreasonable thoughts are identified. Adaptive thoughts blend into the memory in their place. In some cases, these thoughts come from stored memories. In other cases, they are introduced. Distressing emotions can literally be expressed (released) and this time the memory is connected to calmer, more supportive emotions. The unspeakable memory is given words since verbalizing helps to put the memory together and be viewed more logically. Bringing the highly emotionally charged memories under the light of reason settles them down.

We come to see the memory in clearer perspective. The distressing energy of the memory is neutralized. We re-evaluate the triggers and see them simply as reminders, not a repeat of the trauma. The traumatic event is viewed as part of the past, not the present. Now the memory can take its place in long-term memory, one memory alongside all other memories.

The traumatic memory no longer seems to be the only one on file, but just one in an entire life history. As with other memories, it can be recalled but without overwhelming emotion and arousal.

Integration means more than just thinking about memories. Intrusions are thought about, but that is not sufficient to heal. In fact, simply thinking about traumatic memory may simply reinforce the memory. Integration means that memories are transformed and reorganized in a meaningful way. We process the dissociated trauma memories until we come to terms with them, make sense of them, and can put them to rest. This healing process is referred to in many ways, including:

- integrating
- processing
- assimilating
- digesting or metabolizing (becoming aware of memory fragments and then neutralizing and assimilating each part)
- coming to terms with the memory
- making sense of the memory
- reframing (changing the way we view the event)

3. *Healing occurs when confronting replaces avoidance.* Avoidance is a hallmark of the anxiety disorders. It seems natural to avoid pain and suffering. However, without awareness, integration does not occur. When we avoid we do not master. We never learn that we can triumph over our fears. We never learn new coping skills and we remain controlled by the past. So we shall confront in a safe and orderly way that which we find distressing.

4. *Healing occurs in a climate of safety and pacing.* When you were traumatized you were not safe. This time, however, you will always remain safe and in control. You will progress steadily, but as slowly as you need to remain in control. Steady progress is more beneficial than going too fast. In fact, Kluft has stated, "The slower you go, the faster you get there."[66] You will only start when you are ready, and always move at a comfortable pace.

5. *Healing occurs when boundaries are intact.*

6. *Kind awareness and acceptance of feelings aid the healing journey.* Acceptance of feelings begins with compassionate acceptance of self. In various ways, trauma therapist Beverly James communicates to traumatized children early in treatment: "There are parts of you that are funny, heroic,

strong, smart, warm, angry, gross, tender, weak, and tricky that make you wonderfully special. I like the whole, big, warm, smelly, alive package of you."[67] This is the view we strive for: "Even though I am imperfect, nevertheless, I am worthwhile; I matter."

7. *Balance in our lives is necessary to heal.* Healing is work. You can't work constantly on difficult material. You will need a break, a time out from your healing work. You will need to nourish your mind and body. You'll need to permit time for recreation, laughter, play, and beauty.

BOUNDARIES[68]

Think of yourself as a beautiful house, lovely outside and in. The house is a place of joy and comfort—a secure place from which you explore the world. Around the house is a sturdy fence with a gate. You also have strong doors and windows. You can open the doors and gates to invite in welcomed guests—neighbors, friends, and family. You keep them closed to keep out danger. Trauma blew open your doors and burst into your house. It may have convinced you that you are powerless to close the doors. Perhaps the door has remained open and danger has walked in too often. Or you may have locked the door so tightly that no one can get in anymore. Perhaps you no longer open the windows, so stale air remains trapped and no light and fresh air can enter. Maybe you have stopped beautifying the inside of your home and your health is declining because you stay so confined.

Your boundaries are like doors, gates, and windows. Healing occurs as you learn to put into place very strong, secure boundaries. These boundaries allow you to feel safe. They open and close at your choosing. You are in control. You will learn to keep out dangerous people, and you will again invite in safe people to enjoy. You will choose when to open your windows to express feelings that need to be confided/shared, and permit the light of friendship, love, and healing ideas to enter.

Building strong boundaries also means that you know what you are responsible for; you do not assume responsibility when you are not responsible. You can see clearly that you are responsible for your house and all that is in it (sometimes you need to call in the plumber for help). You will probably choose to assist your neighbors because that makes the neighborhood nicer, but you realize that they are responsible for their own houses. You can't personally fix all the houses in the neighborhood. The best you can do is bring your tools and offer to help.

You will beautify and take care of your own house, at a pace that is right for you. You will never berate yourself because your house is unique or because yours has not progressed as far as someone else's. In this way you enjoy your house.

Boundaries give us a feeling of inner strength. Ultimately they enable us to enjoy ourselves and the world. They empower us to love and relate to others better.

FEELINGS

Life is feeling. Not to feel is to be dead. To be at peace with all feelings is to heal. Nominated for the Nobel Peace Prize, the exiled Vietnamese monk Thich Nhat Hanh has put this in beautiful perspective in *Peace Is Every Step*. With permission, I wish to share his insights on feelings:[69]

> In us, there is a river of feelings, in which every drop of water is a different feeling, and each feeling relies on all the others for its existence. To observe it, we just sit on the bank of the river and identify each feeling as it surfaces, flows by, and disappears.
>
> There are three sorts of feelings—pleasant, unpleasant, and neutral. When we have an unpleasant feeling, we may want to chase it away. But it is more effective to return to our conscious breathing and just observe it, identifying it silently to ourselves: "Breathing in, I know there is an unpleasant feeling in me. Breathing out, I know there is an unpleasant feeling in me." Calling a feeling by its name, such as "anger," "sorrow," "joy," or "happiness," helps us identify it clearly and recognize it more deeply.
>
> We can use our breathing to be in contact with our feelings and accept them. If our breathing is light and calm—a natural result of conscious breathing—our mind and body will slowly become light, calm, and clear, and our feelings also. Mindful observation is based on the principle of "non-duality"; our feeling *is* not separate from us or caused merely by something outside us; our feeling *is* us, and for the moment we *are* that feeling. We are neither drowned in nor terrorized by the feeling, nor do we reject it. Our attitude of not clinging to or rejecting our feelings is the attitude of letting go, an important part of meditation practice.
>
> If we face our unpleasant feelings with care, affection, and nonviolence, we can transform them into the kind of energy that is healthy and has the capacity to nourish us. By the work of mindful observation, our unpleasant feelings can illuminate so much for us, offering us insight and understanding into ourselves and society.

(Like surgeons, some helpers) want to help us throw out what is unwanted and keep only what is wanted. But what is left may not be very much. If we try to throw away what we don't want, we may throw away most of ourselves.

Instead of acting as if we can dispose of parts of ourselves, we should learn the art of transformation. We can transform our anger, for example, into something more wholesome, like understanding. We do not need surgery to remove our anger. If we become angry at our anger, we will have two angers at the same time. We only have to observe it with love and attention. If we take care of our anger in this way, without trying to run away from it, it will transform itself. This is peacemaking. If we are peaceful in ourselves, we can make peace with our anger. We can deal with depression, anxiety, fear, or any unpleasant feeling in the same way.

Transforming Feelings

1. *The first step in dealing with feelings is to recognize each feeling as it arises.* The agent that does this is mindfulness. In the case of fear, for example, you bring out your mindfulness, look at your fear, and recognize it as fear. You know that fear springs from yourself and that mindfulness also springs from yourself. They are both in you, not fighting, but one taking care of the other.

2. *The second step is to become one with the feeling.* It is best not to say, "Go away, Fear. I don't like you. You are not me." It is much more effective to say, "Hello, Fear. How are you today?" Then you can invite the two aspects of yourself, mindfulness and fear, to shake hands as friends and become one. Doing this may seem frightening, but because you know that you are more than just your fear, you need not be afraid. As long as mindfulness is there, it can chaperone your fear.

3. *The third step is to calm the feeling.* As mindfulness is taking good care of your fear, you begin to calm it down. "Breathing in, I calm the activities of body and mind." You calm your feeling just by being with it, like a mother tenderly holding her crying baby. Feeling his mother's tenderness, the baby will calm down and stop crying. . . . So don't avoid your feeling. Don't say, "You are not important. You are only a feeling." Come and be one with it. You can say, "Breathing out, I calm my fear."

4. *The fourth step is to release the feeling, to let it go.* Because of your calm, you feel at ease, even in the midst of fear, and you know that your fear will not grow into something that will overwhelm you. When you know that you are capable of taking care of your fear, it is already reduced to the minimum, becoming softer and not so unpleasant. Now you can smile at it and let it go, but please do not stop yet. Claiming and releasing are just medicines for the symptoms. You now have the opportunity to go deeper and work on transforming the source of your fear.

5. *The fifth step is to look deeply.* You look deeply into your baby—your feeling of fear—to see what is wrong, even after the baby has already stopped crying, after the fear is gone. You cannot hold your baby all the time, and therefore you have to look into him to see the cause of what is wrong. By looking, you will see what will help you begin to transform the feeling. You will realize, for example, that his suffering has many causes, inside and outside of his body. If something is wrong around him, if you put that in order, bringing tenderness and care to the situation, he will feel better. Looking into your baby, you see the elements that are causing him to cry, and when you see them, you will know what to do and what not to do to transform the feeling and be free. (In looking, you might) uncover causes of suffering that stem from the way (you) look at things, the beliefs (you) hold about (yourself), (your) culture, and the world. . . . After recognizing the feeling, becoming one with it, calming it down, and releasing it, we can look deeply into its causes, which are often based on inaccurate perceptions. As soon as we understand the causes and nature of our feelings, they begin to transform themselves.

The above beautifully expresses an important concept of healing. Feelings are not to be feared or avoided. As we calmly look into our negative feelings—without judging them, but accepting them with compassion—we discover the cause of our suffering and better see the pathways to healing, recovery, and growth. Healing is permitting feelings into awareness in a safe and paced way, while always retaining control.

CHAPTER 6

Treatment Approaches

Professional, Medication, Group, and Self-Managed

> There is always an easy solution to every human
> problem—neat, plausible and wrong.
>
> —*H.L. Mencken,* **A Mencken Chrestomathy**

In recent years, researchers have learned much about PTSD and its successful treatment. The prospects of overcoming or lessening your symptoms today are quite hopeful, especially with *skilled, appropriate* treatment.

Many ask whether or not they should treat PTSD, since some people seem to recover on their own. A point to remember, though, is that untreated PTSD can worsen and needlessly lead to problems like depression, anxiety, substance abuse, chronic pain, or personality disorders. Treatment can be very helpful and is suggested if:

1. Symptoms are causing considerable suffering.

2. Symptoms are interfering with your capacity to work, enjoy life, and connect to others.

3. Symptoms are causing physical illness.

4. Symptoms do not lessen within one to three months. This is a rule of thumb. In many cases, immediate treatment might prevent worsening of symptoms, and is recommended if symptoms are extremely disturbing. Treatment is a good idea even if symptoms have diminished but are still disturbing.

5. Suicidal thoughts, hallucinations (seeing or hearing things), or fear that you will hurt yourself or others occurs.

6. You are taking any medication for your symptoms.

The saying, "That which doesn't kill me makes me stronger," is not always accurate. Some traumatic wounding severely weakens people, and the symptoms can worsen with time. Treatment can help these persons heal and grow stronger. Because PTSD sometimes runs its course, people might urge you to:

- Just don't think about it
- Just get on with your life—be like you used to be
- Get over it
- Stop dwelling on the past

Everstine writes[70] that it is a myth that PTSD will go away and be forgotten if you don't talk about it, if you pretend it did not happen, or if you don't tell anyone. If willpower alone has not helped you dissipate dissociated traumatic material (it rarely does), then seeking treatment would be a wise choice—a way of caring for yourself.

We will explore many approaches that have been found to foster recovery. Research has not yet established one approach as vastly superior to any other. Rather, people are unique and respond differently to specific strategies. So the principles will be presented for each strategy. This will empower you to determine if the particular strategy is suited to you and decide when or if to apply it.

CAUTION

Treatment is not easy. It generally does not provide a quick fix, although some gains might occur fairly rapidly. Homework is usually needed to heal. Be prepared to encounter feelings of depression and anxiety as you encounter difficult memories until they are resolved. You might initially experience the worsening of some symptoms and a desire for unhealthy comforts. However, the work of healing progresses with each appropriate effort and eventually becomes easier.

PRINCIPLES OF TREATMENT

The following principles optimize treatment success:[71]

1. *Transcend your fears of treatment in order to facilitate treatment.* Under-

stand that your fears of treatment are normal. There are good reasons for them, and they are shared by many others, at least initially. Fears might include:[72]

- *The fear of discovering the cause of the disturbance.* Although it may feel like you are the only one to have gone through an experience like yours, in fact many have. We learn that many people react in ways similar to the way we have. Feelings of disgust, humiliation, fear, and self-dislike are typical. They don't mean that you are inadequate. Understanding the root cause of the symptoms will help dissipate the symptoms.

- *The fear of alienating the therapist.* An experienced therapist knows that PTSD reactions are normal and understandable. She is not shocked by the symptoms, and this response will help you realize that you are not crazy or abnormal.

- *The fear of being overwhelmed or going crazy.* You will learn how to cope effectively with difficult thoughts and feelings so that you are less likely to feel overwhelmed.

- *Fear of losing good memories.* In actuality, when negative memories are processed the good ones come to awareness and/or become stronger. Treatment just allows a negative memory to take its place properly in the past.

2. *Understand the treatment options and the reasons behind them.* Know what to expect, then formulate a plan in conjunction with your counselor. Be open to various treatment possibilities.

3. *You must be willing to give up harmful "retraumatizing behaviors" like drugs, violence, self-destruction, or dangerous thrill seeking.* These all keep you in the survivor mode (vigilance, minimizing risk, detachment from feelings) or the avoidance mode (isolation, numbing).[73] Both are contrary to recovery. You will learn to understand the purposes of these behaviors and substitute constructive behaviors that better meet your needs.

4. *Stay in control as you gradually learn to trust the healing process.* Many strategies have demonstrated effectiveness. If you work with a helper, recognize that it may be difficult to trust. You might have learned from experience that other people are not trustworthy. Part of the role of trauma therapy is to teach the survivor how to relate in a relationship. Over time, if the therapist is constant, and models good boundaries, the survivor will learn to trust. You may decide to give her a chance to earn your trust,

gradually letting her know of difficulties you are having so that she will know how best to help.

5. *Be willing to confront traumatic memories in a therapeutic, controlled way—if and only when you are ready.* Do not dig. Memories will come to the surface as a natural part of therapy.

6. *You must be willing to give up secondary gains.* Secondary gains are desirable payoffs for being sick. Thus, the person is unwilling to be well. Sometimes the payoff is not obvious. In order to heal, the person must be aware of any secondary gains, and then be willing to release them. "Will you miss the problem when it's gone?" If you hesitate, you may have secondary gains.[74] We ask ourselves, "Would any bad things happen if we recover?" Then we formulate a plan to address these needs.

Below are a few secondary gains and their challenges to recovery:[75]

- For a vet, recovery must be more important than keeping a disability check.

- An abused teenager will have to find a new place to live.

- A vet who has the identity of a wounded hero must expand his way of seeing himself.

- A member of a support group must find other ways to meet his social needs.

- A vet fears that an end to his pain will mean that he'll forget his dead comrades. He later learns to better honor the dead with a productive life. Releasing intense pain does not mean forgetting or being disloyal to comrades.

- A police officer who fears losing his edge must realize that constant vigilance degrades performance.

- A person with PTSD fears losing something that has been "a part of me for years." She must learn to see herself as more than her symptoms.

- A survivor of abuse fears giving up her justification for years of failure. She must learn to replace it with a gradual, achievable plan for success.

- A son of a Holocaust survivor with PTSD feels it would be disloyal to become different from his parents. He must learn that he can be happy *and* loyal.

The following questions can help to clarify secondary gains so that a plan to address the secondary gain can be formulated.

- What will I give up if I get better?
- What new challenges will I face if I recover?
- Who am I without this problem?
- Who will I disappoint if I recover?
- What would happen if I were happier or more successful?
- What would happen if I weren't experiencing these symptoms?

Try completing this cost/benefit analysis.

The benefits of having PTSD are:	The disadvantages of PTSD are:

The ultimate questions are, "Is PTSD a problem in terms of its costs?" and "How can I meet my needs without PTSD?" This book will suggest various ways to meet your needs without PTSD.

WHEN NOT TO TRY MEMORY WORK

An important part of treatment is the work of processing traumatic memories, or memory work. This requires that you be stabilized and functioning reasonably well. It should not be tried if any of the following conditions are not under control:

- substance addiction
- self-destructive behavior (self-injury, suicidal tendencies, eating disorder)
- threats of violence or homicide
- life chaos (the likelihood that the trauma will be repeated, abuse is ongoing, no home or income, etc.)
- mental illness, especially schizophrenia, bipolar disorder (manic depression), or other illness needing medication
- the threat of mental health being overwhelmed. Flannery states,[76] "Some victims appear so overwhelmed by the recall of such episodes that in some cases it is better to leave the event sealed in memory and to work on the other steps toward a more normal life. This would leave the victim subject to possible intrusive memories in the face of threat or loss, but given our current understanding of treating these events, this might be a better trade-off in some few victims." A number of steps can help this person manage the stress in their lives. At some point it may be appropriate to explore traumatic memories, perhaps in a controlled environment such as a hospital ward.

Matsakis[77] adds that memory work should not be undertaken if:

- there is not a strong therapeutic alliance with a mental health professional
- there is no support system
- severe rage, nightmares, flashbacks, and irritability are uncontrolled
- the individual is not ready

Remember, you are the one who is in control. You determine when to begin. You set a safe pace and say when to stop. Stop or ease up at any time you feel overwhelming or dangerous emotions, such as extreme or dangerous anger or panic. Likewise, ease up if you dissociate, experience psychotic episodes, or encounter strong physical upset—such as nausea, pain, dizziness, or panic attack.

APPROACHES TO TREATMENT

There are many treatment approaches with demonstrated effectiveness.

Professional Treatment

A skilled mental health professional can be an invaluable resource in helping you treat PTSD. If the PTSD is severe or long lasting, a psychotherapist will probably be needed to guide you through the process of healing. Think of psychotherapy as crisis counseling for stress and anxiety, not counseling for mental illness. An important aspect of psychotherapy is that it provides a supportive relationship while you work through difficult material and learn new coping skills. A good therapeutic relationship will also help the individual learn to trust again.

Psychotherapists include psychologists, psychiatrists, clinical social workers, psychiatric nurses, clinical mental health counselors, certified pastoral counselors, and marriage and family therapists. Certified pastoral counselors consider both psychological and spiritual needs. All of these can be helpful if they are specifically trained to treat PTSD.

As Ochberg observes:[78] "There are not enough therapists in the world to treat the millions of men, women, and children who have been assaulted, abused, and violated as a result of war, tyranny, crime, disaster, and family violence. When people do seek help, suffering with posttraumatic symptoms, they may find therapists who are ill equipped to provide assistance." It is important, then, for a person with PTSD to be a good consumer. The resources listed at the back of the book will help you locate a psychotherapist who treats PTSD. However, not all clinicians are equally skilled. You must find one whose skills you respect and who you feel comfortable working with. You will want to select one whose values you are comfortable with, who is trustworthy and ethical. It is advisable to discuss the principles of therapy before you begin treatment. Before settling on a psychotherapist, ask questions such as the following (a therapist who is unwilling to discuss these important issues is not likely to be a good match for you):

- What is your training and experience in treating PTSD?

- What is your approach to treating it? (You will get a sense for the types of approaches you prefer by reading later sections of this book.)

- What are your views about dissociation and its treatment?

- Do you have experience treating those who have encountered traumatic events similar to mine?

- Are you experienced in treating the associated conditions that I experience (such as drug addictions, eating disorders, depression, generalized anxiety, or panic disorders)?

- What are your views about the use of medication in the treatment of PTSD? If needed, can you prescribe it, or do you have a working relationship with someone who does?

- Do you provide family counseling or have a working relationship with counselors who do?

- What are your policies about calling you during the week should I need to?

The psychotherapist will ideally bring a number of attributes to counseling:

- *He will put you at ease and share control—you will hold primary control.* He will be comfortable in allowing you to set the pace and will work to ensure that you are as comfortable and safe as possible. He might remind you that "you don't have to tell anything you don't feel ready to or feel safe disclosing," or to feel free to control the timing or back away from uncomfortable material.[79]

- *She will explore your fears of treatment.* Everyone feels weak and helpless at times. After trauma most people fear being overwhelmed. Emotions are temporary, not a permanent reflection of character. She will understand your fear of bringing up material that causes more pain, and will work to help you replace that fear with trust and understanding.

- *He will be skilled in forging a strong therapeutic alliance.*

Early in the course of treatment the therapist will make a thorough assessment of your trauma and your life history. This will be useful to both of you. This process helps you to see that you will not go crazy talking about the trauma. The process begins to name the pain. The assessment also helps the therapist to plan the course of treatment. If, for example, you have a history of distrust in your family where it was not okay to express feelings or needs or take care of yourself, treatment might start by addressing these issues before addressing the trauma.

The assessment will also identify factors that could impede treatment. For example, a treatment plan for drug addiction would be implemented before PTSD is treated (if you are addicted to any substance, be sure to find a therapist experienced with treating addictions).[80]

Expect the counselor to be respectful and supportive but not infallible. She will not always be available nor able to fill all your needs. Some days will be less productive than others. Don't worry about expressing your secrets. Keeping secrets is part of the problem of PTSD. Experienced counselors will not be uncomfortable with such material. Keep going to therapy even after you feel better since return of symptoms is likely at some point.

It can prove helpful to involve family members of the survivor in counseling since they can be troubled by the victim's symptoms. The therapist will help them understand PTSD, and realize the real cause of the symptoms. Family members will learn what is helpful and what is beyond their capacity to fix. They might learn new ways to take care of themselves. If they are unwilling or unable to provide support to the survivor, then other social supports would be recruited. Of course if the family member is the perpetrator he would be excluded as a social support.

Remember that you will form a working team with your therapist but you are the one in control. You will learn to be more tolerant of distressing feelings that may arise. You will learn to watch them come and go. Pay attention to how you are feeling. If you experience any of the following, stop and talk to your therapist:[81]

- feeling that you are losing touch with reality such as experiencing flashbacks, hallucinations, or derealization

- feeling disoriented, spaced-out, or loss of control

- hyperventilation (rapid, irregular breathing), uncontrollable shaking, pounding or irregular heartbeat, panic attack, gasping for air

- extreme nausea, diarrhea, bleeding, new or intense pain, exacerbation of existing medical conditions (e.g., diabetes)

- desire to hurt yourself (e.g., cutting or suicide)

- desire to perform self-defeating behaviors (vomit, use drugs, overspend, inappropriate sexual activity)

- thoughts of hurting others

- emotions so overwhelming that you fear you are going to die, go crazy, or lose control

Medication

Medications do not cure PTSD. However, they may be useful under certain situations to lessen symptoms so that other forms of treatment can work. For example, medications might help reduce symptoms of depression or anxiety when these symptoms are severe and blocking treatment success. Psychiatrists and other medical doctors prescribe medications. Seek a psychiatrist who is skilled in working with people with PTSD. General practice physicians will be unlikely to have such experience. Psychiatrists do not usually provide psychotherapy, although some do. All medications have side effects. A wise consumer will discuss these considerations with the prescribing physician. Appendix 8 discusses other medication considerations.

Survivor Groups

The use of groups to treat PTSD was pioneered with Vietnam war veterans. Survivor groups typically include five to ten people meeting weekly to provide support and encouragement as you process your experiences and learn coping skills. Some groups are run by or advised by mental health professionals. Others are self-help groups organized and directed by nonprofessionals. Groups can prove a useful adjunct to individual counseling and individual efforts, once symptoms are stabilized. Experience has taught that groups accomplish a number of critical steps in healing:[82]

- *Alienation and estrangement are countered.* The group member comes to realize that others can understand what he has gone through because they have had similar experiences themselves. Survivors realize that they are not the only ones to react as they did. They see that others are struggling too, and that others can understand. They feel less abnormal, less weird, less different.

- *Groups provide a sense of community, a feeling of security that is akin to family.* This is important since safety and security are needed for recovery. This breaks down further the feeling of isolation and helps people transition back into society.

- *Groups destigmatize the experience.* Members can assure the victim that they are not abnormal for what they experienced. Seeing the worth of those who have experienced a similar trauma helps counter feelings of worthlessness.

- *Groups facilitate the disclosing of secrets thus unburdening the secret keeper and countering the idea that "my story is too horrible to tell."*

- *Group members will challenge each other to take a more realistic view.*

- *Groups help survivors to talk and process their traumatic memories in a supportive climate.*

- *Groups permit the sharing of coping ideas.* Members see coping attempts modeled and can try out new ideas and behaviors.

- *Groups are especially empowering when they are not run by therapists* (the disadvantage here being that needed clinical skills may be absent).

- *Groups combine the strengths of many individuals not just one or two.* Thus, members might brainstorm ways of coping, ways to assign meaning, and ways to grow.

- *Families can be involved to increase social support.*

- *Groups create an environment where members can learn to trust others and repair their ability to relate to others.* The group format allows members to create relationships that simulate the world, but are in some ways safer. In that controlled environment, then, group members can practice necessary skills while learning how to relate to people in healthy ways.

Certain cautions apply. The frank discussions of groups might trigger troubling dissociated material. An individual should not, therefore, enter a group until he is in fairly good control of his symptoms. He might, for example, seek individual psychotherapy until he is comfortable confronting traumatic memories. He then might prefer a group with an experienced mental health professional. Obviously, group work is inadvisable for one who has never talked about his traumatic memories, or for one whose life is chaotic. Groups are also inappropriate for people who are suicidal, homicidal, violent, abusing drugs, self-mutilating, or borderline, at least until these are controlled. Groups for dissociative identity disorder can be a useful adjunct when secondary to one-on-one psychotherapy (see Appendix 4).[83]

Self-Managed Treatment Approaches

There are many steps that people with PTSD can take to help themselves, especially with regard to managing symptoms and restoring balance, stability, and health to one's life. Should people with PTSD try to treat themselves? As a general rule, professional help is suggested since, by definition, PTSD means that one's present coping abilities have been overwhelmed. While a minority of survivors seem to fully recover on their own, most will continue to experience troubling symptoms for a long time afterward without treatment. Properly trained specialists can help the survivor along the road to recovery faster, much like a skilled coach can help an athlete improve performance. Mental health professionals can help survivors develop new coping skills and process material that is "stuck." Acknowledging the need for help and seeking it is a sign of self-esteem.

Be Aware of Your Choices

Unfortunately, many of those who need help will not find it. Sometimes skilled professionals are not readily available. Sometimes individuals cannot afford treatment or feel embarrassed to seek it. Sometimes people with PTSD do not know where to look for help or don't realize how useful it can be.

This book will guide you to finding and facilitating the correct treatment. As much as possible, specific instructions for treatment strategies are provided since an informed client will progress better in treatment. Use the book as a resource. Discuss it with your mental health professional. Together, you might decide to practice certain treatment strategies at home as part of your comprehensive treatment plan. Some people who do not have a formal diagnosis of PTSD but are nevertheless troubled by symptoms might find some of the strategies herein useful. In some cases, the originators of certain techniques indicate that they can be used without supervision. However, these should be used with caution. The main principle to remember is that dissociated material can be more troubling than needed if it is not managed in a controlled and safe way. If in doubt, consult with a mental health professional skilled in treating PTSD before using any of the treatment strategies in this book. Take responsibility for your recovery. Seek to be as self-reliant as possible, but also know when to ask for help.

FINDING THE BEST HELP

Various organizations listed in the Resource Section, Appendix 10, will help you find the right mental health professional and/or group. Remember to be a good consumer. Check out credentials and experience. Make sure that you are comfortable with a therapist before committing to therapy.

PART III

Preparations

CHAPTER 7

Stabilization and Balance

Before beginning treatment, restore as much equilibrium in your life—balance, order, and health—as you can. You can't concentrate on recovering if you don't feel reasonably safe and strong. Treatment is more like a marathon than a sprint. Recovery may take months or longer, depending on the amount of upheaval in your life. So you'll need to have your life in good balance. This section will help you regain control of your life and prepare for the work of healing. Many of the steps are themselves healing. They send a soothing signal that you are willing to rebuild damaged boundaries and take care of yourself. Don't feel like a failure, though, if you feel a need for professional help in getting started.

PHYSICAL SAFETY

You have the right to be safe and protected from harm. Building physical safety includes protecting against harm:

- *From others.* Take all necessary precautions to insure your safety. Steps might include:
  - *Removing yourself from an abusive partner or causing the partner to be removed.* Shelters or crisis centers will advise you of your rights and assist in obtaining protective or restraining orders (which are not always well enforced) or other legal protections. Know how to summon the police to quickly report battery (being attacked or beaten up).
  - *Making an emergency escape plan.* Plan in advance how you will find shelter or safe relatives/friends. Pack a bag or make a seventy-two-hour emergency preparedness kit (see Appendix 5). This can provide a tremendous sense of security should you need to flee criminals, abusive

partners, civil unrest, or natural disaster. If you live with an abuser, keep emergency supplies elsewhere such as at a trusted friend's or at an airport storage locker.

- *Checking the security of the house.* It is quite normal for people who have suffered a traumatic event to make frequent checks of locks and windows, or to look under beds and closets. If your house has been violated, you might put up protective bars, install dead bolts on doors, or change locks or telephone numbers. Join a neighborhood watch group or form one with help from the police.
- *Learning self-defense.*
- *Being fully mindful of the environment.* Trauma victims might temporarily lose their protective instinct, becoming stunned and feeling helpless. Take control of your safety again. Carefully scan for signs of danger. Look around parked cars, for example, or inside your car before entering it. Do this with a sense of confident anticipation. That is, if you detect potential danger, you will have a sensible action plan (e.g., run away, blow a whistle, loudly call for help).
- *Avoiding risky places and/or arranging for companionship* (e.g., a college student calls for a security escort before walking to a dark parking lot).

- *From self.* Commit not to harm yourself in any way. Drugs, mutilation, and other self-destructive acts are ways you might have learned to deal with painful dissociated material. They undermine treatment. Seek professional help if you need assistance in controlling these practices. It is an act of self-caring to arrange for hospitalization if you anticipate the need for protection.

- *To others.* Violence must be halted and anger must be controlled (see chapter 16). Family crisis centers often provide anger counseling for individuals and couples. Hospitalization might be necessary if you suspect that you might harm others. Some family members might simply be harmed by your withdrawal or mistrust. You might explain, "I went through a rather difficult experience some time ago. I have my ups and downs. If I seem distracted or unreasonably upset sometimes, it's not because of you. I will recover, but it will take some time." You may or may not choose to disclose the details of the traumatic event. People can be known emotionally without disclosing private facts. The important point is that feelings can be openly communicated so that family members can make sense of their world.

EMOTIONAL SAFETY

A strong therapeutic alliance with a mental health professional that you respect and feel comfortable with can be a crucial component of healing. Social support can also be provided from family and friends (if they are available and willing) and/or support groups. Fight the tendency to isolate yourself following exposure to a traumatic event. Do choose your social supports wisely. Be sure that you disclose information only to people whom you discern to be safe and trustworthy. That is, you will be reasonably confident that they will keep confidences and will not negatively judge you or harm you. Again, recognize the limits of family members. They may not understand the nature of PTSD. Perhaps they won't understand why you just can't bounce back to normal. You might let them read this book. They themselves may be overwhelmed or unavailable for other reasons. In such cases it will be wise to cultivate additional social supports.

CONCERNS OF LIVING

These include food, shelter, employment, medical and legal care, bills, and time management (see Appendix 6). Most counties have organizations to help people find employment and low-cost or free shelter. Medical care may be needed to help heal physical wounds, check for sexually transmitted diseases or pregnancy, or clear you for physical exercise. A thorough medical exam can also detect physical conditions that can increase symptoms of arousal and anxiety. For example, thyroid disorders can create a wealth of anxiety and depression symptoms. An inexpensive test called the TSH test can frequently detect subtle abnormalities that normal blood tests will miss.[84] You might have to specifically request this test from your doctor. A biopsychiatrist specializing in PTSD might be more likely than a primary care physician to look for such conditions. Sleep apnea can also lead to fatigue, depression, and loss of sexual interest. Sleep apnea is signaled by loud snoring, followed by silence and gasping for air. It is very treatable but frequently goes undiagnosed.

Learn how not to be harmed by the legal system. National Organization for Victims Assistance (NOVA) helps victims of crime, for instance, navigate the criminal justice system, including the risks of police investigations (giving details might be traumatizing), precourt appearances, trials, and sentencing hearings (see Resources, Appendix 10). Be prepared for messages from insensitive lawyers or police who might suggest that you caused the crime or asked for it, or did not respond "correctly." Personal details of your life history will also become a matter of public record should you choose to prosecute an offender.

See Appendix 10 for additional resources which can help you get back on your feet following a traumatic event. Some services will not apply if you let too much time elapse after the trauma, so act as promptly as you can.

PROBLEM SOLVING

Serious problems of immediate living will need to be solved, or at least reasonably controlled, for recovery to progress. During times of extreme stress we often get tunnel vision, so focused on fear and so desirous of a quick solution that we fail to consider all of our options. Problem-solving skills enable us to explore our options and enact a plan. Problem-solving skills have been taught even to children, resulting in less anxiety and stress. Solving problems is more satisfying than escaping them with drugs. When a problem arises, tell yourself, "This is an opportunity for growth, not a stumbling block." The procedure is:

1. Clearly identify the problem. Some people find that writing the problem down on paper helps to focus their thinking.

2. Determine what the desired outcome is. (What do you wish to see happen?)

3. Brainstorm a list of possible solutions. When we brainstorm, we think of as many ideas as we can, as fast as we can. We don't judge, at this point, whether possible solutions are good or bad, possible or not possible. We simply list. Being critical of ideas stifles the creative process.

4. Appraise the list of solutions. What are the strengths and weaknesses of each? Can any solutions be combined? Are there any solutions that have not been thought of? Do you need more information?

5. Pick what seems like a sensible solution.

6. Make a thorough plan

7. Try it out.

8. Reevaluate and make adjustments.

You need not attempt problem solving alone. The resource list in Appendix 10 suggests many sources of help. Trusted acquaintances can be especially helpful in brainstorming. However, studies have suggested that the best creative problem solving occurs when people alternate between working in groups and working alone. Thus, it might be wise to solicit ideas and information from sensible people, but rely on yourself to think through all aspects of your plan. It is unlikely that you will find a perfect solution; it is likely you'll find one or more reasonably good solutions.

You can use this problem-solving process for the immediate problems of living. Later, you can use it when stressful situations arise or when you wish to manage troubling PTSD symptoms.

HEALTHY PLEASURES

Your physical and mental well-being depend on a healthy balance between work and play. Plan to incorporate a variety of healthy pleasures into your lifestyle to sustain your mood and literally recreate (i.e., *re*-create). Perhaps you'll want to try things that used to be pleasurable. Perhaps you'll wish to try new things that might prove enjoyable. Remember activities such as warm baths, gardening, getting together with friends and family, pleasant reading, or other forms of recreation that you found enjoyable in the past. At this point, you might not feel capable or worthy of pleasure. These ideas will wane over the course of treatment. For now, set some simple, modest goals to regularly engage in pleasant activities, and then experiment. Try some events alone and some with others. On a one-to-ten scale, predict how pleasurable you expect an event to be. Then rate how pleasant it was afterward. The latter might be slightly higher than you predicted. Don't get down on yourself if events don't seem as pleasant as they used to. This is a normal symptom of PTSD. This will change. Avoid violence in the media—movies, videos, television—that will trigger arousal.

CHAPTER 8

Taking Care of Your Health

The mind and body are connected. The condition of your body will profoundly affect your moods, energy level, performance, and symptoms, including sleep quality. Developing a healthier body will help you through the course of treatment.

EXERCISE (CONDITIONING OR BODY PLAY)

Note: If you hyperventilate, do not begin an exercise program until you are skilled in automatic, slow, regular, and rhythmic abdominal breathing. Complete chapter 11 before proceeding with this one. If physical activity is a trigger, see chapter 18 before beginning an exercise program.

Virtually everyone who engages in a *regular, moderate* exercise program knows how remarkably effective it is in reducing stress. Exercise has been shown to measurably reduce muscle tension and other stress symptoms without the side effects of medication, improve self-esteem and mental health generally, reduce blood pressure, increase energy levels and stamina, reduce resting heart and breathing rates, strengthen the heart, improve the quality of sleep, promote weight loss, strengthen the immune system, and reduce PMS symptoms.

The stress response is designed to culminate in physical movement. Exercise allows the body to expend the energy of the stress response and return to a more restful state. It also gives the mind a break, time to distract and spin free, so that we return to work mentally and physically refreshed. This is why the exercised person can accomplish more in less time. Some think they are too busy to exercise. It helps to think of exercise as an important investment. It enables people to be more productive, accomplishing more in less time. It also enables people to remain more relaxed and in a better frame of mind *while* they cope with problems.

What Kind of Exercise Is Best?

Any kind of exercise is better than none. There are three kinds of exercise:

1. *Aerobic exercise.* This is rhythmic, continuous exercise, such as walking, swimming, low-impact aerobics, jogging, biking, stair climbing, and some racket games.

2. *Strength training* (lifting weights, calisthenics, or similar activities).

3. *Flexibility exercises such as yoga or stretching.*

   If you are limited for time, aerobic exercise is generally recommended at a gentle pace, most days for at least twenty minutes. Daily, longer, gentle exercise (e.g., walking for forty minutes daily rather than running for twenty minutes three times a week) is best for stress reduction and weight loss. However, these are just goals to strive for. Even a ten-minute energy walk can bring ninety minutes of energy, elevated mood, and stress reduction. Try a quick energy walk to get away from your desk for a few minutes every hour or two. And don't overlook the other two types of exercise. Yogic postures can slow the effects of aging and stiffening, and the improved muscle tone from weight training facilitates weight loss and greatly reduces anxiety.

   Start your exercise program gently and build up gradually. You are not in a race. Exercise should leave you refreshed and energized. It should not hurt or exhaust you beyond a pleasant fatigue. If you eventually work up to twenty minutes or more on most days, great. If not, do what you can to start. Do make a plan for regular, moderate exercise. If you have trouble falling asleep, try exercising before dinner, or earlier. Allow five to ten minutes before and after exercising for warmup and cool-down. If you are older (age forty for men; fifty for women) or have any health risk factors (being overweight, symptoms or family history of high blood pressure, heart disease, or diabetes) have a physical examination first and discuss your exercise plans with your doctor.

SLEEP HYGIENE

Poor sleep can be both a cause and effect of anxiety. Two considerations are crucial: (1) *Amount.* Most sleep researchers believe that almost all adults function and feel at their best with at least eight hours of sleep. Many do better on considerably more. (2) *Regularity.* Regular sleep and wake-up times are needed to keep the body's sleep cycle consistent. Retiring at irregular hours (e.g., getting to bed much later on Friday and Saturday nights than on weekdays) can lead to insomnia. In this century, a number of developments have interfered with sleep: the light bulb permits people to stay up later and do shift work; worldwide communication allows people to work or be entertained around the clock; twenty-four-hour shopping promotes irregular sleep patterns. It is no wonder that today's American is sleep-deprived but does not realize it.

The idea is to get a little more sleep than you think you need, and to keep sleep and wake-up times as consistent throughout the week as possible, varying no more than an hour from night to night. This will probably take considerable discipline, given all the temptations of modern society. The payoffs will surprise you.

Beyond the major issues of amount and regularity, the following tips can also improve sleep:

- *Use the bedroom only for sleeping.* Sex is an exception when it is enjoyable and relaxing. Remove phones and television. Don't pay bills, work, or read arousing material in bed. All can condition you to be aroused in bed.

- *Reduce light and noise, which can disturb sleep.* If your clock emits light, cover it or turn it away from you. Be sure that early morning light does not enter through the window.

- *Don't eat a big meal within four hours of retiring.* A light carbohydrate and/or low-fat dairy snack before bed can help you fall asleep quicker (e.g., warm milk, crackers and cheese, sweetened yogurt, bread).

- *Avoid stimulants, like caffeine, for at least seven to ten hours before bedtime.*

- *If you are having difficulty sleeping, either eliminate naps altogether,* or try them regularly each day for fifteen to ninety minutes around 1:00–2:00 P.M.

- *Once in bed, try slow breathing and/or progressive muscle relaxation to unwind* (see later chapters).

- *If you wake up and cannot fall back to sleep within fifteen to twenty minutes, get out of bed and do something quiet.* Do not reward yourself for not sleeping with television or something else enjoyable. Rather, try something like paying bills. Some people prefer to meditate to calm down.

- *If you are afraid to go to sleep because of nightmares, read chapters 10 and 28.*

- *If the bedroom itself is a trigger (e.g., for a rape victim), try the arousal re-duction techniques in Part IV.*

EATING PRACTICES AND NUTRITION

Sensible eating habits are essential in managing stress. Simply stated, good nutrition raises resistance to stress and anxiety, while poor nutrition is a stressor. (See Figures 8.1–8.4.) If you visualize a plate where less than one-fourth of the plate comprises meat products, and plant foods fill the rest of the plate, then you have a pretty good idea of eating goals which include:

- *Get most of your calories from complex carbohydrates, which come from plant foods* (e.g., fruits, vegetables, breads, rice, pasta, cereals). Foods that are fresh, frozen, or minimally processed are usually better choices because they tend to have less added sugar, salt, fat, but more fiber.

- *Reduce meats, which contain saturated fats and cholesterol, to about 6 ounces daily.* Use mainly lean meats, poultry without skin, fish, or meat alternates such as dry beans and peas, or nuts.

- *Reduce fats, sugar, salt, caffeine, processed foods, and alcohol.* If sleep is troubled, avoid caffeine altogether or for at least seven to ten hours before bedtime. (Nicotine and recreational drugs can also increase anxiety, so gradually reduce or eliminate these too, over a period of several weeks.)

- *Take adequate calcium.* Adults age nineteen to fifty need 1,000 mg of calcium each day. A glass of skim milk provides 300 mg. Even if they drink three glasses of skim milk each day (or yogurt or cheese equivalents), then additional calcium would still be needed from sources like spinach, broccoli, or tofu.[85] Adults age fifty-one and older need 1,200 mg daily. Do not exceed 2,500 mg daily.

Additional guidelines which can improve health generally, help control weight, and/or help stabilize the mood include:

- *Keep blood sugar steady throughout the day.* This can be done by eating breakfast, not skipping meals, and eating smaller, more frequent meals. There is evidence that five or six smaller meals will reduce fatigue and irritability while also facilitating weight loss. "Meals" can include mid-morning and mid-afternoon snacks such as a half-sandwich, yogurt, or fruit. Avoid concentrated sweets, which cause blood sugar fluctuations.

- *Shift food, so that some of the calories that would normally be eaten at a big dinner are eaten at breakfast, lunch, or as snacks.*

- *Choose foods often that are less than 30 percent fat.* To quickly estimate fat content, multiply the grams of fat by ten and divide by the total calories. The result should be less that 33 percent. A candy bar contains 250 calories, and 14 grams of fat. Thus:

$$\frac{14 \text{ grams fat} \times 10}{250 \text{ calories}} = 56\%$$

This choice is quite high in fat. The sugar would also tend to give a momentary energy lift, but would make people more tired and tense an hour later (a brisk walk would give a similar energy lift that would be sustained). Similar calculations for bread, potatoes, or almost all other plant products (before adding butter or oil) would show these to be healthy choices. Although meat can exceed the 30 percent fat goal, meats can be mixed with vegetables to reduce overall fat (e.g., meat stir-fried in a little oil).

- *Drink lots of water.* Drinking too little water can lead to low-grade dehydration, fatigue, and hunger. At least two quarts of fluid are needed per day so drink water throughout the day. Stop by the fountain when you pass it.

Figure 8.1

MY PLAN TO TAKE CARE OF MY BODY

There is power in making a written plan and committing to stick to it. Please make a realistic plan that you can follow for life. It is alright to give yourself several days to "work up" to the goals in your plan.

1. **Exercise.** At least three to five times per week; at least twenty minutes aerobic exercise. Describe your plan below:

2. **Sleep.** _____ hours/night (a little more than you think you need—most adults require about 8¼ hours of sleep or more per night to feel and function at their best) from _____ (time you'll retire) to _____ (time you'll wake up)

3. **Eating.** Eat at least three times a day using healthy choices. Make a written one-week menu using the worksheet on the next page and check it against the eating goals and guidelines, including the dietary guidelines on page 83.

Figure 8.2
SAMPLE MENU: A WEEK OF MEALS

(Write down what you plan to eat each day, with corresponding amounts.)

	Mon.	Tues.	Wed.	Thurs.	Fri.	Sat.	Sun.
Breakfast							
Snack							
Lunch							
Snack							
Dinner							
Snack							

Figure 8.3
DIETARY GUIDELINES

Check to see if your sample menu meets the following guidelines for healthy eating:

1. Does your plan provide the daily recommended servings from each food group as indicated below? (Someone trying to control their weight would use the smaller figure for servings.)

Food group	Servings needed per day	Examples of one serving
Breads, cereals, rice, pasta	6–11	I slice bread I oz. ready-to-eat cereal ½ bun or bagel ½ cup cooked cereal, rice, or pasta
Vegetables	3–5	I cup raw leafy greens ½ cup other kinds of vegetables ¾ cup vegetable juice
Fruits	2–4	I medium apple, banana, orange ½ cup fresh, chopped, cooked. or canned fruit ¾ cup fruit juice
Milk, yogurt, cheese	2–3	I cup milk or yogurt (skim or low-fat best) 1½ oz. natural cheese 2 oz. processed cheese
Meats, poultry, fish, dry beans, peas, eggs, nuts	2–3	Amounts to a total of approximately 6 oz. per day, where one serving is 2–3 oz. of cooked lean meat, poultry, or fish. Count as I oz. meat: I egg; 2 tbs. peanut butter; ½ cup cooked, dry beans or peas; ⅓ cup nuts; or ¼ cup seeds

2. Does your plan provide variety? That is, do you vary your choices within each group (e.g., instead of an apple each day, try bananas or strawberries as alternatives)?

3. Does your plan follow the other guidelines stated on the previous pages?

Figure 8.4
DAILY PROGRESS RECORD

Keep a record to see how well you stick to your plan for two weeks. Throughout this period, make whatever adjustments are necessary, and then continue the plan.

Day	Date	Excercised (minutes)	Number of Meals Eaten	hours	Sleep time to bed	time out of bed
1						
2						
3						
4						
5						
6						
7						
8						
9						
10						
11						
12						
13						
14						

PART IV

Managing Symptoms

CHAPTER 9

Affect Management

The most damaging feelings are
those that are never discussed.
—Dr. Don R. Catherall[86]

Throughout the course of your recovery, you will likely encounter times of high emotional and physical arousal, especially when you experience intrusive recollections. This part of the book will describe approaches that help to manage these symptoms so that they become less troubling.

Remember the caution about trying to do too much, too fast, or too much by yourself. You'll likely find better success if you read and apply the skills in this part under the guidance of a skilled therapist, who can act as a coach and help ensure that you do not become overwhelmed. A therapist's guidance is especially important for the skills in chapters 17 and 18 (and for any skills involving imagery or hypnosis or that might trigger dissociation). And discuss with your therapist the best order for reading the chapters in this part. You might find that the present order makes the most sense. However, if intrusions are so troubling that they interfere with symptom management, you might wish—again under your therapist's guidance—to start with chapters 17 and 18, in order to permit you to succeed with the other chapters. Again, if you have any questions, discuss them first with your therapist before proceeding.

Before we discuss learning to control your physiology let's begin by discussing emotional or feelings skills. Often, people who have experienced very painful emotions have learned to control their pain by shutting down their emotions. It is as if they think, "Feelings are too painful—I refuse to feel." They might also have picked up messages along the way that reinforce this decision not to feel.

- *Family messages*. Perhaps members were mocked if they cried or expressed tenderness or anger (big boys don't cry; ladies don't get angry). Perhaps they grew up in a family where feelings simply were not expressed. In some families, people were too preoccupied with survival to feel.

- *Occupational messages*. Perhaps there is an occupational mindset that does not permit feelings (soldiers, policemen, firefighters, doctors, nurses shouldn't cry—they'll be sissies, unable to perform).

- *Fear messages*
  - I won't be respected if I show my feelings.
  - If I feel at all I will lose control and not be able to regain it.

Certainly some people lose control of their emotions in unwholesome ways. This is the case with violence and uncontrolled anger. It is the case with those who say things in the heat of emotion that they later regret. It might be the case with those who repeatedly give in to their fears. We'll advance here the proposition that the *wholesome* experience and expression of feelings is necessary for mental health, peak performance, and relationships that go deeper than mere superficiality. We are referring here to being aware of our feelings, distinguishing between appropriate and inappropriate behaviors, and knowing how to constructively channel and express our feelings. Feelings make us human. Wisely schooled, they elevate us to a higher level of humanity. I think, for example, of combat veterans shedding tears at their fallen comrade's funeral. The tears signaled their love for their friend and validated their sadness. It showed that it was okay to feel sadness at the loss. The commander's tears revealed a heart. Respect for him increased. It is easier, perhaps, to follow such a leader than one who has little regard for human life, or for the feelings of his people.

The wholesome release of emotions returns our system to equilibrium, better prepared to react to the next emergency. Those who remain on constant alert are often the ones who blow up or burn out. In PTSD, while people seem to feel little, there are often many intense emotions that have been numbed. They remain under the surface, though, ready to explode. Often anger is the closest to the surface. However, anger usually covers up more primary emotions such as fear and hurt. As long as only the anger is experienced and expressed, the other emotions will never heal. So our goal is to be fully aware of the range of feelings, and their gradations, so that we can channel them constructively. A person who can view her feelings without judgment is in the strongest position to control them.

All feelings serve a protective purpose. Without fear we don't take wise precautions. Without anger some protective acts would not be initiated. If we pay attention to it, grief tells us where healing is needed. Uncomfortable feelings tell us that something is wrong so that we can take appropriate action. Even numb feelings protect us from overwhelming emotions at first and signal a need for healing later. It is said that the difference between a coward and a brave person is that one acts despite fear. Feelings make life interesting. Without fully feeling, we do not fully respond to life. To shut down some feelings is to shut down others.

Our goal, then, is to learn to experience and express feelings as normal, constructive, and wholesome. If we don't, we are more likely to experience intrusions, rage, bodily complaints, fatigue, and self-destruction.

Relax and ask yourself, "What am I feeling right now?" It is normal for victims to have a tough time identifying their feelings.

Realize that all feelings are valid and a normal part of life. Don't judge them. Feelings change. Tears do not last. They are expressed, and then we return to normal. The idea is to first recognize feelings so that we can control what we do with them. It is a beautiful thing to see a child with joyful feelings so openly expressed. Likewise, it is comforting to see an adult who feels—joy, love, tenderness, even negative emotions if they are directed constructively and lovingly. Again, we can't shut down the negatives without shutting down positive emotions. Perhaps you weren't permitted to grow emotionally. That was then. Now the goal is to feel comfortable with all emotions, identify them, and channel them constructively.

SKILLS

1. *Learn to name your feelings and recognize gradations.* For example, there is a difference between rage, anger, irritation, and frustration. Naming emotions gives us a sense of control over emotions; it helps us to express them verbally rather than needing to act them out inappropriately. You might consult the list below for the varieties of emotions (see page 90).

2. *When you notice yourself feeling, just observe the process without judging.* Do not think, "This is awful to feel such things. I shouldn't feel like this. How dare she make me feel like this." Just notice the feelings arise and notice them subside.

WORDS OF EMOTION

accepted	ecstatic	interested	safe
affectionate	edgy	irritable	satisfied
afraid	elated	isolated	scared
aggressive	embarrassed	jealous	secure
aggrieved	enthusiastic	joyful	sensitive
agitated	envious	lonely	serene
alienated	excited	loved	shocked
alive	exhausted	love struck	shy
ambivalent	fearful	manipulated	silly
amused	friendly	mischievous	sorry
angry	frightened	miserable	stubborn
annoyed	frustrated	misunderstood	stupid
anxious	furious	moody	supportive
apathetic	generous	negative	sure
appreciated	glad	nervous	surprised
ashamed	gloomy	old	suspicious
awkward	graceful	optimistic	tender
bashful	grateful	outraged	tense
beautiful	grouchy	overjoyed	terrified
bored	grumpy	pained	threatened
brave	guilty	panicky	torn up
calm	happy	paranoid	touchy
cautious	hateful	passionate	unappreciated
confident	helpless	peaceful	uncertain
confused	hopeful	persecuted	uncomfortable
courageous	hopeless	pessimistic	undecided
curious	horrified	playful	understanding
cynical	hostile	pleased	uneasy
daring	humiliated	possessive	uptight
defeated	humorous	preoccupied	used
dejected	hurt	pressured	useless
delighted	hysterical	protective	victimized
depressed	impatient	proud	violated
desperate	inadequate	puzzled	violent
determined	incompetent	quiet	vulnerable
devastated	indecisive	rejected	warm
disappointed	inferior	regretful	weary
disconsolate	inhibited	relieved	withdrawn
discontented	innocent	remorseful	worthwhile
discouraged	insecure	resentful	
disgusted	insulted	sad	

3. *Feelings always make sense.* Like a scientist who observes with detachment, see if you can identify the cause of the feelings. Something happens. You think about it. Then you feel. You might with curiosity try and identify the thoughts that led to your feelings. If you can't determine what brought on the feeling, try to discover if there was a trigger related to the trauma. Distinguish between feelings and actions. You don't have to do anything with feelings if you choose not to. On the other hand, you might constructively express your feelings in a journal or drawing, or you might talk it over with a trusted friend or relative.

If becoming aware of your emotions in any way becomes overwhelming or causes you to fear harming yourself or others, do not try these skills for now. The skills will become easier as the dissociated material is digested.

CHAPTER 10

Reducing General Arousal

Many PTSD symptoms are caused by your sensitized nervous system. Trauma overwhelmed the brain's arousal center and sent it into a condition of high alert. The alarm center has since remained on alert, overreacting to stressful situations and keeping your body aroused. In turn, bodily arousal feeds back to the brain, keeping it sensitized. A vicious cycle now exists between anxiety and arousal. Reducing general arousal in the body is an important step in desensitizing the nervous system. Although it may take from several weeks to months to desensitize the nervous system, this section can help you notice relief from many of the symptoms of arousal fairly rapidly. When arousal symptoms do occur, they will often be less severe, and you'll learn how to relax *into* them to prevent additional arousal from becoming alarmed at the symptoms.

RELAXING INTO THE SYMPTOMS

Let's consider panic attack as a worst-case scenario of arousal. In a panic attack the brain's alarm center goes off full blast. Every pathway of the stress response is triggered to a maximum degree. The pounding, racing heart, dizziness, air hunger, and other physical reactions are bad enough for the person affected. But in his terrified state, the panic attack sufferer also feels that he might do something drastic (like run or hit someone) or lose control. This is a normal response to a threat and would make sense provided there was a real threat and provided there was a physical outlet for the energy of the stress response. We might consider a panic attack, then, as a normal physical (stress) response when there is little or no threat. It is simply an alarm response caused by sensitized nerves. The body is designed such that the maximum stress response can only be maintained for five to ten minutes. After peaking, the symptoms begin to subside of their own accord, often quite rapidly—especially if we relax so as not to induce further arousal.

Even in panic sufferers, reducing general arousal can reduce the number of attacks. However, a goal more important than *avoiding* symptoms of arousal is learning how to *master the fear* of arousal. As we master the fear of symptoms, anticipatory fear and general arousal also decrease.

Dr. Claire Weekes is sometimes referred to as the "Grandmother of Anxiety" because she has helped so many people learn to deal with the symptoms of nervous arousal from sensitized nerves. She has given four principles of recovery from sensitized nerves. Although these principles are designed for panic, they also apply to any anxiety symptoms.

1. *Face the symptoms.* Confront them until they no longer matter. A little girl is invigorated by facing into the wind and learning that she can stand up to it without being defeated. Even panic will not defeat you. The body is designed to adapt to the stress response. The mind becomes sharper under stress. Arousal does not cause people to act crazy. Indeed a certain amount of arousal sharpens reactions. It is dissociation, not arousal, that impairs performance.

2. *Willingly accept the symptoms.* Relax, let go, and invite in the body's "rattling." Let the body go loose as much as possible, then go toward, not withdrawing from, the feared symptoms and experiences. Go with the symptoms, "bending like the willow before the wind—rolling with the punches."[87] Realize that with time the arousal and the intensity of the symptoms will diminish because the secretion of chemical messengers of stress decrease. As Weekes says, "so many people allow an electric flash to spoil their lives by withdrawing from it in fear."[88] Go into it; never withdraw. At their worst, symptoms will pass.

3. *Float.* With a deeply relaxed body (the paralysis in panic is simply from overtensing the body), breathe gently and peacefully and see yourself floating forward as in a cloud or on the water. There is no struggle, grim determination, or clenching of muscles—these increase arousal. Likewise, trying to erase or forget memories also creates tension. Accept them as ordinary. Act and do anyway what you want to do. As you read more in this section, you will learn how to more deeply relax your breathing and your body.

4. *Let time pass.* A sensitized nervous system will not be cured overnight. So allow time for chemical readjustment and to learn new ways to react to stressors.

It is important to learn that anxiety symptoms will not defeat you. Under professional supervision in clinical settings, panic attack sufferers are often helped to induce their own panic attack (by intentionally hyperventilating, spinning around, or exercising too intensely) and then float through the symptoms. This helps them in two ways: They realize that there is a reason for the attacks—there is not something drastically wrong with their bodies; they are not having a heart attack; it is not a brain tumor causing the symptoms. They also learn as they relax and stifle the urge to run away that the symptoms subside on their own. It's not as bad as they had feared. They don't die. They can tolerate the symptoms of anxiety. This is a major step in reducing their fear.[89]

REDUCING CAFFEINE, NICOTINE, AND OTHER ANXIETY-PRODUCING DRUGS

Even the caffeine in two cups of coffee can be enough to trigger intense anxiety symptoms. You might, therefore, consider reducing or eliminating caffeine gradually over the course of several weeks to reduce withdrawal symptoms. If you are having difficulty sleeping, avoid caffeine for at least seven to ten hours before bedtime. Caffeine is also found in tea, chocolate, certain soft drinks, and various nonprescription medications and weight control aids. Check the label. You might consider switching to decaffeinated coffee, herbal teas, or soft drinks without caffeine.

A variety of other substances can cause arousal and anxiety symptoms. Recreational drugs (nicotine, alcohol, marijuana, PCP, LSD, cocaine, etc.) and a variety of prescription and nonprescription drugs can also trigger anxiety. Discuss this with your doctor. You might consider their discontinuation, reduction, and/or replacement.

EXERCISE, SLEEP, AND NUTRITION

Exercise, sleep, and nutrition are all extremely important foundations in your plan to reduce anxiety. Exercise directly reduces arousal by expending the energy of stress. Exercise also strengthens the body and builds resistance to stress-related disease. Sufficient sleep and sound nutrition also helps us to be more stress-resistant. Diets high in white sugar (found in processed foods) and white flour (which is handled by the body like sugar) have been linked to anxiety and arousal. Eating more fresh, frozen, or minimally processed foods in accordance with the food pyramid discussed in chapter 8 can help reduce anxiety symptoms.

CHAPTER 11

Breathing Retraining[*]

BREATHING AND HYPERVENTILATION

Many people are surprised that very subtle shifts in breathing can cause anxiety symptoms ranging from muscle tension to migraines, panic attacks, and high blood pressure. The highly respected researcher and physician Chandra Patel sums it up:

> Behind the simple act (of breathing) lies a process that affects us profoundly. It affects the way we think and feel, the quality of what we create, and how we function in our daily life. Breathing affects our psychological and physiological states, while our psychological states affect the pattern of our breathing. . . . Hyperventilation causes not only anxiety but also such a variety of symptoms that patients can go from one specialty department to another until a wise clinician spots the abnormal breathing pattern and the patient is successfully trained to shift from maladaptive to normal breathing behavior.
>
> It has long been known that slow, rhythmic, diaphragmatic breathing can soothe our inner storms and make us feel calm and composed. It is difficult to apportion the benefit contributed by breathing exercise, but I now believe it is likely to be larger than I had originally imagined.[90]

Hyperventilation is seen in many, and perhaps most, people with anxiety disorders. It accounts for many visits to primary-care physicians and most of the calls for ambulances.[91]

---

*The author wishes to express appreciation to Dr. Ronald Ley, University of Albany, for reviewing this section, which has drawn much from his work: B. H. Timmons and R. Ley, eds. 1994. *Behavioral and Psychological Approaches to Breathing Disorders*. New York: Plenum.

WHAT EXACTLY IS HYPERVENTILATION?

Hyperventilation, or overbreathing, means that you expel carbon dioxide (CO_2) faster than your body is producing it.[92] This usually occurs with rapid, shallow "chest" breathing, but can also occur with deep breathing.

WHY IS IT A PROBLEM?

When blood CO_2 drops, at least two major changes occur in the body. First, certain blood vessels constrict, causing less oxygen to reach the brain, heart, and extremities. Second, the blood acidity changes, causing less oxygen to reach the tissues[93] and certain ions to flood body tissues.[94] These changes account for a wide array of symptoms that are virtually identical to the symptoms of anxiety (see page 98). The change in blood acidity is thought to play a role in sensitizing the nerves.

WHAT CAUSES HYPERVENTILATION?

When stressed or worried we tend to tense the muscles of the neck, throat, chest, and abdomen. Especially when we tighten the abdominal muscles, we begin to breathe with rapid, shallow breaths primarily in the upper chest region. As the drop in CO_2 causes distressing symptoms, we become afraid of the symptoms. Arousal remains high and a vicious cycle of worry and arousal occurs.

Hyperventilation is more likely when one becomes stressed and remains immobile such as when driving or watching an upsetting television show. If worrisome thoughts trigger hyperventilation, one might learn to manage such thoughts. Learning to relax while one faces these thoughts will reduce the arousal.

In addition to stress, hyperventilation is also caused by:

- *Lung or airway disorders* (e.g., asthma, bronchitis, interstitial lung diseases).

- *Impaired breathing caused by problems of the nose, throat, or ear.* Some of these problems only appear during sleep. If nothing else accounts for your symptoms, an ear, nose, and throat doctor experienced in rhinomanometry and nasopulmonary testing might be able to detect disturbed or impaired breathing.[95]

- *Certain postures.* Under stress, some people seem to assume an "attack posture" (hunched shoulders, head and neck thrust forward, clenched teeth). Others puff up their hard, firm chests on inhalation, and underdeflate

SIGNS AND SYMPTOMS OF HYPERVENTILATION
(breathlessness and chest pain are most common)

Cardiovascular: palpitations, missed beats, tachycardia, sharp or dull atypical chest pain, "angina," vasomotor instability, cold extremities, Raynaud's phenomenon, blotchy flushing of blush area, capillary vasoconstriction (face, arms, hands)

Neurological: dizziness, unsteadiness or instability, faint feelings (rarely actual fainting), visual disturbance (occasional blackouts or tunnel vision), headache (often migraines), parethesiae (i.e., numbness, deadness, uselessness, heaviness, pins and needles, burning, limbs feeling out of proportion or "don't belong"), commonly of hands, feet, or face, sometimes of scalp or whole body, intolerance of light or noise, large pupils (wearing dark glasses on a dull day)

Respiratory: shortness of breath (typically *after* exertion), irritable cough, tightness or oppression of chest, "asthma," air hunger, inability to take a satisfying breath, excessive sighing, yawning, sniffing

Gastrointestinal: difficulty in swallowing, globus, dry mouth and throat, acid regurgitation, heartburn, "hiatus hernia," flatulence, belching, air swallowing, abdominal discomfort, bloating

Muscular: cramps, muscle pains (particularly occipital, neck, shoulders, between scapulae; less commonly, the lower back and limbs), tremors, twitching, weakness, stiffness, or tetany (seizing up)

Psychic: tension, anxiety, "unreal feelings," depersonalization, feeling "out of the body," hallucinations, fear of insanity, panic, phobias, agoraphobia, catastrophizing

General: weakness; exhaustion; impaired concentration, memory, and performance; disturbed sleep including nightmares; emotional sweating (axillae, palms, sometimes whole body); woolly head

Allergies

Source: From personal communication from Lum, Dr. L. C. (1991) in B. H. Timmons and R. Ley, eds. 1994. Behavioral and Psychological Approaches to Breathing Disorders. *New York: Plenum. Copyright © 1994 Plenum Press. Used by permission.*

during exhalation.[96] Relaxing the body and roughly equalizing the inhalation and exhalation phases of breathing helps.

- *Excessive, fast, breathless talking and taking large breaths of air can maintain hyperventilation.*

- *Tight clothes.*

- *Heat, humidity, or a steep fall in barometric pressure can trigger symptoms.*

- *Blood sugar in the low-normal range in combination with hyperventilation can aggravate symptoms.* The antidote is a) multiple meals, and b) avoiding refined sugars.

- *Progesterone causes CO_2 to drop.* Hyperventilation can contribute to PMS or pregnancy symptoms such as fatigue or headache.

- *Strong perfumes or smells.*

- *Uncontrolled diabetes (acidosis), kidney or liver failure, heart disease, excessive caffeine, other stimulants.*

- *After hyperventilating for about ten days, the body makes certain accommodations to adjust to low CO_2 and restore the blood's acid-base balance.* Breathing may slow down, but when it increases (as under stress), the symptoms of anxiety will be even more pronounced. Even a deep breath or sigh can then trigger symptoms.[97] Some people may be symptomatic most of the time. Some are symptomatic only during stress.

HOW DO I KNOW IF I HYPERVENTILATE?

There is great relief that comes from knowing that hyperventilation is contributing to your distressing symptoms and that it is treatable.

- *Rule out medical causes.*

- *Observe breathing rate and other signs.* Simply paying attention to your breathing can help you breathe correctly. Notice if any of these indications of hyperventilation exist:
  - A rate in excess of fourteen breaths per minute usually indicates hyperventilation.
  - Breathing is mostly chest (thoracic) breathing. Little use is made of the diaphragm, the muscle below the lungs that normally moves down when inhaling while pushing the abdomen out. So the chest breather will show little abdominal movement. Instead, the breastbone (sternum)

moves up and out, with little lateral expansion.[98] Sometimes, you'll also see the neck, shoulders, and clavicles (collar bones) move up and down.

- Once established, low blood CO_2 can be maintained by normal breathing plus occasional deep breaths or sighs. So look for other signs: occasional deep breath or sigh, repeated sighs, air hunger, inability to take a satisfying breath, coughing, frequent yawning, clearing the throat, sniffing, or nasal drip.

- Other possible indications: Moistening lips (excessive breathing dries out the airways), occasional spasmodic twitching of facial muscles, tenderness of chest wall,[99] or irregular inhale/exhale ratio.

- *Provocation Test.* An expensive but useful test in a lung function laboratory or other specialty clinic, this involves intentionally breathing fast (thirty to sixty times per minute) and deeply or thoracically for two to three minutes. The appearance of symptoms or the inability to complete the test indicates that hyperventilation is the cause. Determination of low blood CO_2[100] and decreased acidity of the blood confirms the diagnosis. By demonstrating to the person that symptoms are only the result of breathing and that they are safe and reversible, this test can be very reassuring.[101] In some cases, as little as twelve rapid breaths while standing will produce symptoms.

- *The Think Test is often used along with the Provocation Test. Sometimes just thinking about and recalling a stressful time when great physical distress was experienced will bring on hyperventilation and anxiety symptoms.* After the provocation test, persons close their eyes and recreate the situation at the time of a panic attack. That is, they think about circumstances (such as disturbing topics they were thinking about at the time of the attack), feelings, sensations, and symptoms. The combination of the two tests is more likely to create hyperventilation symptoms, thus confirming the diagnosis.[102]

HOW DO I TREAT IT?

The effects of stress-induced hyperventilation can be reversed by altering the breathing so that CO_2 is conserved, or by increasing through exercise the amount of CO_2 produced by the body. The first approach is called breathing retraining, a most important skill which we'll discuss next.

Breathing Retraining[103]

Normal breathing is slow, effortless, regular, fluid, and quiet with virtually no movement above the diaphragm. Some master breathing retraining quite rapidly, while others may require months of practice. The goals are to change from erratic breathing to slow, regular, rhythmic abdominal breathing and to make this kind of breathing automatic. This shift in breathing results in long-term changes in the nervous system and anxiety symptoms. Here are the steps:

1. *Loosen your clothing* (belts, ties, collars, clothing around waist and abdomen). Remove contact lenses or glasses if you wish.

2. *Lie on your back or in the half-lying position with pillows under back and knees to relax the abdominal muscles.*

3. *Relax your entire body.* Especially warm and relax the abdomen. Also release tension in the chest, shoulders, neck, face, and jaw. Using the upper body's muscles to breathe wastes energy.

4. *Place a telephone book over the abdomen* (the area below the diaphragm down to the pelvis; practically, this means putting the book below the ribs and over the navel). The book provides resistance to strengthen the diaphragm and encourages abdominal movement.

5. *Bring your lips together.* Breathe comfortably and rhythmically, *not* deeply, through your nose. As you breathe in, let your stomach rise slowly, gradually, quietly. Think of your stomach as a balloon easily filling gently with air. Move smoothly into the exhalation without pause. Expiration is quiet, passive, and relaxed. The in-breath and out-breath are approximately equivalent in time, the out-breath perhaps a little longer. Transition smoothly between the out-breath and in-breath, with little pause between phases.[104] Keep all of your body above your diaphragm relaxed and still, moving only your abdomen. You'll see the book gently rise as you breathe in and fall as you breathe out, while the upper body remains still.

6. *Practice.* It might take a few weeks until abdominal breathing becomes automatic. Here are the suggested guidelines:
   - Practice twice a day or more, for five to ten minutes each time.
   - For the first few days, just breathe at your regular rate. If at any point you feel dizzy or faint, or if your diaphragm cramps, stop immediately.

You might need to build up gradually to five to ten minutes over the course of days or weeks, beginning with only a few seconds of practice. Generally, dizziness and faintness result from improper breathing. These symptoms will disappear if you get up and walk (e.g., up stairs) to increase the body's CO_2 production. When you resume practice, *be sure that you are not breathing fast or deeply, only slowly and regularly.*

- After about a week, begin to gradually slow your breathing rate. Perhaps you'll eventually reach a rate of six to ten breaths per minute (i.e., about six to ten seconds for each complete breath cycle). *However, don't worry about the rate. Focus on achieving a rate that feels comfortable.*

- After the second week, progress to the seated position, then to standing and leaning against a wall, standing unsupported, slow walking, and fast walking. Remember, first relax your entire body, warm and relax your abdomen, then breathe slowly, regularly, abdominally.

- Try rebreathing in a variety of situations (e.g., in bed as you wake up or before sleeping, walking down the hall, jogging, watching TV, on the train).

- As you gain confidence, try consciously rebreathing in slightly stressful situations before anxiety symptoms appear (e.g., in a traffic slowdown). Then try it in situations where anxiety symptoms have already begun to appear. Just notice the symptoms. Think to yourself, "My breathing is causing this. I'm not going mad or having a heart attack. These symptoms are harmless and reversible. I know how to breathe." Then relax your body, warm your abdomen, and breathe slowly and regularly. Watch your symptoms come and watch them subside, like a scientist watching an experiment.

- Do not attempt breathing retraining without first discussing this with your doctor if you have diabetes, kidney disease, or other disorders which might cause metabolic acidosis. In such cases, breathing may have become rapid to normalize the metabolic acidosis, and slowing down your breathing could be dangerous.

Tips for Breathing Retraining

- If you can, breathe through your nose which increases resistance and helps to slow breathing. If you can't, breathe through pursed lips.

- Don't be too concerned with technique. Just be aware of your breathing and attempt to breathe in a manner that is restful for you. Simple awareness of how you're breathing is often all that is needed to slow down and encourage abdominal breathing.

- Visualizing air being drawn through the toes into the abdomen and pelvis helps to slow down. As you practice, think "Low and slow."

- Some find it helpful to visualize being on the beach, breathing in refreshing air and likening the breath to the easy rhythm of the waves.

- When first practicing, use a mirror to check for tension or movement in the face, jaw, shoulders, or chest. Insure that the abdomen, or belly, is moving up and down rhythmically.

- Wear looser clothes around the neck, chest, and abdomen.

- When you feel confident, move on to Progressive Muscle Relaxation to learn how to further relax.

- Don't sigh or yawn, which will expel more CO_2; suppress coughs and sniffles. Instead of sighs or yawns, swallow. Or hold the normal breath for a count of five, then breathe out slowly, hold to five, then resume easy abdominal breathing.

- Learn ways to express feelings constructively. You might have learned to smother your feelings. This can be unlearned. We can school our feelings, thus giving them constructive outlets. More about this later.

- When speaking, relax your muscles. Go more slowly and smoothly. Use short sentences with gentle breathing through your nose; no gasping or gulping air. Seek natural pausing places to breathe gently.

Troubleshooting

- If you can't relax your abdominal muscles while seated, Weiss advises putting your fists on the back of your hips and trying to bring your elbows together behind you. Someone behind you can assist. Getting on all fours with the abdomen relaxed is another way to learn to relax and move only the abdomen.[105]

- If rebreathing frightens or frustrates you, and you find that anxiety increases or you tune into the physical symptoms:
  - Relax into the symptoms. Let them happen. Keep practicing until the nervous system is desensitized. Remind yourself that the symptoms are harmless. Or consider enlisting the help of a mental health professional

specializing in anxiety and breathing retraining (call the Anxiety Disorders Association of America listed in Appendix 10 for referrals).

- In an emergency, should all else fail, hold a paper bag over your nose and mouth with thumbs and forefingers of both hands. Take six to twelve easy natural breaths, then breathe abdominally. Breathing into and from a bag recaptures CO_2. The bag should have a capacity of about one liter.

Physical Activity

Recall that *fight or flight* is designed for activity. When the muscles move, more CO_2 is produced. The breathing increases just enough to expel the appropriate amount of CO_2. So hyperventilation does not usually occur with exercise. Regular, moderate exercise is recommended to decrease arousal. This type of exercise also decreases resting heart and breathing rates. However, those with a pattern of hyperventilation need to learn first to breathe abdominally before engaging in exercise. Warning: Slow down *gradually* after exercise. Suddenly stopping can produce acute hyperventilation. Cool down for several minutes by walking, perhaps followed by stretching.

Yoga is a form of exercise that improves the physical condition of people of all ages and promotes breathing control. However, deep breathing that fills the entire lungs, holds the air, and then emphasizes long exhalations should be avoided by overbreathers.

CHAPTER 12

About Relaxation

In stress, both the mind and body are aroused. Muscle tension in the chronically anxious body keeps the nervous system sensitized. Relaxation is the opposite of stress. Relaxation means that the mind and body are calm. As the mind and body remain in a calm state of reduced arousal, they become restored. In particular, the nervous system is allowed to desensitize.

As Harvard's Benson notes,[106] four to six weeks of relaxation training typically result in reductions in anxiety symptoms, stress, headaches, insomnia, and blood pressure; prevention of hyperventilation; control of panic attacks; greater inner peace and enhanced creativity.

He notes that relaxation training is particularly useful for those who feel their worries are justified and reasonable. Among the many other advantages of relaxation training are greater feeling of control; better mood; enhanced immune system functioning; ability to think more rationally; better judgment; improved work efficiency, and fewer errors.

Because the mind and body are connected relaxation can be achieved in two ways: First, the body can be relaxed, and the mind follows. Second, the mind can be relaxed, and the body follows. We'll explore both approaches. Regardless of the form of relaxation, the following general guidelines apply.

1. *Regular practice.* Relaxation is a skill that improves with practice. Most forms recommend practicing once or twice each day, for ten to twenty minutes each time. If possible, find a quiet place free from distractions. Soon this place—through association—will become a cue to relax.

2. *Concentration.* Each form of relaxation asks that you focus on one thing rather than scattering your attention. A singular focus allows the mind to

calm down. You might wish to develop a way to "store" your worries during relaxation sessions. Some people put their worries in an imaginary box outside of the room or house. Some write down their worries first. Some simply say, "I'll deal with you later, but right now I wish to relax."

3. *Relaxation training works well after exercise or yoga, when the body is calming down and the mind is clear.* However, digestion seems to interfere with relaxation so don't practice right after a meal.

4. *Relaxation techniques work very well for people wanting to fall asleep at night.* You will probably want to use these techniques for this purpose at times. However, as a rule, try to keep your mind alert and focused when you practice to gain the most benefit.

5. *Trust that the technique will bring benefits.* Develop a confident attitude. Also, develop a passive attitude that simply allows whatever is to happen with each practice session to happen. Don't force or hurry relaxation. Just accept and enjoy whatever happens. It is the process, not the immediate outcome, that matters.

6. *Some people need less medication when practicing relaxation, so speak with your doctor about the need to monitor dosages.* Requirements may lessen for insulin or medications for high blood pressure, epilepsy, depression, or anxiety.

7. *Rise slowly after relaxation training, allowing ample time for your blood pressure to return to normal.*

8. *For each form of relaxation you will find a script which you can read to yourself, have someone read to you, or put on an audio cassette.*

9. *Some people feel as if they are floating or losing track of time as they relax.* Most people feel this is pleasant. If it is not, simply stop.

WHAT IF I FEEL MORE ANXIOUS AS I TRY TO RELAX?

Occasionally, you might be surprised to find that your anxiety actually seems to increase as you try to relax. This is understandable. First, as we relax our awareness increases, so we are usually more aware of our physical symptoms, such as tension. Some feel like they are vulnerable and out of control when relaxing. For example, if one had been abused while prone, lying down might understandably feel frightening. If we are carrying around suppressed fears or worries, relaxing will let down our guard, allowing them to come into awareness. This is similar to the person who suppresses worries all day by keeping busy but then becomes preoccupied with them at night when he wants to sleep. Others might worry that they should be accomplishing something tangible.

There are a number of ways to deal with these concerns:

1. *Remind yourself that you are safe now.* Look around. Make sure you are safe. Is the door locked? Remind yourself that a frightening event from the past was then; this is now. If you wish, sit up and/or practice with your eyes open.

2. *Remind yourself that anxiety symptoms are just a result of sensitized nerves.* Stay with the practice and notice how they subside. Allow time for this to happen.

3. *Write out your worrisome thoughts in a journal before you try to relax.* For about twenty-five minutes write down facts and feelings about what worries you.

4. *Persist and counter the belief that bad things will happen if you relinquish control.* This is a step toward confronting fears and learning to master them.

5. *Remind yourself that people who take a relaxation break (or exercise) usually accomplish more.*

Remember this important point: any relaxation practice is helpful. It does not matter whether perfect relaxation is attained. Each attempt is an effort toward desensitizing your nervous system.

If you still are not having a good experience practicing relaxation, don't despair. You might wish to try some of the other strategies in this book to increase your sense of control, and then return to the chapters on relaxation.

CHAPTER 13

Progressive Muscle Relaxation

This relaxation technique is generally tried first because it is so effective for almost everyone who tries it. Developed in the 1920s by Dr. Edmund Jacobson, progressive muscle relaxation (PMB) is so named because you tense and then relax the muscles in the body from toe to head, relaxing increasingly deeper as you go. The point of focus in this technique is the tension and then relaxation in your muscles.

Jacobson showed that you cannot relax your muscles and still worry at the same time. He demonstrated that just thinking about throwing a ball increased tension in the throwing arm. Conversely, relaxing that arm quieted worries in the mind. There is a paradox in muscle tension in that simply willing oneself to relax leaves residual tension in the muscles. So even bedrest is not necessarily relaxing. The brain becomes used to chronic muscle tension. It takes an *increase* in muscle tension to jolt the brain's arousal center into relaxing unnecessary tension. In this technique we purposefully tense our muscles, then relax deeply. As we concentrate on the contrast between tension and relaxation, we retrain our brain to recognize tension when it starts. This can aid us greatly in warding off tension headaches and backaches.

The instructions for this relaxation technique follow. You may read the script to yourself as you practice, use the summary at the end, or place these instructions on an audio cassette. They are easily adapted to the sitting position, if you prefer that position.

PROGRESSIVE MUSCLE RELAXATION SCRIPT

Note: The tensing in PMR might be a trigger for some people. If so, you might view practicing it as a way to challenge your fears, using calming self-statements such as, "Tension is just a reminder of an old memory. I am safe now. It's okay to relax now." Try keeping your eyes open as you practice, and start initially with briefer periods of practice.

We are about to progressively tense and relax the major muscle groups in the body. This is a very effective way to reduce general arousal and muscle tension. I'll explain first the exercise for each area, and then ask you to tense by saying, "Ready? Tense." Tense relatively hard, but always stop short of discomfort or cramps. Tense until you are aware of tension in the area. Fully pay attention to it, and then study its contrast, relaxation. You'll tense for about five to ten seconds and then relax for about twice as long. For areas that are injured or sore, simply avoid tensing those areas or else tense very gently and slowly.

To prepare, please loosen tight clothing. Remove glasses, contact lenses, or shoes if you wish. Lie down comfortably on a firm mattress, or on the floor with a small pillow under the head and another under the knees. Rest your arms at your sides and let your legs lie straight with your feet relaxed.

1. *To begin, please let your eyes close.* As you distract from visual stimuli, it is easier to notice the pleasant rhythms of your breathing. Just pay attention to your breathing. Breathe gently and peacefully, noticing a slight coolness on the air entering your nostrils on the in-breath and a slight warmth on the out-breath. Throughout this exercise just breathe normally—slowly, rhythmically, abdominally.

2. *When I say tense, I'd like you to point both of your feet and toes at the same time, leaving the legs relaxed.* Notice the pulling sensation, or tension, in the calves and the bottoms of the feet. Form a clear mental picture of this tension. Now relax all at once. Feel the relaxation in those same areas. When muscles relax, they elongate, and blood flow through them increases. So you might feel warmth or tingling in areas of your body that you relax. Just let your feet sink into the floor, feeling completely relaxed.

3. *Next, pull your toes back toward your head.* Ready? Tense. Observe the tension in the muscles below the knee, along the outside of the shins. Now relax all at once and see and feel the difference as those muscles fully relax and warm up.

4. *Next, you'll tense the quadricep muscles on the front part of the leg above the knee by straightening your leg and locking your knees.* Leave your feet

relaxed. Ready? Tense. Concentrate on the pulling in these muscles. Visualize it clearly in your mind. And relax. Scan your quadriceps as you relax. Sense them loosening and warming, as though they are melting.

5. *Imagine now that you are lying on a beach blanket.* Keeping your feet relaxed, imagine pressing the back of the heels into the sand. Ready? Tense. Feel and see the tension along the backs of the entire legs. Now relax as those muscles loosen and relax.

6. *A slightly different set of muscles, those between the upper legs, are tensed when you squeeze your knees together.* Ready? Tense. Observe the tension. Then relax and observe the relaxation as you deeply relax, and keep relaxed, all the muscles in the legs as we progress upward. Just let the floor support your relaxed legs.

7. *Next you'll squeeze the buttocks or seat muscles together while contracting your pelvis muscles.* Leave your stomach relaxed as you do this. Ready? Tense. Visualize the tension in these muscles. Then relax and observe what relaxation in those muscles feels like—perhaps a pleasant warm and heavy feeling.

8. *Next you'll tense your stomach muscles by imagining your stomach is a ball and you want to squeeze it into a tiny ball.* Ready? Tense. Shrink your stomach and pull it back toward the spine. Notice the tension there and how tensing these muscles interferes with breathing. Now relax. Let the abdomen warm up and loosen up, freeing your body to breathe in the least possible fatiguing way. Continue to breathe abdominally as you progress.

9. *Now leave your shoulders and buttocks down on the floor as you gently and slowly arch your back.* As you do, pull your chest up and toward your chin. You'll observe the tension in the back muscles along both sides of the spine. Now gently and slowly relax as your back sinks into the floor, feeling very warm and relaxed. Study that feeling. Notice where relaxation is experienced.

10. *Tense the lower back muscles by pressing the lower back against the floor.* Ready? Tense. Observe the tension there, then relax and observe the relaxation in that area.

11. *Prepare to press your shoulders downward, toward your feet, while you press your arms against the sides of your body.* Ready? Tense. Feel the ten-

sion in the chest, along the sides of the trunk, and along the back of the arms. You may not have been aware of how much tension can be carried in the chest or what it feels like. Relax and feel those muscles loosen and warm. Realize that you can control and release the tension in your upper body once you become aware of it.

12. *Now, shrug your shoulders.* Ready? Tense. Pull them up toward your ears and feel the tension above the collar bones and between the shoulder blades. This is where many headaches originate. Now relax and study the contrast in those muscles.

13. *Place your palms down on the floor.* Pull your relaxed hands back at the wrists so that the knuckles move back toward your head. Observe the tension on the top of the forearms. Relax and study the contrast.

14. *Next, make tight fists and draw them back toward the shoulders as if pulling in the reins on a team of wild*

SUMMARY: TENSE, OBSERVE; RELAX, OBSERVE

1. Point feet and toes

2. Pull toes and feet back toward head

3. Straighten legs; lock knees

4. Press back of heels down

5. Squeeze knees together

6. Squeeze buttocks together; tighten pelvis

7. Squeeze stomach

8. Arch back

9. Flatten small of back down against floor

10. Press shoulders down, arms against body

11. Shrug shoulders

12. Bend hands back at wrists

13. Make fists; pull back to shoulders

14. Rotate neck

15. Press head back against floor while raising chin

16. Lift eyebrows up

17. Wrinkle nose; squeeze eyes shut; squeeze eyebrows together

18. Frown

19. Clench teeth

20. Smile

horses. See the tension in the fists, forearms, and biceps. Relax and notice the feelings as those muscles go limp and loose. Just let your arms fall back beside your body, palms up, heavy and limp and warm. Pause here to scan your body and notice how good it feels to give your muscles a break. Allow your entire body to remain relaxed as you move on.

15. *Let's learn how to relax the neck muscles, which typically carry much tension.* Right now, gradually, slowly turn your head to the right as if looking over your right shoulder. Take ten seconds or longer to rotate the neck. Feel the tension on the right side of the neck pulling your head around. The sensation on the left side is stretching, not tension. Hold the tension for just long enough to observe it. Then turn around slowly back to the front and notice the difference as the muscles on the right side of your neck relax. Pause. Turn just as slowly to the left and watch the left side of your neck contract. Rotating back to the front, see the left side relax.

16. *Now press the back of your head gently against the floor, while raising your chin toward the ceiling.* Do you notice the tension at the base of the skull, where the skull meets the neck? Much headache pain originates here, too. Study the tension. And relax. Allow those muscles to warm up and elongate. Relax the neck completely and let it remain relaxed.

17. *Lift your eyebrows up and furrow your brow.* Feel the tension along the forehead. Relax. Imagine a rubber band loosening.

18. *Wrinkle up your nose while you squeeze your eyes shut and your eyebrows together.* Observe the tension along the sides of the nose, and around and between the eyes. Now deeply relax those areas. Imagine pleasantly cool water washing over the eyes, relaxing them. Your eyelids are as light as a feather.

19. *Frown, pulling the corners of the mouth down as far as they'll go.* Feel the tension on the sides of the chin and neck. Relax. Feel the warm, deeply relaxing contrast.

20. *The jaw muscles are extremely powerful and can carry much tension. When I say tense, clench your jaw.* Ready? Tense. Grit your teeth and study the tension from the angle of the jaw all the way up to the temples. Observe the tension. Now relax and enjoy the contrast, realizing that you can control tension here, too. Relax the tongue and let the teeth part slightly.

Figure 13.1
RELAXATION RECORD

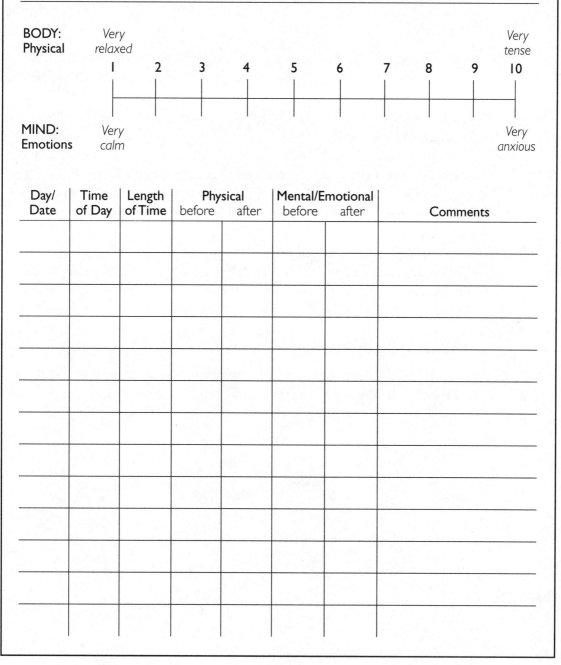

BODY: Physical — Very relaxed (1) ... Very tense (10)

MIND: Emotions — Very calm ... Very anxious

Day/ Date	Time of Day	Length of Time	Physical before	after	Mental/Emotional before	after	Comments

21. *Make a wide smile. Open the mouth wide.* Ready? Tense. Grin ear to ear and feel the muscles around the cheekbone contract. This really requires little effort. Now relax and let all the muscles of the face become smooth and completely relaxed.

Allow a pleasant sense of relaxation to surround your body. Imagine that you are well supported and floating on a favorite couch, bed, or raft—all your muscles pleasantly relaxed. When you are ready to end this session, count slowly to five, send energy to your limbs, stretch, sit up slowly, and move your limbs before standing slowly.

Practice this twice a day for two weeks or more. At first you might be more aware of aches or tension in your muscles. This tends to disappear with practice as those tense muscles get a break and your nerves desensitize. With practice, you'll notice that you can relax your muscles passively, just by reminding yourself to relax them. Some people use a reminder, like a dot on their watch or a picture on the wall, as a cue to relax their muscles throughout the day.

When you feel that you are aware of the first signs of tension and can cause those muscles to relax, then progress to the next relaxation exercise. Or if you wish to stay with this one, keep practicing daily as you move on to chapter 16.

RELAXATION RECORD

Keeping track of your practice and progress can be very motivating and revealing. Keep a record for several weeks on the form in Figure 13.1.

CHAPTER 14

Autogenic Training

While progressive muscle relaxation was being developed and researched in the United States, autogenic training was being developed and researched in Europe. It is also very effective for reducing general arousal. It was developed by the German physician, psychiatrist, hypnotist, dermatologist, and neurologist Dr. Johann H. Schultz. Like Jacobson, Schultz was ahead of his time in understanding the mind/body connection. From his experience with hypnosis, he knew that hypnotized people frequently felt relaxed, and that their limbs felt warm and heavy, as though they'd been in a warm bath. He reasoned that people could simply give themselves the suggestions of warmth and heaviness to induce deep relaxation.

Practice it daily, for a week or two. As you practice, you'll find that you're getting better at relaxing, irrespective of the type of relaxation that you use.

AUTOGENIC TRAINING SCRIPT

1. *Sit or lie quietly and comfortably.* Loosen tight clothing and remove glasses, contact lenses, and shoes if you wish. Imagine that you just returned from a pleasant walk. You sit or lie in your favorite soft chair or couch. You feel peaceful and pleasantly fatigued after your walk. Relax your body. Just let it sink into the chair or couch. Starting with your feet and progressing upward, relax each part of your body. Take a few moments to do this. Breathe abdominally for a few moments—gentle, rhythmic, regular, slow breaths.

2. *You notice that across the room is an inviting stairway that leads downward.* You walk over and go down the first step, noticing the beautiful wood on that step. You step down to the next step, the ninth step. It also has unique textures and colors. And down to the eighth, and so on, noticing each unique step as you step down. (Pause.) At the foot of the stairs you see sliding

glass doors that lead outside to a beautiful spring day. You walk across the lush green grass and see an inviting hammock (lawn chair, float in the pool, or boat lined with cotton, whichever you prefer). You lie down in it, looking up into the sunny sky with beautiful clouds. The temperature is just as you like it. While lying there suggestions come into your mind. Repeat each suggestion to yourself three times slowly. With each repetition, imagine that the suggestion is happening and allow it to happen.

Suggestions of Heaviness
With each suggestion, allow your body to feel pleasantly limp and heavy:

- My right arm is heavy.
- My right hand is heavy.
- My fingers are heavy.
- My left arm is heavy.
- My left hand is heavy.
- My fingers are heavy.
- My right leg is heavy.
- My right foot is heavy.
- My left leg is heavy.
- My left foot is heavy.
- Both arms are heavy.
- Both hands are heavy.
- All my fingers are heavy.
- Both legs are heavy.
- Both feet are heavy.

Suggestions of Heaviness and Warmth
With each suggestion, allow your body to feel heavy and warm, as if you are relaxing dreamily in a warm bath.
(Repeat the script above, replacing "heavy" with "heavy and warm.")

- My right arm is heavy and warm.
- My right hand is heavy and warm, etc.

Form a little sparkle smile, with a little twinkle in your eye. Tell yourself that you are alert, amused, and refreshed.

See, in the clouds, the purple and white clouds are forming the number one. The one begins to change to a two, and so on until five. With each count, your limbs receive energy, and you feel more alert and refreshed, and entirely relaxed.

Practice this script for a week. Thereafter, try adding some or all of the following suggestions, perhaps one or two each week:

1. My abdomen is warm and relaxed.
2. My chest is warm and soft.
3. My breathing is calm and regular like branches swaying in the gentle breeze.
4. My heartbeat is calm and regular like a swing swaying back and forth in the breeze.
5. My forehead is pleasantly cool.
6. My mind is calm. Things will work out.

CHAPTER 15

Meditation

Meditation may be thought of as awareness of our true, happy nature. We do not need to get rid of fear; we only need to be aware of love and compassion. We need not flee pain, but notice it with full awareness. As we penetrate pain with peace and acceptance—not fear or avoidance—we find that pain lessens. Thus, we can be comfortable in any situation with full awareness, knowing that avoidance degrades consciousness and erodes physical and mental health.

Meditative practice has been recorded throughout history. Modern science has shown that meditation measurably calms the brain and reduces arousal. At the same time, it leads to heightened concentration, efficiency, job performance, health, and life satisfaction. And it can be practiced independent of lifestyle or philosophy.

WHAT IS MEDITATION LIKE?

Recall a time that was pleasurable: sunset on the beach, a peak athletic performance, holding a sleeping child or someone you love. In each, the commonality is that you were absorbed in the moment, just being you. Meditation is like a mini-vacation that leaves you refreshed.

TWO MINDS

We might think of each person as being of two minds. The ordinary mind surrounds the wisdom mind, which represents our true nature. The wisdom mind is peaceful, dignified, kind, compassionate, peaceful, joyful, good humored, self-respecting, expansive, humble, and accepting. Surrounding the wisdom mind like muddy water, the ordinary mind clings to negative emotions, such as sorrow, hurt, worry, anger, bitterness, unkindness, and false pride. Just as water that is left unagitated becomes clearer, so does resting peacefully in your mind allow you to more clearly experience your true nature. The wisdom mind is simple, dramaless and pleasant to experience. In meditation, we generously accept the ordinary mind. As we rest in the wisdom mind, it is as if our true nature breaks through the ordinary mind and unites with the light of the sun.[107]

THE PROCESS

In meditation we peacefully focus our full awareness. At the University of Massachusetts Medical Center, meditation is introduced by asking patients to eat a raisin mindfully, with full awareness. They are instructed to slowly feel, smell, and observe it, bringing it slowly to their mouths and noticing how the mouth begins to salivate even before the raisin enters. They let it sit on their tongue and really taste something that is normally eaten automatically. From there it is a very short jump to realize that we may not be fully in touch with many of the beautiful moments in life because we are busy rushing somewhere else, physically or figuratively. As we practice meditation, we become more aware of the simple beauties and peaceful pleasures existing moment by moment.

THE ATTITUDE

A receptive, quiet, pleasantly expectant attitude is essential. Here we observe without judging, allowing peace to emerge without forcing, competing, or striving for it. One simply allows oneself to be in the present and enjoy it without perfectionism or asking: "Am I doing this right or fast enough?" Such questions create tension.

In novice meditators, about a third initially are troubled by intruding worries that distract and arouse them. They either want to fight them (which creates tension) or avoid the activity that permits the worries to enter into awareness (which maintains arousal). Meditation teaches an extremely useful skill. Namely, it helps to think of worries cordially, as logs drifting down a river as you watch from a riverboat. You would not jump into the water and struggle with the logs. You simply watch them come into view and then float away without engaging them. You think, "That's okay, that's life." This is a step toward "avoiding avoidance."

WHY IS MEDITATION SO EFFECTIVE?

Several theories account for the benefits of meditation. One is that meditation affords a restful, restorative distraction from worrisome thoughts, like a good night's rest. Another refers to the log metaphor. As we realize that we can look like a scientist at anything, without getting sucked into the pain, and are able to experience things with peace and detachment, we become more confident "copers." Yet another theory likens the mantra (the word on which we focus) to a broom that sweeps the mind of surface cares and permits us to descend to the quieter regions of the mind where creative and healing thoughts originate.

AM I READY TO START?

Meditation works best for those who are reasonably prepared. If you have practiced abdominal breathing and progressive muscle relaxation such that you are automatically breathing correctly and can relax your muscles quickly, then you are probably ready. Some find that beginning meditation helps them to better accept life's inevitable lack of total control. Some need to build self-esteem before starting (see chapter 36). It takes reasonably good self-esteem to enjoy meditation because meditation assumes that you can permit yourself to stop striving for a few moments, realizing that you will not lose your worth as a human if you are not constantly achieving. On the other hand, some find that reconnecting with one's true nature provides the needed boost for their self-esteem. People are different. If in doubt, experiment. If you find that you dissociate when you meditate, avoid it for now. If you decide to skip this for now, do return later. You won't want to miss this one.

KEY POINTS IN REVIEW

1. *The purpose is to experience your true, happy nature.* This you can do if you are not busy rushing about and worrying about things.

2. *When intrusive thoughts/worries enter your mind, remember the analogy of watching logs floating by.* Greet them cordially—"these thoughts are okay; that's life"—and let them pass by. Let your mantra ride in after the log and return to paying attention to it. Think of an unwelcome house guest. You can say hello cordially, let them in for awhile, give them your attention, and then let them out the back door. They don't have to stay. Just practice noticing concerns casually.

3. *Tell yourself the world won't end if you're not accomplishing something for twenty minutes.* Just allow yourself to enjoy being in the moment without letting worries pull you away.

4. *Patiently expect a quiet, peaceful experience, not drama or fireworks.* It is a little like eating a meal. It can be very enjoyable when you slow down and enjoy it, and some are better than others, but each can be delightful, satisfying, and nourishing.

THE MEDITATION SCRIPT

1. Go to a quiet place where you will be free from distractions for fifteen to twenty minutes. Loosen clothing. Remove glasses/contacts or shoes if you wish.

2. Sit quietly and comfortably. Place both feet flat on the floor. Use the back of the chair to support your whole back so that your spine is comfortably erect. This frees the diaphragm and disinhibits energy flow through the spinal column. Think of a bamboo pole that goes from your head to the base of your spine. Two holes at the bottom release all tension from your body. Your chin is neither up nor down, but resting comfortably, perhaps slightly back to straighten the neck. Rest your hands in your lap. The shoulders, neck, and chest are very relaxed. Sit like a dignified mountain.

3. Gently close your eyes. Relax your entire body. Start at your feet and relax each part in turn. Especially warm and relax your abdomen. Let your facial muscles be smooth and relaxed in a pleasant peaceful expression. Breathe gently and peacefully through your nose, if that is possible. Take regular, rhythmic, slow, abdominal breaths.

4. Notice the gentle coolness of the air going into your body, and the pleasant, relaxing feeling as it leaves. As you concentrate on breathing, allow external stimuli to fade into the background. Much as the sound of the waves at the beach begin to fade into the distance until you barely notice them, so the sounds of the world around you gently fade until you hardly notice them. Like the raisin, notice that the simple act of breathing is pleasant. Just be aware of your breathing and enjoy its pleasant rhythm. Notice that in closing your eyes and paying attention, your breathing tends to slow down and become more regular on its own. Don't try to make this happen. Just notice whatever the breath does.

5. Imagine the breath to be like gentle waves on the shore. Ride the waves of the in-breath. Ride the waves of the out-breath.

6. Now begin to concentrate on the word "one." See it rolling in on the in-breath, and say it silently to yourself. See it roll out on the out-breath, and say it silently to yourself as you exhale. Let the word "one" fill your mind.

7. Should distracting thoughts (worries) enter your mind just remember to view them cordially, and as you get weary of them watch them float by, using them as a reminder to return to repeating the word "one" as you breathe in and as you breathe out. So, it's breathe in . . . "one." Breathe out . . . "one." Continue quietly and peacefully for the next few moments. Let the word "one" fill your awareness, reverberating peacefully in your mind. Eventually you, your breathing, and the word "one" become one. Most of your attention focuses on the peacefulness of resting in your true nature. In time, you might simply stop focusing on breathing and the word "one," and simply rest in your mind, noticing that it becomes whole and peaceful. (If your mind wanders to distracting thoughts, then simply return to the method of counting and focusing on the word "one.")

8. End your meditation rather slowly, allowing peaceful feelings to spread to the rest of your life.

Practice meditation once or twice daily for at least a week. Initially, you might wish to practice for about five minutes each time, increasing gradually to about twenty minutes each time. After practicing this form for a week, you might also try this beautifully simple approach to meditation described by Dr. Weekes:[108]

Just sit quietly. Close your eyes and listen with as little thought as possible to noises around you. Do this for a few minutes twice a day.

Note: An advantage to this approach is that it encourages focusing on the environment, not the physical sensations of anxiety. This perspective is central to the treatment of panic attacks.[109]

CHAPTER 16

Managing Anger

He who gives way to violent gestures will increase his rage.
—*Charles Darwin*

Intense anger is common in PTSD for reasons that all make sense. Normal day-to-day living rarely demands intense, extreme emotions. But during traumatic events raw emotions are often unleashed. For example, a soldier in combat for the first time encounters a destructive rage at the enemy who killed his comrades. A victim of rape for the first time encounters intense bitterness and desire for vengeance. It is said that PTSD is "lots of fire temporarily numbed." Such highly charged emotions are likely to erupt repeatedly until they are resolved—often the anger will be misdirected at loved ones or colleagues. People with PTSD live with pain and frustration. Anger is usually the least painful emotion to acknowledge because the focus of anger is outside of yourself. You can focus outwardly in anger without acknowledging inward feelings of sadness, shame, fear, or self-dislike. In fact, anger tends to distract from such feelings. Angry aggression overrides fear. That is, for a little while we no longer feel as helpless and out of control.

People with PTSD might be angry at any or all of the following:

- A perpetrator of a crime or accident—especially if the offense was sense-less, intentional, or preventable (e.g., a drunk driving accident is not really an accident because the person chose to drink and then chose to drive).

- God or life for letting the traumatic event happen.

- Everyone (e.g., a man who was struck by an oncoming car now views all drivers as enemies).

- "Normal people" who are still happy and act like nothing has happened.
- Self—for being unable to function better or "get over it," for hurting one's family.
- The imperfections of people (e.g., a victim who was hurt by the weaknesses of another is now impatient with all imperfections in others).
- People who don't understand or know how to help.
- Family members for annoying or disappointing you.
- Firefighters, police, parents, or others who failed to protect you.
- The criminal justice system for failing to find or punish the offender.
- Secondary wounders—people who are hired to help you but end up offending you further.
- Everyday stressors.

Intense, uncontrollable anger from the past will likely be reduced as traumatic material is fully processed and the concerns underlying the anger are addressed. In the meantime, this chapter will furnish you with the skills needed to control present anger so that your health and relationships are not damaged.

WHAT IS ANGER?

Anger is a negative, uncomfortable feeling that follows from specific thoughts about something that we view as threatening or frustrating. Along with this feeling, anger leads to physical arousal (increased heart rate, breathing rate, muscle tension, blood pressure, and stress hormones in the blood; flushed face) and certain chosen behavior responses. For example, when angry you might choose to clench your fist, raise your voice, become quiet, or leave the room. Some people become physically violent. Others become critical or sarcastic. Such behaviors are learned habits that become reinforced through repetition. Just as ineffective ways for coping with anger might have been learned during or after trauma, so can effective coping styles be learned or relearned.

Varieties of Anger

Table 16.1 lists the varieties of angry feelings, metaphors, and behaviors that we sometimes use to describe the experience of anger.

Table 16.1
VARIETIES OF ANGER

I feel . . .	Metaphors	Behaviors
aggravated	angry enough to kill/shoot you/cut you	argue
agitated	off/cry/strangle you/explode	attack posture, body tightens
angry	blew a fuse/gasket	avoids eye contact
annoyed	blind with rage	backbite
churning	blood boiling	becomes quiet
defensive	boiling mad	blaming
disappointed	breathing fire	clench fist
embittered	burning mad	clench teeth
enraged /rage	couldn't see straight	criticism, put downs, sniping
exasperated	fighting mad	cry
frustrated	flew off the handle	destroy property
fuming	flipped his wig	drink, use drugs
furious	hit the ceiling	glare
hostile, hate	hopping mad	harassment
hot	hot potato	insults
hurt	hot under the collar, hot as a firecracker	interrupt others
incensed	icy cold	makes demands
indignant	loaded and ready to fire	physically attack or harm
infuriated	mad as a bat out of hell	pout
irate	madder than hell	raise voice
irked	madder than a mad hatter	sarcastic comments
irritated	madder than a wet hornet	silent treatment
livid	madder than a wet hen	sneer
mad	popped his cork	sulk
malicious	raging bull/maniac	threats
offended	ready to explode	throws things
out of control	seeing red; red hot	vulgar language
outraged	sizzling	walk away, storm out,
peeved	slow burn	withdraw
perturbed	smoke coming out of ears	yell
pissed off	so angry I could explode/bust	
royally pissed off	so angry I could spit	
riled up	so angry I couldn't speak	
seething	spitting nails	
slamming	steaming mad	
spiteful	went through the roof	
steamed, steaming		
teed off		
ticked, ticked off		
upset, uptight		
vengeful		
vexed		
violent		

UNDERSTANDING ANGER

Anger is something we experience as we try to control our world and avoid pain. Some people are troubled by their difficulty in managing anger better. Others feel completely justified in their anger and see no reason to change it. Anger provides some distinct payoffs. If it did not we would probably experience it far less often. Before deciding, then, if anger management is something you'd like to work on let's sharpen our understanding of anger and its impact on our lives. Please list below all the advantages and disadvantages of anger that you can think of:

BENEFITS. The good thing about anger is . . .	COSTS. The bad thing about anger is . . .

The following are benefits that people have identified over the years:

- Anger honestly communicates my feelings about other people's faults.
- Others might quickly comply with my demands.
- It shows that I care.
- It gives the feeling that I am in control and viewed with respect.
- Anger clears the air—it vents my frustration so that I don't explode.
- Anger protects me from injustice.
- Anger lets me at least feel something—I feel more alive; a sense of self.
- Anger is a cue that something is wrong and in need of fixing.
- Anger energizes me.

On the cost side, people have identified these:

- Communication suffers.
  - People hear only my anger, not the issue.
  - They're afraid to have a dialogue with me, so all useful ideas don't surface.
- Anger sours relationships—people distrust me; see me as mean.
- I feel out of control—humiliated because I can't control my own emotions.
- When I am not cool, my job performance suffers. I don't think clearly.
- I get fired when I blow up at work.
- Conflict increases. Some people don't cooperate with me; some argue more.
- My kids are learning violence from watching me.
- I feel guilty for blowing up at my family.
- Some of the people I've offended have sabotaged me.
- As long as I'm angry I don't heal underlying hurts.
- I avoid learning better coping skills.
- My health suffers (heart disease, ulcers, high blood pressure, higher death from all causes).
- I don't give people the chance to show me that some people are trustworthy and good.

- Anger is unpleasant; I've lost my sense of joy and peace.

- Anger escalates. The more I lose patience, the angrier I get.

As we consider the pros and cons, it is apparent that anger sometimes makes sense. Anger has a number of apparent payoffs, at least in the short-term. People who get angry are not bad people. They are behaving in a way that makes sense to them. Perhaps they have not learned other ways to meet their needs. On the other hand, anger has many disadvantages, especially in the long run.

Perhaps anger is a long-term habit that has worked for you in many ways. Before considering changes you might consider:

- "Is anger a problem for you in terms of its costs?"

- "Are you getting what you really want when you are angry?"

- "Could you get your needs and wants met with less anger?"

- "What are the positive consequences of being less angry?"
  People have suggested:
  - I'll be cooler, more in control, more powerful.
  - I'll have relationships based on more trust; better friendships; better relationships with my wife and kids.
  - I might see that some people will respond to me because they want to, not because they fear me.
  - I'll see myself as more patient, tolerant, kinder, cooler, more in control of my emotions.
  - Others would probably view me as calmer and more in control.
  - I'd be more respected.
  - I'd give people a chance to do good things because they choose to.
  - Communication with others will improve. People will be more open and creative.
  - I'll be able to funnel my energy more effectively and work more logically.
  - I'll be more relaxed; healthier.

ANGER MANAGEMENT SKILLS

Everyone has a limbic system and so will experience anger at times in his or her life. The question is how you experience it, and how often. Do you hold anger in at work and then explode at home? Does anger build until you let it out at work and then get reprimanded or fired? Many people debate whether it is better to hold in anger or let it out. At times, both approaches can be useful choices, but there is a third option: the choice to be angry. We'll explore a number of ways to be less angry and to be in greater control of the anger we do experience.

1. *Take responsibility for your own anger.* The first principle taught in military spouse abuse programs is that no one *makes* us angry. We choose who we let under our skin and how we will express the anger that results. We can choose to talk calmly rather than scream or become violent. We can choose to walk away from a fight rather than give in to conflict. Giving others control of our lives—by choosing to let them annoy us—places us in the victim role and reinforces the feeling of powerlessness. Violence to self or others is not an option. It only temporarily relieves tension, while destroying inner peace and relationships.

2. *Put your anger into words.* Refer to the feelings list in Table 16.1. Select the four that represent your most intense anger levels (or include your own). Also select the four that describe your lowest anger levels, and the four that represent mid-range anger. Within each category, rank in order these feelings from most to least intense. This helps to reinforce the idea that there are gradations of anger. That is, there are many ways to experience anger between having none and being out of control. It will help you to later be able to calmly describe your feelings in words rather than to act them out physically. If you prefer to draw, place the variety of angry feelings on a thermometer from cool to hot.

    Try writing about your anger in a journal. Describe the event that triggered your anger. Then describe the emotions and body sensations. Then identify why you felt the anger. Remember this important point: Anger is a secondary emotion. Under the anger is the primary emotion: Hurt or fear of being hurt. Try to calmly identify what the underlying hurt is and put it into words. Perhaps you felt that you were not respected or treated fairly. Perhaps people were not as loyal as you would have liked. It's okay to identify and feel that hurt. You realize that you can identify it, and just watch it. You will learn ways to soothe the hurt rather than retaliate. If you can think of another way to view the hurt, write that down too.

3. *Soothe the hurt.* Anger in the present is often just a button that is pushed, where the button symbolizes an unhealed hurt from the past. This imagery

technique developed by Klein provides practice to soothe yourself.[110] It is described from the perspective of the therapist who acts as a guide.[111]

- Hear the complaint. Help the client identify the present unwanted and/or inappropriate behavior and the associated feelings of anger that occur in these situations.

- The therapist will require that the client is desirous and motivated to change.

- Have the client recall a time when they were supportive and comforting to someone else, and/or engaged in an activity where they were competent. Assist the client to experience fully the feelings and the details of being resourceful in that situation. Ask the client to describe these feelings in a word or phrase, which becomes ANCHOR A (e.g., "secure, affectionate, here, and/or competent").

- Instruct the client to imagine sitting in a movie theater or in front of a TV with a blank screen waiting for the movie to start. Tell the client that they can move the screen as far away as desired, the picture can be brightened or darkened, and the volume of the sound can be adjusted from their seat. When the client feels a sense that the picture is at a safe distance, a word describing this distancing becomes ANCHOR B (e.g., "safe; screen over there").

- Ask the client to access a recent example of experiencing the unwanted behavior, *but* to watch the scene unfold as if it were on the imaginary screen. While the client watches this situation play out as a motion picture the therapist helps the client to remain comfortable by utilizing ANCHOR A and ANCHOR B.

- When the scene has reached some sort of completion, ask the client to evaluate what resource(s) the younger self needed in that situation—resources that would have allowed the client to have responded favorably, such as self-acceptance, humor, or curiosity. Next, direct the client to remember and to access an example of being resourceful in this fashion. Instruct the client to associate into the resourceful experience and to describe the related resourceful feelings with a word that becomes ANCHOR C.

- The therapist repeats ANCHORS A, B, and C as needed, while requesting that the client access earlier and earlier representations of the unwanted behavior on the screen until they come to the one that appears to be the earliest experience. Remind the client that they are a full grown adult, that they have many resources that the younger self needed and that the younger self is having the experiences *over there* on the screen.

- As the therapist continues to utilize ANCHORS A, B, and C, the client watches the younger self go through the above earliest scene until it reaches completion. Ask the client to then imagine going over to the younger self as an older, and more resourceful adult. The client is in effect a "VISITOR FROM THE FUTURE" who can comfort and encourage the younger self to express and relieve the emotions (such as loneliness, fear, sadness, shame) present in that old scene, for example, by telling the younger self that it's "okay to feel what you feel."

- The client is directed to suggest to the younger self that he/she did his/her best at that time; that he/she survived that unhappy event and went on to have many positive experiences in his/her future. Tell the client to send, by mental projection and/or imaginary touch, the appropriate resources, insights, and understandings that were needed (therapist again utilizes ANCHORS A, B, and C).

- The client now is asked to start the scene from the beginning and to watch as the younger self goes through the decisive experience again, *but this time* with protection, the new resources and understandings that have been conveyed from the older self. Tell the client to observe the changes the younger self makes at the conclusion of the scene.

     Suggest that the client congratulate and embrace the younger self. That they bring the younger self into the body and experience the integration as positive energy and vitality. Give the client permission to take a few moments to feel the body making adjustments as these new ways of being are assimilated.

- Ask the client to imagine going through three or four situations from the past, *but to realize* that they are behaving and feeling differently in each of them. The therapist uses all three ANCHORS as needed.

- Future mental rehearsal. The client mentally constructs a situation in the future like the ones that *used* to generate the unwanted behavior and/or feelings. Have them imagine going through the experience to test that they can now do so resourcefully.

- Personal impact considerations. Invite the client to think through the consequences of the changes that have taken place and to make any adjustments if needed.

4. *Communicate.* Tell your loved ones that the anger comes from hurts you are trying to heal—that they are not the reason for the anger's intensity. Tell them you love them at every opportunity and whenever you experience even the smallest positive feelings. Focus more on complimenting what they are doing well rather than criticizing what is wrong.

- *Communicate preventively.* Rather than waiting for problems to develop, set aside an hour a week with your partner. Sit down with your calendars and "Wish Lists." Identify what is going well. Then anticipate problems and plan to solve them. For example, an Army officer got very angry when his wife would bombard him with problems as he came home from work. He and his wife found that a weekly meeting enabled them to calmly anticipate most problems and plan solutions. If something came up in the meantime, they would wait until he had had a few minutes to relax and then discuss them.

- *If someone verbally attacks you, you might feel the urge to fight back. Instead, try this.*

  - Put your ego on the shelf and just listen. Don't defend yourself, just notice that you can absorb the speaker's information without undue arousal. Quietly think, "This is not an emergency situation. It's just useful feedback. I'll calmly listen and evaluate it. I'm still worthwhile even though he is angry now." Try to see things from the speaker's point of view.

  - Gently ask questions to show the person that he is being listened to and respected. ("Are there other ways I have offended you? When did I do that? Would you help me better understand how that upset you?")

  - Paraphrase to check for understanding. You might say, "Let's see, it sounds like I offended you by doing such and such. Do I have that right?"

  - If possible find a point of agreement. "I understand what you're saying and I agree. I wasn't as sensitive as I'd have wished to be." If he has called you dumb, you might agree, "I certainly feel dumb sometimes." Or you might try, "I see your point and I'll correct X, Y, or Z."

  - Only then try to solve the problem. You might ask, "What would help?" You might want to negotiate a solution. Remember to compromise ("How about a compromise. If I do X, would you do Y?").

This technique works nicely with someone who is fairly reasonable, but not with someone who is abusive. For such a person, you might say, "I'll discuss this with you, but not until you calm down."

- *Constructively express your feelings and preferences.* Remember the three-step formula: 1. Make a positive statement; 2. Describe your feelings related to another's behaviors; then 3. State your preferences. Bob was a combat vet who got angry and frustrated that his teenagers would not clean the truck after using it. He learned to firmly but without anger assert, "I really love you guys and I don't want to be nagging you. But I get upset when you return the truck without cleaning it. I'd like you to pick up the trash inside and hose it down after you take it out. Will you do that?" They responded, "Sure Dad. We didn't realize that mattered to you." Had they responded differently, Bob could have stated the consequences. "If you don't clean the truck I won't permit you to use it for a month." Then he would have to follow through on these consequences.

- *Take time-outs.* In athletic events teams take time-outs when things start to get out of control. Should anger start to build, take a time-out from the discussion. Explain to your partner that you are trying to manage your anger better. So whenever anger is building either partner can say, "I need a time-out to collect myself. Let's take a break for _____ (specify the time, usually less than an hour) and then meet to continue." This is not a sign of rejection, just a strategy to keep anger from getting out of hand. During the time-out, take a walk, write in your journal, take a bath, or do any of the other things that help you reduce anger (don't drink alcohol, drive, or take drugs).

5. *Channel vengeance fantasies.* It is common that women who have been raped will have a strong and constant desire for vengeance that will not dissipate over time. This can be very upsetting to women who have not previously been violent, or who feel that violence violates their values. So they try to bottle up these feelings and pretend not to feel them. Like dissociated material, however, such intense feelings might intrude in unhealthy ways. It might manifest as physical illness or erupt as anger misdirected at loved ones. One possibility, stated with caution, is the option of verbalizing vengeance fantasies in a support group or with your therapist. The caution is that verbalizing does not authorize or encourage violent retaliation. In one group, women laughed with relief to realize that

others had the same feelings. It almost became a humorous "Well-I-can-top-that-one." The process enabled the safe venting of anger in a setting that formed new associations with the anger. Shame for the feelings was replaced with understanding, acceptance, and humor. Simple venting (e.g., screaming at a loved one) does not put a person in touch with the real cause of the anger. Talking about the underlying hurt in a safe setting can.

6. *Exercise or do physical work.* Exercise is a wonderful outlet for pent-up anger. So is gardening or other physical labor. Such physical outlets reduce general arousal.

7. *Remember the opposites.* Creative problem solvers can conceive many opposites to the problem. Thus, they have many options. What are the opposites of anger? Consider friendliness (stand up to a bully in a friendly way and he might become your friend), patience, understanding, happiness, compassion, acceptance, trust, enjoyment, conciliation, indifference (I don't have to hook into every problem), optimism, happiness, flexibility, or inner security.

8. *View the offender differently.* Compassion is a beautiful word. It means sorrow for the suffering of others and a desire to help. When people disappoint you or hurt you, try to view them with compassion. Longfellow wrote, "If we could read the secret histories of our enemies we should find sorrow and suffering enough to disarm all hostility." When people disappoint you try to ask yourself, "Why would someone do that to another? What need is he trying to fill? How is he trying to protect himself?" You will usually find insecurities and fears. Since overrunning Tibet, China has killed hundreds of thousands of its citizens and destroyed countless beautiful temples. Yet the Tibetan religious leaders have refused to be embittered or loaded down with hate. One of the Tibetan teachers has written that no one in his right mind would knowingly harm another human being. One who behaves unkindly is never completely in his right mind. So instead of becoming embittered we might cultivate compassion and remember that hostile people are hurting people. Instead of condemning the person or taking offense, we might ask ourselves, "I wonder if I could wish him well." If this is too difficult to do just now, remember the idea and return to it when you have healed.

9. *Humor can give problems perspective and provide a certain sense of mastery.* If someone seems unbearable, just think, "That poor fellow must have a

brain tumor." Or see him as a baby dressed in diapers screaming for his bottle. If you think, "He is such a butthead," you might ask yourself what a butthead would look like and try to draw it. We realize, of course, that he is not a total butthead, nor has he got a brain tumor. Rather, he is just a flawed, suffering fellow traveler who is behaving badly at the moment.

10. *Practice relaxing others. In interchanges with others, try to model calmness.* Encourage others to talk, as you listen calmly. Show that you are trying to understand. Practice reassuring others. Help them save face. In many arguments, the real issue doesn't surface because the communication degenerates to attacks and trying to save face. Rather than criticizing the other person for coming home late ("You irresponsible idiot!"), you might get to the heart of the issue by saying, "I'm disappointed because I didn't get to spend time with you last night."

11. *Avoid watching media violence which reinforces the tendency to react aggressively.*

12. *Distinguish the two forms of anger.* Disturbed anger is out of control and disproportionate to the offense (rage, fury, etc.). Nondisturbed anger is functional (e.g., annoyance that stimulates us to rational communication, reasonable action to prevent disrespectful treatment, or problem solving).[112] The question really is not should we give up all anger but can we choose when and how to experience it.

13. *Choose cool thoughts.* Angry feelings follow from our thoughts. During traumatic events, we develop thought patterns that seem appropriate for survival. Getting fighting mad, for instance, might have saved us from harm or spurred us to seek justice afterward. We might call these thought patterns the "Emergency Mode." Once learned, the Emergency Mode can be automatically triggered by everyday stressors, like traffic jams or disrespectful people. Explosive anger follows from our thoughts, even though the Emergency Mode is no longer needed. The Emergency Mode is learned. We can also learn another thinking mode that is more suitable for non-emergency situations. The Non-Emergency Mode lets us respond to stressors more calmly. We think more clearly and thus function better. Let's take a look at some of the most common hot thoughts and how they can be challenged and replaced:

EMERGENCY MODE (HOT THOUGHTS)	NON-EMERGENCY MODE (COOL THOUGHTS)
Catastrophizing	
"This is awful. I can't stand it. I hate this! I can't let myself be helpless again. I've got to do something. I must stay in control."	"This is certainly inconvenient and frustrating. But this isn't combat, rape, or any other present emergency. In fact, compared to the trauma this isn't nearly as bad. No one is now shooting at me or assaulting me. It's okay if I'm not in total control. No one ever has that. But I'm never powerless. I can at least always control my thoughts and actions. This is a problem to be solved, not the end of the world."
Dehumanizing	
In war it was easier to shoot a faceless enemy. If you were abused as a child you know what it is like to be treated as a worthless object. In either case, you might now find it automatic to think of someone who disappoints or hurts you, "That worthless loser deserves my outrage."	"As disappointing as his behavior is, no one is worthless. I don't like it when I'm treated that way. This person is fallible, but he is nevertheless worthwhile."
Angry Demands	
In battle, incompetence lost lives. Now Fred, an ex-Marine, finds himself demanding perfection of his kids ("I must keep them in line at all times"), himself, and most other people.	"No one ever had perfect kids, no matter how demanding they were. If I kindly and gently support, lead by example, and allow them to be fallible, they'll probably turn out to be decent human beings."
Thinking in Extremes	
"He's an enemey—out to get me."	"Maybe he's indifferent. He probably has reasons why he's doing this that makes sense to him. If he really is out to get me, he's just one bad apple among many good ones. Everyone isn't like that, so why should I let him get under my skin?"
"I have to win or I'll lose."	"It's okay to compromise or even yield on many matters. I can bend."
"I won't be respected if I'm not angry and in control."	"Anger might win me victory by intimidation and fear. Respect, however, is earned by respectful treatment."

CHAPTER 17

Eye Movement

At this point we will introduce a very useful skill called the eye-movement technique.[113] Used as a quick distraction and a way to gain temporary relief from distressing thoughts, this technique helps about two-thirds of those who try it. Remember that this and the techniques in chapter 18 especially are best taught and learned in the context of a therapeutic relationship. It is not recommended they be first tried alone.

1. *Identify something that upsets you.* It might be a stressful present situation that triggers intense emotions. Perhaps it is seeing one of your triggers and trying to fight off the intrusive thoughts. It may be thinking about the trauma. In a moment, you will think about it to the point that you feel five to six Subjective Units of Distress (SUDS). SUDS are simply a rating of how distressed you are feeling. 0 means you feel pleasantly relaxed with no distress. 10 means extreme distress, as uncomfortable as you have ever felt or could imagine yourself feeling. When you have identified the upsetting event you wish to work with continue to step two.

2. *Imagine the upsetting event.* Now add worry, the "What ifs . . . Oh nos . . . I can't stand it . . . here we go again." Stew about the event until you get your SUDS to the 5–6 range, but not higher because we don't want this to become overwhelming. A SUDS of 5–6 suggests moderate distress that is unpleasant but tolerable. Although you might notice fear, anxiety, or other uncomfortable physical and emotional states, you are still able to think clearly. (For reference, a SUDS of 3 is the amount of arousal needed to concentrate—it is not unpleasant. A SUDS of 4 suggests mild distress that is easily tolerated; A SUDS of 8 is high distress that can't be tolerated for very long and impairs thinking.)

3. *With your eyes open and your head still, watch as I (the mental health professional) move my hands.* Notice if this works. (The therapist moves his hand back and forth at a distance of about fourteen inches from your eyes. The hands move a horizontal distance of about two feet. About twenty-five back and forth cycles are completed.)

4. *Where are your SUDS now?* A typical drop might be to 4–4½. What happened to your images and thoughts? (Often people will say they are blocked, suppressed, blurred, they shrink or fade).

5. *If your SUDS dropped a little, if your thoughts and images altered somewhat, then this technique seems like a useful skill to practice.* If so, let's put this skill under your control and learn to self-direct it.
   a. Pick two spots in the room, maybe on the wall or your hands on your knees.
   b. Think about something that upsets you, that could take you to the 5–6 SUDS range.
   c. Get a clear image of it.
   d. Add the worry.
   e. Bring yourself to the 5–6 SUDS range.
   f. Complete about twenty-five cycles of eye movements.
   g. Check for any alterations in your SUDS, images, and thoughts.
   h. How easy is it when you self-direct? (Often people find it to be a little easier when the therapist directs, but most people can do it alone.)

6. *You might be in situations when you cannot conveniently move your eyes back and forth.* In such situations, you can do the eye movement technique with your eyes closed. You might even wish to do it with your hand over your eyes, as though you are deep in thought. Are you willing to try it with your eyes closed?
   a. If so, let your eyes close.
   b. Get an image of the stressful event.
   c. Now add the thoughts until you reach the 5–6 SUDS range. Let me know when you reach that level.
   d. Now try moving your eyes back and forth about twenty-five times.
   e. Check your SUDS and notice what happened to the images and thoughts.

If you observe a drop in your discomfort, then the eye movement technique seems like a good skill to practice. Try practicing it several times a day over a one- or two-week period to gain mastery of the skill. You can use this as an effective distraction from upsetting intrusions and as a rapid stress reducer. It might be used later in the course of treatment to calm intense emotions that might arise during processing work.

Note: Thought Field Therapy can also rapidly reduce distressing symptoms of PTSD (see chapter 23). It can be especially useful before one feels ready to talk about traumatic events.

CHAPTER 18

Intrusion Management[114]

FLASHBACKS

The following skills can help defuse the distress of flashbacks, an especially troubling type of intrusion, although the techniques can be helpful for any forms of intrusions.

1. *If flashbacks occur when your eyes are closed, open them and perform about twenty-five cycles of the eye movement technique.* If opening your eyes is not practical, do it with them closed. Although some people find that simply closing their eyes tightly distracts from the intrusive thoughts, most people find they cannot get oriented to the present and away from reliving the past without seeing where they are.

2. *Ground yourself.* This means to do things to bring your awareness solidly back to the present. Rub fabric or the arms of the chair. Notice what your body feels like. Notice colors or other details in your surroundings. Name items in your surroundings. Push your feet down or stomp them. Rub a ring or another piece of jewelry that you associate with someone safe or a safe time in your life. Say to yourself, "That was then, I am here, this is now." Count something, like beads. Repeatedly tell yourself:[115]

   - This is just a memory from the past—old stuff. It will pass.
   - My feelings are understandable. They come and go.
   - I am safe now.
   - That was then. This is now.
   - I'm here now. Today is _____ (think of today's date).

You might also exercise, take a shower, play with pets, focus on breathing, or take a nap.

SAFE PLACE IMAGERY[116]

The object is to create a safe place in your imagination, a haven or place of rest. This skill is very effective anytime that you feel overwhelmed during or between sessions. It is also a pleasant way to start the day, and is frequently used for restoring calmness at the end of a therapy session.

1. *Select an image that evokes calm and safety* (not the safe place yet; just some image that makes you feel safe and calm).

2. *Focus on the image. Feel the emotions.* Identify the location of the pleasant sensations in your body. Just allow yourself to experience and enjoy them. (Therapist allows time and asks you to signal when you feel the soothing emotions and sensations. She asks you to identify where in your body you feel the sensations.)

3. *Now bring up the image of your safe place, the place that feels safe and calm to be in.* Your safe place can be real or imagined, outdoors or indoors. Maybe you have really been there or maybe you've made it up. You may go there alone, or some person that makes you feel safe can be there. You are the boss. If you can't think of a safe place, then imagine the safest place you can think of.[117]

4. *Notice all your physical senses in that safe place.* Notice where you feel the pleasant sensations in your body and allow yourself to enjoy them. Now concentrate on those sensations.

5. *What single word fits that picture* (you might pick a word such as relax, beach, mountain, trees, etc.). Think of that word and scene, allowing yourself to again experience the pleasant sensations and a sense of emotional security.

6. *Self-cueing.* Repeat the procedure on your own, bringing up the image and the word and experience the positive emotions and physical sensations.

7. *Self-cueing with disturbance.* You can use this technique to relax during stressful times. To emphasize this point, bring up a minor annoyance and

notice the accompanying negative feelings. Now use your cueing word and bring up the emotions and physical sensations of peace and safety.

8. *Bring up a disturbing thought once again and access your safe place on your own.*

9. *Practice at least once daily.* Call up the positive feelings, word, and image while you use the relaxation techniques that you like best.[118]

You might wish to be creative. You might envision the safe place nearby with a door you can open and step through into the scene. Take a nice relaxing breath before entering. You might find a couch there, next to which is a feelings dial. You might rush there to tell your concerns to the safe person, or just go to be safely alone.

FEELINGS DIAL

You can use this imagery to gain better control over the intensity of your feelings. With practice, you can learn to "turn down" overwhelming feelings. (This technique is not a way to avoid or get rid of feelings—these must eventually be processed for healing to occur.) Imagine a volume dial, say on a radio. This is like a "feelings dial." It has numbers from 1 to 10, from low to most intense. Notice what the dial is made of. Notice if it is smooth. Think of an unpleasant feeling you sometimes feel. Notice whether you are feeling it right now. What number on the dial reflects how weak or strong the feeling is now? What number is the dial on now? What is that like to be on that number? What would it be like to be at 1? Or 8? How about somewhere in the middle? If you'd like to try turning down the feelings dial, what number would you turn it to? Turn down the dial lower and lower until it goes down a number. And keep turning it lower and lower and lower. Would you like to keep going? Keep going nice and slow until you find your desired intensity. Please repeat several times so that you can master this skill. Do easy deep breathing. Time your breathing so that each time you exhale, you turn the dial a little lower.

Anytime that your feelings are too high, imagine the dial. Turn it down. It can be a revelation to some that feelings can be controlled in this way. This is a good technique if you feel angry, demoralized, anxious, out of control, or depressed. It can be useful for feelings associated with flashbacks or for ending a therapy session.

OTHER CONTAINMENT SKILLS[119]

These are additional steps that help you firmly control intrusive thoughts on a temporary basis, until you are ready to process them. Containment helps you function each day without being overwhelmed. It provides a way to tolerate intense feelings and choose when you wish to work on them. Containment also helps you to keep past separated from present.

- *Split screen.* This skill is like watching a television screen where two sports events appear at once. You divide a mental TV screen, putting the past on one side and the present on the other. You have remote controls that allow you to mute, slow down, shrink, fast forward, turn to black and white, or turn off the past. You download the difficult memories to a videotape as the therapist counts from one to three. You turn off the TV, take out the tape, and store or file the tape in a safe place (wherever you want, maybe a safe with a special key). Place it there until you are ready to take it out.

- *Freezing.* Imagine that the intrusive thoughts, images, feelings, or recollections are ice cubes that you'll store at your therapist's office. Visualize a big scoop that scoops up the ice cubes and drops them into Tupperware containers. Tight-fitting lids on the containers seal in the ice cubes. See the containers safely stored in a freezer outside your therapist's office. You and your therapist can retrieve the ice cubes, one container at a time, and use them in an appropriate way to help your therapy progress.

- *Dirty laundry.* Imagine the intrusive thoughts, images, feelings, or recollections as soiled clothing which needs to go to the laundry. See yourself stuffing the soiled clothing in a laundry bag and calling the laundry service. Imagine that the laundry truck arrives. The laundry bag is placed in the laundry truck, the truck doors are closed, and you watch through a window as the laundry truck drives away. Watch the truck turn the corner and disappear. The laundry is next to your therapist's office. You and your therapist can pick up your laundry together, sort it out, and use it in an appropriate way to help your therapy progress.

- *Shrinking techniques.* Imagine that you are looking at distressing material through a telescope in reverse, so that it becomes very small and far away. Or imagine that you are in a plane flying over the material and looking down. You are in control; you are the boss. You say how high and far away you wish to go.

- *Other containment techniques.* There is no one best way to do this. The best technique is the one that works for you. Create a strategy that you like to get better control of your symptoms. You might, for example, imagine the distressing material written on a chalkboard, then erased; written on a letter and mailed to a safe place; or packed in a suitcase and stored in a locker.

PART V

Treatment

CHAPTER 19

Principles of Memory Work

> I don't want to remember but I can't seem to forget.
>
> —*PTSD sufferer*

A major goal of treatment for PTSD is to integrate dissociated traumatic memory material with your associated memories. Think of a young boy in your neighborhood that you have watched grow up with great enjoyment. Imagine that he is called to war and returns quite shaken. At the airport you notice that much of the sparkle has left his eyes. The town holds a parade and welcome home party to celebrate his return. The neighborhood goes out of its way to integrate him back into normal life. He is embraced again and again. Eventually the life begins to return to his eyes. If the young man is to resume his life again, he hopefully will not be shunned or shamed, but will be made to feel a part of the community again. Now think of a personal traumatic experience. If you are to heal and pick up again, you will need to embrace your traumatic memories and integrate them with the rest of your life experience. You will not try to destroy them or cast them out. To do so would be to disown the part of you that experienced them.

It is normal to wish to flee from painful memories. Yet these memories continue to pursue us, much like a little barking dog chases a person until that person stops, turns, and faces the dog. As Williams notes, "Only a remembered trauma can be worked through and then let go."[120] It is easier to live with a memory when all aspects are remembered and processed.[121] How is this done?

In memory work, you will give yourself the opportunity to call up memories in sufficient detail so that you can accurately see what happened and understand their impact. You will learn to view trauma like a scrapbook of an event that you can store on a shelf and take down as needed. The trauma gives you a unique experience, but you don't have to look at it everywhere you go, and you don't equate the owner of the album with the album.[122] You are more than the traumatic event. Eventually you will see your traumatic experience in the context of your broader life experience, neither exaggerating nor underemphasizing your role or its impact. As you confront rather than avoid traumatic memories, you find that the memories no longer are as frightening.

In the process of healing, you will answer questions like the following:

- What does the trauma mean? Why did it happen?
- How do I make sense of my world again?
- Who or what was responsible and how do I make peace with my actual role(s)?
- Why haven't I adapted better and what coping skills will help me cope better?
- What does it mean to process memories so that I can let them go? How is it done?

In telling your story and recalling memories you will have the opportunity to break the secrecy that maintains dissociation, and correct misinterpretations and unrealistic expectations.

A word of caution is important to reemphasize. During treatment, intrusions (memories, nightmares, flashbacks, reactions to triggers) are likely to increase. This simply signals the need to process traumatic material. Information in the intrusions can be very useful as long as you are not overwhelmed by the intrusions. Remember that you need to be the boss, to dictate the pace of memory work. Remember to work in partnership with your therapist. Communicate if you are beginning to feel overwhelmed. Allow yourself time to prepare for memory work, and time at the end of sessions to restore a feeling of safety and balance. Safety and balance can be restored by safe place imagery, relaxation, and/or containment exercises. Continue to practice the skills you have acquired thus far. You might hear your therapist use the word "titrate" to refer to the process of gradually bringing up enough memory detail to allow processing but not so much that you feel overwhelmed. As a rule, the more aspects of a memory that can be processed, the more effective the integration will be. Eventually as you "tell your story" repeatedly, you will be able to tolerate more and more detail without being overwhelmed. Do not rush the process however. Like building a house, slow and steady progress is better than rushed, sloppy work.

Note that some people choose not to or cannot face traumas. Discuss with your therapist when to do this work, if at all. For example, some people feel the need to be in therapy for a year or two before talking about trauma, because they need to learn the techniques and/or feel safe enough to process memories. Poor health may prevent others from having the strength to do memory work.

Your therapist will explain various ways to do memory work. Some proceed more slowly, others are somewhat accelerated. Some are primarily intellectual, while other approaches involve more emotions and/or behavior. PTSD can be responsive to all of the approaches summarized in this part of the book when they are applied appropriately. Become familiar with the treatment options described herein so that you can create a treatment plan with your therapist that makes sense for you. For many cases of PTSD, treatment could logically follow the general sequence as outlined in this book. However, the treatment plan is usually affected by the skills, resources, and preferences of both the survivor and the clinician, as well as the particulars of the case.

When children face distressing setbacks, they bounce back when embraced with love, faith, hope, humor, and a sense of purpose. You too will recover as you embrace your experience in similar ways.

CHAPTER 20

Cognitive Restructuring[*]

When circumstances don't fit our ideas, they
become our difficulties.

— *Benjamin Franklin*

We remember that a major PTSD treatment goal is to integrate dissociated trauma material with associated memories, so that the fabric of our memory becomes like one continuous memory. The problem is that traumatic memory doesn't mesh with the way we want to look at the world. The dissociated memories often contain misinterpretations and inaccurate conclusions that were formed under great duress, while strong emotions and arousal continue to interfere with processing.

Integration is facilitated by restructuring unproductive ideas that maintain emotional arousal and interfere with processing. Unproductive ideas can relate to the present (our normal assumptions about life, people, and ourselves; thoughts about triggers, symptoms, or everyday stressors), the past (e.g., misinterpretations about the traumatic event), or the future. Each can keep arousal dysfunctionally high. Reworking these ideas is the goal of cognitive therapy, a mainstay in the treatment of PTSD. Cognitive therapy asserts that thoughts significantly influence our reactions to events. Let's see how this works.

---

*This chapter summarizes the ideas and therapeutic strategies of several cognitive theorists. Albert Ellis originated the ABC model, catastrophizing, and shoulds. Aaron Beck originated the concepts of Automatic Thoughts, the term *distortions*, most of the distortions presently used in Cognitive Therapy, the idea of basic (core) beliefs, and the idea of recording thoughts, distortions, and moods. David Burns wrote *Feeling Good*, a very useful application of Beck's theories. The book is recommended for further reading.

Paramedics Harold and Anne received an urgent call one dark, rainy night. A popular teenager who lived in an unfamiliar section of the county was having difficulty breathing after he returned from playing in a basketball game. Reacting quickly, they drove toward the house but found that the bridge en route had washed away. Quickly looking at the map, Anne directed Harold to an alternate route. In their haste, however, they sped past the turn and lost several precious minutes. When they arrived at the house, the teenager had stopped breathing and could not be resuscitated. Harold thought angrily, "Why did such a fine young man have to die? Life is so unfair!" Then sadly, "If only I had heeded my instincts and turned sooner. I could kick myself for being so dumb." Later he worries, "What if something like that happens to my kids?" Harold begins to have trouble sleeping, and can't get the thought of the young teenager out of his mind. He starts worrying about his own children, and becomes overprotective of them. He starts to notice his heart pounding and worries that maybe he'll have a heart attack. He can't seem to unwind, and eventually takes a leave of absence. Jean processed the event differently, however. She thought, "It is so sad that that fine young man died. He had such a bright future. I'll always wonder if we might have saved him had we arrived sooner. But we were in unfamiliar territory with such poor visibility. We did the best we could." Jean grieved at the loss, but returned to her job with a renewed commitment to serving others. Both Harold and Jean were capable, bright, and dedicated professionals. Their responses to the traumatic event, however, were largely determined by their thoughts.

Cognitive therapy enables us to stop, identify unproductive thoughts, and replace them with more functional thoughts. We stop running from arousing thoughts—or only partially confronting them—and begin to persistently confront and challenge them. In so doing, we shift from the helpless victim mode to the action mode, gaining mastery over the one thing we can consistently control— our thoughts. This process usually lessens arousal. Should emotional and physical arousal occur, knowing how to replace unproductive thoughts helps keep it within bounds and allows it to subside more quickly. The model is fairly simple:

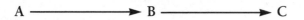

A stands for the Activating (or upsetting) event. B is the Belief (or automatic thoughts) that we tell ourselves about A. C is the emotional and physical Consequences (or arousal). Most people think that A causes C. In reality, it is B, our self-talk, that has greater influence. Productive self-talk would likely lead to appropriate emotional *upset* that allows us to focus and concentrate on functioning. On the other hand, unproductive thoughts lead to emotional *disturbance* that prevents cool thinking and functioning.

AUTOMATIC THOUGHTS AND DISTORTIONS

When an upsetting event occurs, *automatic thoughts (ATs)* run through our minds. Although we're all capable of thinking reasonably about upsetting events, sometimes our automatic thoughts are *distorted*—or unreasonably negative. Distorted ATs occur so rapidly that we hardly notice them, let alone stop to question them. Yet these ATs profoundly affect our moods, our body's arousal, and our ability to process clearly.

Distortions are learned. Sometimes we learn them in childhood. Sometimes they are taught from others; sometimes they are learned from previous traumatic experiences. Distortions are not a reflection of intelligence or strength. They are simply learned habits. When we submit them to new evidence and logic, we can learn new, more productive thought patterns. In this section, you'll improve your skill in catching troublesome distortions, challenging their logic, and replacing them with thoughts that are less arousing.

The distortions that increase PTSD symptoms fall into only thirteen categories. Learn them well. You will use them repeatedly throughout treatment. Beyond PTSD, Cognitive therapy teaches skills that facilitates coping and growth in all people. In addition to being able to quickly spot distortions, the goals are to rebut and replace them as well. Rebuttals generally take the form of three questions: What's the evidence? What's another way to look at the situation? So what if it happens?[123]

The Distortions

1. *Flaw fixation.* Here we tend to zoom right in on what is wrong or what went wrong. This is also called "fear focus" because the mental camera focuses on the fearful. It is like seeing only one aspect of a picture. For example:
   - A firefighter saves twenty people from a fire but dwells on the five that he could not rescue. He ignores the good things that he did before and during the fire, and fixates only on the bad outcomes.
   - On vacation, a paramedic sees a cross on the side of the road, reminding him of a life that he could not save. He stops noticing the beauty of the countryside.

- A rape victim surveys a crowd of people and only notices the face of a man who reminds her of the perpetrator.
- A soldier thinks of his shortcomings in a battle when he recalls his three years of military service. He ignores the fact that he persisted in his duty and showed great skill in surviving many difficult situations.
- A father concentrates on his child's "C" and doesn't praise the "As" and "Bs" on the report card.

The problem with this "worm's eye view"[124] is that it ignores the very aspects that make life satisfying and enjoyable. And through conditioning, related negatives snowball so that many places and events now remind us to feel guilt, anger, fear, sadness, or insecurity.

The antidote is to expand our focus—use a wider lens to see the whole picture. Ask: "What else could I notice? What *isn't* wrong? What's gone well? What is right? What percentage of the time did I perform well? What's here to enjoy?" Notice that the suggestion is not to ignore the negative aspects, but to see *more* aspects.

2. *Dismissing the Positive.* Whereas flaw fixation ignores the good, dismissing the positive actually discounts it, as if it didn't matter. You don't give yourself deserved credit, so you feel badly. When armed terrorists seized her school, a teacher coolly led her class out a basement passage. When complimented on her cool functioning, she replied, "It's not worth thinking about. I was just lucky to survive; there was no skill to it." The teacher might have thanked the giver of the compliment and privately thought, "I am glad that I had the presence of mind to function so well." Good always counts.

3. *Assuming.* There are three kinds:
   - *Mind reading.* Here we assume that we know what others are thinking. Examples:
     - "My colleagues think I'm a wimp for being so stressed about this."
     - "They hate me for letting them down."
     - "God doesn't love me and couldn't possibly forgive this kind of mistake."

     These distortions are challenged by asking, "What's the evidence? Is there another possibility?" Some people will have empathy and understanding for your suffering. Others might be indifferent or curious—not mocking. People may or may not be disappointed in your behavior. On the other hand, some, most, or all of them may find it understandable under the circumstances.

- *Jumping to conclusions.* You hear a noise and assume that a burglar is in the house. You literally jump at this conclusion, which is called the startle response. This is tested by asking, "What is the evidence. Is it possible that this is not a repeat of my trauma?"

- *Fortune telling.* Here we pessimistically predict a negative outcome without testing the evidence. Following are some examples and some replacement thoughts. Fortune telling often starts with a fear focus ("It *might* happen. After all it's happened before. Or, it could happen for the first time."), and subtly shifts to "It will *undoubtedly* happen," which arouses further. To challenge this distortion, we think somewhat tentatively and openly like a scientist. "Certainly bad things might happen, but what's the probability or odds of this happening?" Other antidotes include asking, "Why might this negative *not* happen? Why might something *good* happen?"

4. *Catastrophizing* is making things much worse than they actually are. We assume that something is so horrible, dreadful, disastrous, or awful that we can't stand it. In exaggerating the badness of the situation, we also magnify our arousal and create a feeling of helplessness. Following are some examples:

CATASTROPHIZING	REPLACEMENT THOUGHTS
These intrusions are unbearable.	It's okay. It's just a symptom of dissociation, and a cue to process when I am ready to.
It's awful to feel these bad feelings.	It's a sign that I can still feel. Good feelings will likely return as I heal.
I hate that reminder of my trauma.	Yes, this is difficult, but it is just a trigger, not a repeat of the traumatic event.
I can't stand it when things don't go the way I want.	I can stand it even if I don't like it.
This is hell all over again.	Five years from now maybe this won't seem like such a big deal. It's okay to not get my way all the time.

FORTUNE TELLING	REPLACEMENT THOUGHTS
If I let myself feel, I'll lose control and never stop crying. I'll go crazy.	It's highly unlikely that feelings make people crazy. Tears eventually stop. Bottling feelings is more dangerous than processing them. I'll learn ways to process feelings gradually in a safe and controlled setting.
Talking about it will make me feel worse.	The research shows that talking about it helps most people feel better eventually.
If I express my anger, I'll explode. I'll become violent and beat my kids, just . like Dad did to me.	I can verbalize feelings. That's different from acting on them. In fact, only a minority of adults who were abused as children abuse their own children.[125]
I'll never recover. I'll always be thinking of this bad stuff.	These thoughts are just the effects of trauma. They are understandable when someone has felt helpless and out of control. They are also depressing, frustrating, and unreasonable. The only evidence is that my present methods have not been effective to date. As I learn new skills I'll likely start to climb the staircase to recovery.
If I leave the house the trauma will occur again.	Perhaps, but maybe the trauma was a glitch, an exception to the rule. Rather than constantly worrying and expecting the worst, I'll do all I can to be prepared.
I'll never feel safe again.	Life is never 100 percent safe. If I take reasonable precautions I might feel reasonably safe.
I'll never fit in. No one will understand me. I'll never be attractive to others. No one will love me. They'll shun me if they know what I've been through.	Some might shun me. Some might be unable or unwilling to understand. On the other hand, some might appreciate me, knowing what I have battled to overcome.
If I go to the party I'll have a rotten time.	I might have a mediocre or somewhat enjoyable time. Maybe some aspects will be pleasant. I won't really know until I experiment.

· "What ifs" commonly signify catastrophizing ("What if this awful thing happens!; What if I screw up again! What if I can't recover!"). "What ifs" keep the focus on the worst possible fear, so we remain aroused, while distracting us from what we can resolutely do to maximize the possibility of a good outcome.

There are many rebuttals to this pervasive distortion:

- Ask, "How likely is this to do me in? Will the world really end?"
- Think, "It's not so bad. This is inconvenient, not a catastrophe."
- Think, "Okay, let's assume the worst is really happening or will happen. What will I *do* then?" There is something calming about fully facing the worst, accepting that it could happen or is happening, and then determining what you would do to improve upon the worst. Turn a *What if* . . . to an *If then* . . . (If such and such happens, then I'll do such and such to make the best of the situation and salvage what I can.) For example, "If I were unable to fully recover and were to lose my job, I'll grieve for a while that I can't do some things anymore, but not forever. I'll retool for a job I can handle, and find new ways to enjoy life." Remind yourself that the negative may never happen, but if it does you'll make the most of it. Instead of "What if this negative happens?" ask, "What if it doesn't?"
- Look calmly and fully at your symptoms. Think, "This is common to PTSD. With treatment, they'll most likely improve. I can handle it. Though frightening, arousal is just my normal stress response that hasn't turned off. This is a real opportunity to relax, process my disturbing material, and improve my health."
- Remember to focus on the here-and-now to redirect your focus from catastrophic, arousing thoughts. For instance, instead of focusing on a racing heart and intrusive thoughts, count backward, focus on abdominal breathing, concentrate on what people are saying or wearing, look around the room and notice colors, sounds, smells, and other aspects of your surroundings.
- To realize that there are many coping options, ask what others have done in similar situations.
- Try humor. "Oh, no! I'm losing it. I'm going to blow up like an atomic bomb." Or, "Bad things happen in life. Tough!" Or, "Maybe I can find a certificate guaranteeing me perpetual tranquillity."

5. *All-or-none thinking.* Here we think in extremes that create arousal and often lower self-esteem. Think of a pole vaulter who sets the bar very high and considers himself a loser for not making it over. There is no middle ground and no partial credit in this distortion. Examples are:

- Either I handled the trauma perfectly or horribly.
- I'm a hero or a heel; a success or a failure.
- If I make a mistake I am a complete failure.
- I'm brave or I'm a coward.
- I'm completely competent or I am incompetent.
- I'm not fitting in very well since the trauma. I'm a social retard.
- I'm either a good guy or a bad guy. I performed badly during the trauma. Therefore I am bad, irresponsible, inadequate.
- Either I am symptom-free or I am out of control—strong or an emotional wimp.

In reality, most humans operate in the middle much of the time. (Half of all brain surgeries are below average.) No one excels in all things at all times. Falling short of perfection makes you fallible, not worthless. In some situations, just surviving or performing reasonably well is quite a feat. All you can do is your best. If you are already committed to your best, then worrying or condemning yourself adds nothing to your performance. Rating your performance on a one to ten scale helps correct this distortion. For example, "I performed at about 80 percent today." (Notice, we rate *behavior,* not people, who are too complex to rate.) Also, redefine success as trying your best and progressing, not reaching perfection.

Extreme thinking can also be applied to others. "I must trust you 100 percent or I can't trust you at all" might lead one to trust a person who really is not worthy of trust. Or it might cause one to reject a kind and sensitive person who occasionally acts irresponsibly but is willing to improve. Trust is earned gradually. There can be many shades of gray between complete trust and complete absence of trust. Some people are somewhat trustworthy, honest in certain situations and dishonest in others; sometimes dependable and sometimes not. People are not all good or all bad, but are a combination of bad and good attributes at varying degrees of development. It takes time to build trust and it can be earned and given in varying degrees. If we are willing to patiently walk the middle ground we might make better judgments about people and be disappointed less often.

In addition, extreme thinking might apply to the way we view the world (life was ideal before the trauma, completely good—now it stinks). There is a tendency to forget that some aspects were good and some bad. That's life . . . and this is generally true, even after a trauma. To remember this lessens upset at the parts that are not yet going well.

Another example of extreme thinking is to think that if we are not completely relaxed and calm then we are out of control and back in emergency mode. There are many gradations in the middle and it is okay to be there.

Finally, extreme thinking includes the view that I am either strong or I am emotional. The middle ground might be, "I can be strong *and* have feelings. Having genuine feelings makes me human, not weak. Shedding a tear does not mean that I will become a complete basket case. The constructive expression of feelings will let me bend without breaking."

6. *Shoulds (musts/oughts)* are rigid demands that we make of ourselves or the world. These demands insist that the world be somehow different than it is. The unspoken assumption is that the consequences are dire if the demand is not met. It is clear how this distortion keeps arousal high. Examples are:
   - "I should have handled the traumatic event differently. I should have acted better."
   - "It's not fair. It should not have happened to me. Only good things should happen."
   - "I shouldn't be feeling so distressed. John Wayne never felt this way."
   - "I must be strong."
   - "I must have control over my life. Now. I must no longer make mistakes since mistakes caused me pain in the past."
   - "I should be over this by now."
   - "People should understand what I'm going through." "I shouldn't be afraid, tired, imperfect, etc." "I must be absolutely sure that nothing can go wrong before I risk it. Life ought to be predictable."
   - "I must not allow my kids to mess up—ever."

   A powerful antidote for a should is a *would or could*. Woulds and coulds preserve ideals but in a gentler, more flexible way that accepts the world as it is. For example:
   - "It would be nice to be less distressed during a crisis and perform more coolly. I wonder how I could do this."

- "It would be nice to be recovered by now, but everyone's timetables are different and forcing things will just make me more stressed. In the meantime, I wonder what I could be trying."
- "It would be nice if things were better. But I accept that:
  - People will always be fallible, never perfect.
  - Life will always be unfair and things happen that we don't always deserve.
  - No one can ever achieve total control of events. I won't make myself crazy by insisting that things be perfect. I'll just aim to do a very good job and expect I'll probably improve with experience."

Also, ask, "Why should I? Where is this *should* written?" For example, is it written somewhere that humans should not be frightened when confronted with an overwhelming event for the first time? Or the hundredth time?

A final antidote is to see what happens when you don't do the thing you think you must and realize that the world does not end (e.g., "If I allow myself to be vulnerable, I might learn that people like me better"; "If I allow my children to make some mistakes they might learn some valuable lessons. This is not a combat zone, after all.").

7. *Making feelings facts* is thinking that your feelings represent reality. For example:
   - "I feel so anxious all the time—I must be in danger; I must not be as capable as others; something bad must be about to happen."
   - "Because I feel so anxious, there must be a real and present danger. If not, I'm going crazy." "I feel like I'm going crazy. I must be."

   Remember that feelings result from thoughts. During traumatic events it is easy to formulate inaccurate ideas that don't get challenged. So question your feelings now. Ask, "Is this reality, or just a feeling?" Some common distortions and their antidotes appear on page 160.

8. *Overgeneralizing* is deciding that your negative experience applies to all situations. For example:
   - "People always let you down."
   - "All men want only one thing."
   - "Everything in life is so unfair."

MAKING FEELINGS FACTS	REPLACEMENT THOUGHTS
"I feel so diminished by the trauma, so unworthy, so bad. I must be bad."	Separate the trauma from the resulting feelings of worth. It's the trauma that's bad. Not you. If someone did something offensive to you, you might think, "Something bad *happened* to me." If your behavior fell short of your ideal, you might think, "I made a mistake. That makes me fallible and human, not worthless."
"I feel so dirty."	When people are abused, it is natural to feel that way. Again, separate the event from your worth.
"I feel hopeless."	Are you hopeless, or just in a situation that feels hopeless?
"I feel crazy. I must be crazy."	"This feeling is the result of defending against unpleasant feelings. This doesn't make me crazy. As I learn to gradually process those feelings I'll start to feel better."
"I feel so totally out of control and powerless."	"I was out of control and powerless then. That was then. This is now."
"I feel so numb—like I'm incapable of feeling	"I feel numb now. But feelings will grow gradually as the wounds begin to heal."

- "All new or strange situations are dangerous, especially those that are like situations that frightened me in the past."
- "All authority figures are fearful."
- "I can't do anything right. I never do things right. I always let people down."
- "Nobody has confidence in me."
- "My whole life stinks."
- "Since I was helpless and out of control then, I am that way in all situations."
- "Things always go wrong. It never fails."

Words like *always, never, everyone, nobody, all,* or *none* indicate overgeneralizations. The opposite to these words is *some* (*Sometimes* I do pretty well; *Some* authority figures are safe; *Some* new situations can be exciting and fun.) Ask if a negative event could be an exception to the rule. Maybe the world isn't always like this.[126]

Some people overgeneralize in the positive direction ("All the world is good and safe"; "Good people always make good decisions."). When a traumatic event occurs they cannot reconcile the traumatic memory with this thought. Again, the word *some* helps. For example, Joan was raised in a very close family with a very loving father. She assumed that all men are trustworthy. She could not get over it when her boyfriend raped her. She learned to view reality on a continuum. Between the extremes of *men are totally trustworthy* and *men are untrustworthy*, she viewed a new middle ground: *Some men are mostly trustworthy and some are mostly untrustworthy.* She accepted responsibility to evaluate each individual separately.

9. *Abusive labeling.* Here you give yourself a label, or name, as though a single word could describe a complex person completely. For example, to say, "I am a loser," means that I am *always* and *in every way* a loser. Obviously, this isn't fair or true. Children often internalize spoken or unspoken messages. For example, a child who is repeatedly molested comes to think of herself as just a sex object, a whore—even in adulthood. The antidote is to rate behavior or experience—but not people. Thus, "that was a really difficult experience for me," not, "I'm bad."

Here are some other examples and rebuttals related to trauma:

DISTORTION	ANTIDOTE
I'm damaged goods—worthless.	I was raped. I am more than my wound.
I'm a coward.	I was frightened and unsure of what to do. I made some bad choices.
I'm a slut for climaxing when my stepfather molested me.	Orgasm is an automatic physiologic response to direct stimulation. It means that I am a normally functioning woman.

Notice that labels can be levied at other people as well, which is common in anger reactions. To reduce another human being to an "always and in every way" label is just as inaccurate and unfair as doing it to yourself, even if it feels justified.

10. *Personalizing* is seeing yourself as more responsible or involved than you really are. For example:

DISTORTION	ANTIDOTE
It's all my fault that I was raped. I must have asked for it because of the way I dressed. I deserved it.	This is a faulty way to try to make sense of a crime. Rape is a crime. No one deserves a crime. Dressing attractively is not the same as asking for a crime. The cause was the perpetrator, not me. I'm not responsible for a crime, only my recovery.
There must be something about me that invited the battering, or caused my husband to do it.	Battering is a crime. Perhaps I could learn some social skills, but lack of skills does not justify being criminalized. Crimes happen for reasons outside of my influence.
A firefighter is asked about a fire caused by an arsonist and he replies, "We lost twenty people."	I didn't lose twenty people. They were murdered by an arsonist.
Why did this happen to me? Why was I singled out?	The world is not for or against us. Both bad and good things happen to people.
That driver is out for me.	That driver doesn't even know me. I am not the central figure in his bad day or life. Maybe he hates the world, not me. Maybe he is neutral to me or completely oblivious to me.
In an argument a husband tells his wife, "You are either for me or against me."	People will inevitably disagree about issues. That doesn't mean she is against me, just my idea.
If I worry enough I can keep bad things from happening.	This is trying to be responsible for too much. I accept that I cannot have total control. All I can have is responsibility for what I can control. Instead of worrying and staying aroused, I will make a good action plan, do my best, then release worry.

The antidote to this distortion is to see things accurately. Separate influences from causes. Figure out how much responsibility truly is yours, and keep what is beyond your control outside of your boundaries.

11. *Blaming* is the opposite of personalizing. Whereas personalizing puts all the responsibility on yourself for your difficulties, blaming puts it all on something outside of yourself. For example:
    - "He treated me so miserably. He has ruined my life and my self-esteem."
    - "I'm stressed out today because of _____ (my crummy childhood, Vietnam, the doctor's incompetence, etc.)."
    - "Dogs make me so afraid."

    The problem with blaming, much like catastrophizing, is that it tends to make us think of ourselves as helpless victims who are too feeble to cope. Blaming keeps us stuck in the past problem; we are powerless because the past is unchangeable. The antidote to blaming is to acknowledge outside influences, but to take responsibility for your own welfare. "Okay, I see how these things have influenced my development and/or challenge me. Now, I commit to get back on track and move on." For present stressors we might think, "Nothing makes me do anything—I now choose how I respond."

12. *Unfavorable comparisons*. Here you magnify another's strengths and your weaknesses while minimizing the other's faults and your strengths. So by comparison, you feel inadequate or inferior. For example, you think, "Brian is a bright surgeon. He makes so much money. He was even on the news the other night for treating the governor. Me, I'm just a nurse. I could never get up in front of a camera and talk like he does. Sure, I have wonderful friends and I'm active at the homeless shelter. And it's true that Brian's got a drinking problem and his kids are really struggling. And yeah, he told me he really depends on me in the operating room. But look at what he does!" On a rescue team, Marty is constantly comparing himself to the sharpest, bravest individual. Sometimes he compares himself to movie stars, like John Wayne or Chuck Norris, who never seem to show fear or make mistakes in their scripted settings. A way to challenge this distortion is to ask, "Why must I compare? Why can't I just appreciate that each person has unique strengths and weaknesses? Another's contributions are not necessarily better, just different." Someone humorously noted that doctors have more status than garbage collectors, but one wonders who does more for

public health. We generally function better and with less stress when we focus on doing our personal best, not comparisons.

13. *Regrets.* In looking back, we think, "If only I hadn't . . . (performed so poorly, been so anxious, said what I did)." Beyond a period of introspection where mistakes are acknowledged and courses are corrected, regrets are unproductive because we can't go back and change the past. Regrets are another way to reject our imperfections. We might beat ourselves, thinking, "I deserve to be punished for that." What we actually deserve is the opportunity to try again, improve, and learn from the mistakes. We can think, "I've learned from mistakes in the past and I can do so again. That was then and this is now."

Everly and Mitchell[127] advise the following for dealing with difficult experiences from the past:

- A mistake isn't usually a deliberate act. Ask, "What did I want/intend to happen?"

- If it was an honest mistake, think, "This could have happened to many people."

- Ask, "What did I learn that could prevent this from happening again?" Focus on remedial action.

- How much was I actually responsible for? Were there factors beyond my control?

- What good things are a result of this outcome? What is the possible silver lining?

- Will there be more chances to learn better approaches, new skills, ways to grow?

Note: Turn questions to statements when you analyze your self-talk. For example, asking "Why can't I get over this?" keeps us aroused and provides no resolution. Changed to the statement, "I can't get over this," the fortune-telling error becomes obvious. We can then change this to "I'll probably learn how to come to terms with this."

"Why" questions are intellectual. The intellectual response is straightforward, "I am suffering because I haven't learned how not to yet." However, the real issue is the emotional frustration. It is better to state directly, "I am feeling so frustrated with this pain." Then take steps to soothe yourself as you learn additional skills.

THE DAILY THOUGHT RECORD

Now that you know about distortions, the next step is to use them to help you. When stressed or anxious, thoughts and feelings can swirl in our minds and seem overwhelming. Putting them down on paper helps us to sort it all out and see things more clearly. The daily thought record (please see page 166 and the examples) takes about fifteen minutes each day. It is good to do it right after you notice yourself feeling upset. Or it can be done before you go to bed. Here's how it works:

STEP 1: (THE FACTS)

At the top briefly describe an upsetting event from the past, present, or future and the resulting feelings (such as sad, anxious, guilty, or frustrated). Rate the intensity of these feelings (10 means extremely unpleasant). Remember, getting in touch with disturbing feelings is a way to stop them from controlling us.

STEP 2: (ANALYSIS OF YOUR THOUGHTS)

- In the first column of the Analysis Section, list your Automatic Thoughts (ATs). Then rate how much you believe each. 10 means it's completely believable.
- In the second column, identify the distortions (some ATs might be reasonable).
- In the third column, try to respond, or talk back, to each distorted AT. Realize that your first AT is only one of several possible choices. Try to imagine what you would say to a friend who said what you did, or try to imagine yourself on a good day saying something more reasonable. Ask yourself, "What is the evidence for the reasonable response?" Then rate how much you believe each response.

STEP 3: (RESULTS)

After all this, go back to the Initial Responses column and rate your ATs again. Then at the top rate the intensity of your emotions again. Even a slight drop in your upset feelings is significant. With this process, upsetting events will still probably be upsetting, though not as disturbing.

Remember, work out your thoughts on paper. It is too complex to do it in your head. Be patient with yourself as you learn how to do this. It usually takes a few weeks to become good at this skill.

So each day for two weeks, select an upsetting event and do a daily thought record. You might consider working on symptoms, triggers, feared situations, or past events. Then proceed to the next section entitled "Getting to the Most Distressing Ideas."

DAILY THOUGHT RECORD   DATE: _____

THE FACTS

Event	Impact of Event	Intensity
(Describe the event that "made you" feel bad/ unpleasant.)	(Describe the emotions you felt.)	(Rate the intensity of these emotions from 1 to 10.)

ANALYSIS OF YOUR THOUGHTS

Initial Responses		Thought Fallacies	Reasonable Responses	
(Describe the automatic thoughts or self-talk. Then rate how believable each is from 1 to 10.)		(Find and label the distortions.)	(Talk back! Change the distortions to more reasonable thoughts. Rate how much you believe each from 1 to 10.)	
	Ratings			Ratings

RESULTS

Based upon your thought analysis, rate again how much you believe your initial responses. Then rate the intensity of your emotions again.

Here's an example of a simplified daily thought record. Mark asked his sixten-year-old son as he was leaving if he had mowed the grass yet. The son responded, "Sometimes I feel like a slave around here—I'll do it tomorrow," as he slammed the door. Mark smashed the banister. When asked why, he could not really explain his reaction. His therapist helped him to slow down the action and put his thoughts on paper. By way of background, Mark grew up in a family with a violent alcoholic father. The father was sometimes kind when he was sober. Once he stood up to his father in an attempt to protect his mother. He was brutally beaten. A teacher noticed Mark's bruises and reported the situation. Eventually, the children were placed in a foster home. Mark later joined the Army and tried conscientiously to raise a good family. Here is what the daily thought record looked like.

DATE: June 10

Event	Impact of Event	Intensity
My son was disrespectful as he left the house.	Angry Powerless	9 ➤ 6 8 ➤ 5

ANALYSIS

ATs	Distortions	Reasonable Responses
He shouldn't be rude. 7 ➤ 5	Should	It would be good if he were more civil, but we're both still learning. It's not the end of the world. We'll probably figure out a way to reach an agreement. 9
He should know better than to leave before doing his chores. 9 ➤ 6	Should	It is silly to expect him to always follow my example. His response makes sense to him. Most teenagers prefer being with their friends to doing chores. If he really thought that doing chores makes one wildly happy and successful, he'd do his chores willingly. 8
This disobedience is awful. 9 ➤ 4	Catastrophizing	This is inconvenient, but pretty normal for teenagers. This is not combat. Lives won't be lost. There's time to calmly figure out a solution. 6
He'll get fired from his job. 8 ➤ 6	Fortune Telling	Maybe he won't. 8
People will think I'm a poor dad. 10 ➤ 5	Mind Reading	Maybe I won't be named Father of the Year. But maybe people will just consider him an average teenager. 7

Here's another blank daily thought record to practice on, or to copy.

DAILY THOUGHT RECORD   DATE: _____

THE FACTS

Event	Impact of Event	Intensity
(Describe the event that "made you" feel bad/ unpleasant.)	(Describe the emotions you felt.)	(Rate the intensity of these emotions from 1 to 10.)

ANALYSIS OF YOUR THOUGHTS

Initial Responses		Thought Fallacies	Reasonable Responses	
(Describe the automatic thoughts or self-talk. Then rate how believable each is from 1 to 10.)		(Find and label the distortions.)	(Talk back! Change the distortions to more reasonable thoughts. Rate how much you believe each from 1 to 10.)	
	Ratings			Ratings

RESULTS

Based upon your thought analysis, rate again how much you believe your initial responses. Then rate the intensity of your emotions again.

GETTING TO THE MOST DISTRESSING IDEAS:
THE QUESTION-AND-ANSWER TECHNIQUE[128]

So far you have learned to use the daily thought record to identify and replace distorted ATs. While replacing distorted ATs can reduce distressing symptoms, uprooting *core beliefs* provides an even greater benefit. Core beliefs are deeply held beliefs that lead to many present distortions. Because they are usually learned early in life, they are rarely challenged. We discover core beliefs by starting with an AT and using the question-and-answer technique. In this approach, you take an AT and keep asking the following questions until you reach the core belief:

Assuming that's true: What does that mean to me?
                          Why is that so bad?

For example, on the daily thought record Mark expressed feelings of anger and loss of control because of his son's disrespect. He decided to apply the question-and-answer technique to the AT: "He shouldn't be rude." It went like this:

He shouldn't be rude.

Question: What does that mean to me?
Answer: He'll get fired!

Question: And what else?
Answer: He'll repeat my mistakes and be like me.

Question: What does that mean?
Answer: If I hadn't provoked my father my family would still be together.

Question: Assuming that's true, why is that so bad? What does that mean?
Answer: I did something pretty shameful.

Question: And what does that mean?
Answer: I was a bad son.

Question: And what does that mean about yourself?
Answer: I'm a bad person.
           (= CORE BELIEF!)

In reaching this core belief, we did not pause to challenge the ideas. Now let's go back and look for distortions along the way, responding reasonably at each step. The following shows what the whole process looks like, using the three columns of the daily thought record. The "Q" represents questions, which need not be written down.

INITIAL RESPONSES (ATs)	DISTORTION	REASONABLE RESPONSE
He'll get fired.	Fortune Telling	Most of the time he's quite responsible.
Q		
He'll repeat my mistakes and be just like me.	Fortune Telling Catastrophizing	Maybe he won't. If he does, that will be too bad, not a catastrophe
Q		
If I hadn't provoked my father, my family would still be together.	Fortune Telling Personalizing	I don't know that. My dad had a history that went well beyond one incident.
Q		
I feel so ashamed for what I did.	Making Feelings Fact	What I did was to try to protect my mother. This is not a shameful act.
Q		
I was a bad son.	Label	I was trying my best.
Q		
I'm a bad person. (Core Belief)	Label	I am a fallible person.

SOME COMMON CORE BELIEFS

Here are a number of core beliefs common to PTSD, and their more reasonable alternatives. As a drill, cover up the alternatives and see how you would talk back to each. There are no perfect or "right" answers. What matters is that the response works for you.

CORE BELIEF	POSSIBLE ALTERNATIVES
I am weak.	I am a combination of weaknesses and strengths. I am strengthening the weaker areas.
My weaknesses/flaws will be exposed— how horrible!	Everyone is fallible; each person has flaws. To have them exposed makes me human. That's not awful, just life. Actually, some flaws are endearing.
My worth equals my behavior during a traumatic event.	My worth as a unique individual is far too complex to reduce to isolated performances. Mistakes reflect our skill level or development at the time. A mistake does not totally and irrevocably define a person.
I am no good since the trauma.	My life does not equal my trauma.
If I am not respected by others, I have no value; I cease to exist.	Nobody's opinion determines my worth.
To lose control is awful.	Loss of control is inevitable. Many things in life are beyond my control. Sometimes all I can control is the way I look at the loss of control. Paradoxically, to accept loss of control helps me control my stress. I *can* endure loss of control.
I shouldn't need to work at recovery. I shouldn't need help. I should be able to cope like normal people.	I really should be just as I am, given my present skill level and sensitized nerves. No one is entirely self-sufficient. It's okay to seek skilled help.
If I don't worry it will more than likely happen.	Since most bad things don't happen, I'm just reinforcing this belief. Instead of worrying, I'll make a good plan, take reasonable precautions, and remain cautious but relaxed.
If I obtain perfection nothing fearful will happen.	Perfection is not possible. Trying to be so will just keep me frustrated and aroused. I can commit to doing a very good, steady job.
Bad things won't happen if I am good enough and careful enough.	Rain falls on the good, the bad, and the in-between. Some things happen randomly and are not indicative of divine disfavor. The best we can do is to be prepared.

CORE BELIEF *continued*	POSSIBLE ALTERNATIVES *continued*
I must always prepare for the worst.	Certain precautionary measures might lessen the likelihood of some negative outcomes. Constant worry doesn't. I'd rather take reasonable, intelligent, thorough precautions, and then release the worries.
I can only function if I have a strong individual to depend on. I must lean on a strong individual because I am so helpless.	Nonsense. While everyone needs to rely on others at times, I can learn to be become self-sufficient, or at least, as self-sufficient as most others.
I should judge and punish myself for my shortcomings and failings.	I can greet myself cordially and with encouragement—this is a better way to grow and develop. I'll leave the judgment to others.
My past failures mean I'm incapable and out of control.	Mistakes mean I am human and fallible—just like everyone else. I have every right to try again, to grow from the level where I am.

For a week, use the question-and-answer technique once a day to find your core beliefs. Use previously completed daily thought records or a newly completed thought record.

CHAPTER 21

Confiding Concealed Wounds[*]

Give sorrow words: The grief that does not speak
whispers the o'erfraught heart, and bids it break.
—*Shakespeare in* Macbeth[129]

Traumatic wounds are complex. For some, the damage is quite obvious. Sometimes it is not apparent on the surface. Sometimes we anticipate the trauma's recurrence, or worry about the consequences of the event. Sometimes it is just the memory that keeps us aroused after the actual threat has passed. All these aspects need to be processed so that traumatic material can be filed away like other memories.

Those who bounce back quickly, "rolling with the punches," seem to figure out a way to process the experience, bringing it to closure so that it no longer matters. Many, however, remain troubled by past events. Concern for this latter group led a psychologist at the University of Texas at Austin, Dr. James W. Pennebaker, toward an extraordinary line of research.

Pennebaker initially asked students to write their deepest thoughts *and feelings* about events from the past that they would not even share with their close friends. They wrote fifteen minutes a day for four days while a control group of students wrote about neutral subjects such as what their living rooms looked like where they grew up. The results were surprising.

---

*This chapter summarizes the work of Pennebaker, Dr. James W. 1997. *Opening Up: The Healing Power of Expressing Emotion*. New York: Guildford Press. Copyright © 1997 James W. Pennebaker. Instructions for confiding in writing, cautions, and summary of supporting research are adapted with permission.

First, Pennebaker was surprised about the range of traumas that had been experienced by a seemingly normal group of college students. These are some of the traumas that they related:

- A ten-year-old girl failed to clean up her room when asked in preparation for her grandmother's visit. The grandmother slipped on a toy, broke her hip, and died.
- A boy taught his sister how to sail. The sister drowned on her first solo outing.
- A father announced to a nine-year-old that he was leaving his mother, and that the problems in the marriage were caused by the birth of the children.
- A drunken father beats the mother, then the child.
- Rape, molestation, and sexual abuse by relatives were not uncommon. Suicide attempts were also reported.

Among those who confided their feelings in writing, as expected, there was a short slip in mood during the days of the study. Some cried as they wrote or dreamed about the past events. However, after the study those who confided were significantly happier and *less* anxious than the controls. They often reported that they understood their experience better after writing; it no longer hurt to think about it. The writers also showed stronger immune system functioning immediately after the experiments and became ill less often over the ensuing months than the controls. The greatest improvements were observed in those who had wanted to confide, but never had.

Surveying working adults, it was found that traumas from childhood are least likely to be confided. Those who had experienced childhood traumas were more likely to be ill as adults, especially if they had not confided the experiences. Among survivors of the death of a spouse, those who had talked about the death felt better afterward and ruminated less than those who had not. The more they spoke, the better they felt.

Pennebaker repeated his research with subjects among various populations. He found, for example, that persons fired from their jobs were more likely to be rehired if they wrote about their feelings surrounding their job loss. Apparently, expressing the feelings of frustration, humiliation, and shame helped people to rebound quicker compared to those who just "pressed on." Similar findings were observed among Holocaust survivors: low disclosers were found to be the least healthy.

Pennebaker concluded that confiding is healthy. It can help people to confront, understand, and organize traumas.[130] If you have lost a loved one, broken up, moved, or had some past trauma, find a quiet place and write continually for four to five days about the trauma. Confronting often quells the devastating effects of trauma. If not, seek professional help. A therapist can help you pace and maintain safety as you process trauma-related memories.

TRAUMA AND AVOIDANCE

It appears that suppressing powerful emotions requires such effort that it takes a devastating toll on health. Following a trauma, such as sexual trauma or the suicide of a spouse, people might find ways to avoid the topic by:

- Staying occupied with trivial distractions such as work, cleaning, or exercise.
- Avoiding people who might broach the subject.
- Being with people but saying, "I'm not upset by that." Or, "I was upset, but I'm not anymore."
- Not crying as a way to block out the pain.
- Ruminating, worrying, or mentally rehearsing the event. This is done, however, without feelings or tears. Thus, it is a way to avoid the emotional pain of the trauma.

Pennebaker identified what he called low disclosers, people who inhibited their emotions. These people wrote about superficial topics, or were less emotional and self-reflective, showing less emotional awareness. Some in this group were rigid, chronic, high-level worriers. These people used the *mental* process of worry as a way to avoid contact with their *feelings*. Consistent with other research on repression, the low disclosers were the least healthy.

We might ask why, then, one would choose to inhibit emotions? There are several possibilities.

1. *Concern with image.* One may believe that he'll be perceived as weak or incapable if he is troubled by events (e.g., a policeman or soldier after witnessing a shooting death). Or, he might be ashamed or embarrassed by the trauma (e.g., a transgression or abuse).

2. *One might be too involved with coping with present demands to allow feelings to arise.* This may become a habit.

3. *One might have been punished or discouraged from expressing feelings in the past.*

4. *One might have learned that feelings are futile.* For example, a child finds that feelings are ignored by her distant, distracted parents.

5. *Society might not encourage grief related to certain traumas.* Many modern cultures do not acknowledge grief for miscarriage or provide a way to mourn. People may be reluctant to talk to those whose family member has committed suicide or been imprisoned.

6. *One might fear being overwhelmed by feelings.* Paradoxically, allowing one-self to be "overwhelmed" by feelings, and realizing that the world doesn't end, is usually an extraordinarily effective way to liberate oneself from this fear.

7. *One might simply have never learned to express feelings.*

Pennebaker observed that intrusive thoughts commonly surface after a trauma or when reminded of traumas. The more people dwelled on them or tried to suppress them, the larger and more threatening they became. The intrusive thoughts included thoughts about sex or sexual trauma, aggression (e.g., hurting a baby), illness, death, failure, relationship problems, dirt and contamination, and food.

RESILIENT COPING

Those who cope well with trauma seem to have at least two factors in common:

1. An outlet for their feelings.

2. A way of viewing the trauma in a way that brings it to closure, so that they can view the event and think, "It no longer matters." Notice the striking parallel here with Dr. Weekes's counsel to face and accept anxious symptoms until they no longer matter.

Psychologist Mardi Horowitz has described three stages for the resolution of grief for trauma: (1) denial; (2) working through; and (3) completion. Typically, people good at coping with trauma feel they can communicate about the trauma in some form. They can confide to a spouse, friend, or diary. Some use prayer or religious confession. This overcomes denial and facilitates completion of the second and third stages described by Horowitz.

Disclosing with emotional awareness and expression leads to the many benefits already mentioned. Pennebaker cites several theoretical reasons why communicating feelings, especially in writing, is so useful.

1. *Language unifies and completes our conscious experience.* Lewin and Zeigarnik[131] explained that we remember interrupted tasks until they are completed. Once resolved, we cease thinking about them. That is, understanding, seeing clearly, sorting out and/or organizing our thoughts settles issues. It appears that different aspects of a memory are stored in different parts of the brain. Language appears to unify the diverse elements of experience. Writing increases our focus and understanding. As teachers often discover, they know that they understand something once they can teach it. Putting a complex issue into words helps us organize it, understand it, and then remember it with less stress. For example, once we organize complex material the mind remembers it with less work. It relaxes and stops rehearsing the material. This is the principle behind a "To Do" list. Once we have done the work of sorting out what needs to be done and put it on paper in a clear, meaningful way, the mind relaxes without swirling confusion. So writing helps bring order, detachment, and meaning.

2. *Because writing is slower than talking, it promotes more detailed thought.*

A pattern emerges. The goal is flexible engagement. That is, we willingly face the pain as needful. We face the worst and see it clearly, without fear. Sometimes we see a way to improve upon the worst. Sometimes we see a new way to interpret the event. Sometimes we simply accept life with more peace and understanding.[132] We look until it no longer matters. *Then* we distract and focus on other aspects of life.

SHOULD I TRY CONFIDING IN WRITING?

If you are still anxious or depressed by a past event, writing could help. If you still think about it or spend significant energy trying to avoid thinking about it, you will likely find this strategy helpful. It may be difficult and stressful at first until you get used to disclosing. Once the gates finally open, it usually becomes easier. The instructions for this strategy follow.

Instructions

1. *Find a place where you won't be interrupted for fifteen to thirty minutes.* A neutral place (a table placed in the corner of the room) works well.

2. *Write continuously for fifteen to thirty minutes on four or five consecutive days.* Pennebaker's original instructions are:

   I want you to write continuously about the most upsetting or traumatic experience of your entire life. Don't worry about grammar, spelling, or sentence structure. In your writing, I want you to discuss your deepest thoughts *and feelings* (italics added) about the experience. You can write about anything you want. But whatever you choose, it should be something that has affected you very deeply. Ideally, it should be about something you have not talked about with others in detail. It is critical, however, that you let yourself go and touch those deepest emotions and thoughts that you have. In other words, write about what happened and how you felt about it, and how you feel about it now.[133] Finally, you can write on different traumas during each session or the same one over the entire (period). Your choice of trauma for each session is entirely up to you.

3. *It isn't necessary to write about the most traumatic event of your life.* Remember to pace your healing. If a topic makes you overly distraught, ease up. Approach it gradually or try a different topic.

4. *Especially write about topics that you dwell on and/or you would like to talk about but are embarrassed.* Write mostly about your feelings. Avoid wishful thinking (e.g., I wish he weren't dead; I'd like to get even), which is a way to avoid the underlying feelings. Instead, focus on your feelings and what they mean.

5. *Write continuously for fifteen to thirty minutes.* If you run out of words, repeat yourself.

6. *Write just for yourself.* If you worry about someone reading it you may not write what you honestly feel.

7. *Expect sadness immediately afterward.* This usually dissipates within an hour or, rarely, within a day or two. Most people then feel relief/contentment for up to six months afterward.

8. *Balance writing with action.* Don't let writing be a method of avoidance.

9. *Use any comfortable medium.* Talking into a recorder, writing, and speaking to a therapist are similarly effective.[134] (Talking to a therapist was found to elevate the mood somewhat quicker over the four-day period, and is recommended for difficult problems. Other media can be used for home assignments.) Art can be a useful medium if verbal expression is used to interpret the art and the feelings it conveys.

10. *You can try this before bed if insomnia is associated with intrusive memories at bedtime.* This is a useful way to accept the worries, rather than fight them, and then clean out the mind. (Some with severe PTSD must stop writing several hours before bed or they'll feel worse. You might also find it useful to set a timer to help pace yourself. Monitor your feelings and stop writing if you become too uncomfortable.)

Cautions

1. This is not a substitute for therapy for intractable problems.

2. This is not a substitute for remedial action. For example, you'll probably still need to tell others if they hurt your feelings and you want them to stop. Don't merely complain, which is a way to keep things the same and avoid action.

3. Confiding to friends might change the relationship if:
   • they are threatened by the content
   • they become burned out themselves by listening
   • the listener feels a need to confide what you have told them to unburden
   • your motive is to hurt the listener
   If any of these is a concern try writing or talking to a counselor.

4. Look ahead after discharging and analyzing your traumas. Don't stay in a wallowing stage.

Pennebaker explains that grief and infatuation follow similar courses. The first four to six months typically involve intense feelings, followed by a six- to eighteen-month plateau that is less emotionally charged. After eighteen months what endures is friendship and fond memories. (With traumas this may mean remembering the good along with the bad as well as other good memories not related to the trauma.) We begin new experiences and get on with life. One might consider counseling, then, for grief without trauma, if getting on with life is difficult after about eighteen months.

ISN'T IT BETTER TO LEAVE THE PAST ALONE?

Perhaps. If the past no longer troubles you and feels completed, then revisiting the past might not help. However, if the past is truly settled, revisiting it does not usually hurt, and may often lead to even greater insights and resolution.[135] Most people feel that confronting traumatic material is the hardest but most helpful part of treatment. As a rule, if you can express and reframe it, you'll replay it less.

If you feel that your life is now extremely chaotic, you might wish to regain some control first. (See chapter 7.)

ASSISTANCE

1. Some people find it difficult to express feelings because they have not learned words for feelings. What people typically find is that as they express negative feelings, they become more comfortable with their emotions in general. It then becomes easier to experience and express positive feelings as well. If you feel the need for help in identifying feelings, you might again refer to the list of emotions on page 90.

   When writing you might use direct statements, such as "I feel sad about . . . "; "I'm so frightened"; "I'm feeling so . . . "; "I was so scared that . . . "

   You might also use metaphors such as, "I feel like the weight of the world is on my shoulders"; "I felt like the roof is caving in on me and that makes me feel . . . "; "I felt like a used shoe"; "I felt torn up inside"; "I feel like my life is out of control, like a runaway train."

2. Bruno Bettelheim wrote: "What cannot be talked about can also not be put to rest; and if it is not, the wounds continue to fester from generation to generation."[136] Thus, we might view confiding as an opportunity to stop transgenerational wounding.

3. James likens unresolved trauma material to carrying around a bag of smelly garbage throughout life. Instead of carrying it around, she suggests briefly identifying traumatic events on separate pieces of paper and placing these papers in a plastic trash bag, which is left at the therapist's office. At each

session, a piece of paper is taken out for processing. In this way, trauma material is contained and processed in small, manageable steps.[137]

4. Matsakis[138] advises recording as many details as possible before, during, and after the event, including what others were thinking, or what you thought they were thinking, regarding your experience. To make material less threatening, she advises imagining that you are watching the event through a one-way mirror or imagining that the trauma is happening to someone else, not you. Prompts, such as photos of yourself before, during, or after might help recall, as might a visit to the scene of the event (if that is not too upsetting).

5. Memory work with your therapist should not be done until you have developed a trusted therapeutic alliance. Your therapist will be like a traveling companion as you view old sights, someone who will help you surround the memories this time with respect and calmness. Use enough emotion to evoke the memories,[139] but not so much that you overwhelm feelings of mastery and control.

FINAL THOUGHTS

Cermak and Brown have observed that "No pain is so devastating as the pain a person refuses to face and no suffering is so lasting as suffering left unacknowledged."[140] In support, van der Kolk and Saporta have stated, "numerous studies for the past one hundred years have established a causal relation between the inhibition of expression of traumatic experience and psychophysiological impairment. These studies have demonstrated a marked increase in symptoms of the respiratory, digestive, cardiovascular, and endocrine systems in people with PTSD."[141] It appears, then, that confiding past wounds is an important skill to cultivate. Remember, however, not to rush. Slower is faster.

CHAPTER 22

Resolving Guilt

**It is a human prerogative to become guilty and it is
a human responsibility to overcome guilt.**

—V. Frankl, concentration camp survivor

Your progress in treatment will be blocked by unresolved guilt. So it is fitting that
we turn our attention now to its resolution.

Guilt is an unpleasant feeling. As with other feelings, it arises from our
thoughts. In guilt we feel responsible for what happened. Our conclusion is that
our role in the event resulted in the negative outcome. Guilt is not, as some assert, a useless emotion. Guilt affirms morality. We would be concerned, for example, about a drunk driver who felt no remorse for injuring someone. We
would hesitate to form a relationship or enter into business with someone who
had no conscience. Guilt is a motivator for change. If we hurt someone we care
about, guilt helps us to improve our behavior. Guilt is an ally when it leads directly to a satisfactory resolution. We see clearly what did happen so that we can
make needed adjustments, make those adjustments, and then put the guilt to
rest. Unresolved guilt, however, keeps memories emotionally charged and in active memory.

To integrate memories, we must recall the memory fragments in sufficient detail to put them back together again, and then emotionally defuse the whole
memory so that it can be stored in long-term memory. To begin this process, let's
begin by considering how we might be experiencing guilt.

WHAT DO WE FEEL GUILTY ABOUT?

- What we do, think, or feel. Examples are:
  - drinking too much
  - feeling afraid
  - going along with the demands of the perpetrator (rapist, terrorist, batterer, abusive parent, robber)
  - feeling relief for surviving when others did not
  - causing the offender to commit the crime (e.g., by making oneself attractive, wanting attention)
  - saving myself but not others; abandoning others
  - killing (as in combat), which violates cherished values
  - resistance fighting that leads to the enemy's retaliatory killing of civilians
  - errors in judgment (e.g., permitting a teenager to travel with an irresponsible driver)
  - identifying with the victimizer (seeing good points, trying to win favor or privileges, becoming a participant in the offense)
  - wanting to die and be released from pain
  - living a life that we think is so imperfect as to warrant traumatic events
  - feeling ambivalent about those who died
  - carelessness; thoughtlessness
  - an innocent mistake or accident
  - hating the perpetrator; wanting to harm him
  - enjoying aspects of sexual abuse
  - acting unkindly to someone who was later injured or killed
  - trusting someone's judgment or decisions, which later resulted in harm to people
- What we fail to do, think, or feel. Examples include:
  - failing to save or protect others (parent doesn't stop kidnapping, firefighter does not save burn victims)
  - failing to take suitable precautions

- freezing and doing nothing; didn't fight harder
- failing to leave a relationship with a batterer who severely injures a child
- failing to stop chronic abuse
- wishing that you could have done more
- failing to live up to my ideal or normal expectations
- failing to control symptoms or recover
- failing to say "I love you" or tell the deceased how much you valued them
- not having a proper way to say good-bye to someone who has died
- not pressing charges or reporting a crime to the police
- not feeling sympathetic to others' suffering

- Unreasonable accusations that we internalize ("I feel guilty, so I must be.")
  - police don't believe your story and imply you are making it up or asked for it
  - the lawyer defending the perpetrator attacks your character
  - people think that the crime against you was your fault

STAGES OF RESOLUTION

The successful resolution of guilt follows a course similar to other intense feelings common to PTSD:

1. *Denial.* Because guilt is so uncomfortable, we may deny responsibility at first. We may be shocked and numb.

2. *Processing.* In time we accurately assess the harm done and legitimately assess our responsibility. We learn our lessons and neutralize emotions by clarifying faulty thinking.

3. *Resolution.* Here we express appropriate sorrow for the hurt we have caused, and make amends as appropriate. Guilt and self-punishment are released. The focus transitions to constructive change and growth. We again look ahead, concentrating on elevating humanity—self and others.

Integration is blocked if we get stuck prior to the completion of any stage. We can't process what is not adequately retrieved from memory. If we avoid thinking about the event, then memory fragments will intrude, but not sufficiently for processing. Thus, unresolved guilt continues to be replayed like a broken record. In attempts to kill the pain, we numb our conscience and sensitivity to the pain of others while becoming unable to emotionally connect with them.

Many inaccuracies can enter our memories during the stress of a traumatic event. During the event, it is typical to develop tunnel vision: being so narrowly focused on survival that we do not see the whole picture. We may assume an exaggerated sense of responsibility and underappreciate mitigating circumstances. These views are never effectively challenged as one tries to "just forget the past and move on."

Without complete processing, many other unkind ideas remain unchallenged. Shame often rides in on guilt's coattails. Shame goes one step further than guilt, saying, "Not only did I *do* something bad, but I *am* bad to the core." Shame is frequently a pattern learned in childhood. Perhaps the survivor felt worthless when she was abandoned, or was constantly given messages of badness. The child does not think to question these messages, and so remains vulnerable when a traumatic event later occurs. A variety of other unkind ideas can be learned and connected to the trauma. Again, if they remain unchallenged they retain their ability to disturb the survivor. Notice that the list below is a sampling of distortions and core beliefs that are often associated with guilt.

- I am either all responsible or not at all. I cannot be partly at fault.

- I don't deserve to live or to live happily because of my behavior.

- I should have done better.

- The more I punish myself the more I show I care.

- The more I suffer and punish myself, the more I will ease another's suffering.

- The more I suffer the less likely I will be to repeat the mistake.

- If I give up guilt I will be disloyal to my values, God, or those who have suffered.

- If I suffer enough I will somehow restore fairness and justice.

- I should be able to fix all problems, right all wrongs, save all who are in trouble, vanquish all evil.

- I shouldn't have been afraid.

- I am somehow responsible—even totally responsible—for a crime committed against me.
- There is absolutely nothing I can do to improve upon the past.
- My character is flawed and unchangeable (everyone's character is flawed, but not unchangeable).

These ideas create further pain and increased attempts to wall off the memories. Instead of relief, more intrusions occur.

HOW IS GUILT RESOLVED?

PTSD authority Dr. Charles Figley[142] has presented five questions that need to be answered in a kind, sensitive, and healing way in order to come to terms with traumatic events. These apply particularly well to the processing of guilt. In order to begin the processing of the guilt aspects of your traumatic memory, please respond to the following questions. This is now just a fact gathering exercise. You might think of yourself as a reporter researching a story. I suggest writing the answers because writing tends to make the processing slower and more deliberate. However, you might prefer to speak your responses to your therapist.

1. *What happened?* (Describe the event. List all the facts. What did I do that was good and bad? What did I fail to do that was good and bad?)
2. *Why did the event happen?* (Why did it happen to me? Was it a random act of nature or of God? Was it something about me?)
3. *Why did I act the way I did during the event?*
4. *Why have I acted the way I have since that time?* (How and why have I changed as a result of the event for good and bad?)
5. *If something like this were to happen again, what would I do differently to cope and survive?* (What strengths and knowledge would lead to a more optimistic outcome?)

THE TECHNIQUE TO DETERMINE PERCENTAGES OF RESPONSIBILITY[143]

Dr. Raymond M. Scurfield developed this impressive technique to help Vietnam combat veterans accurately assess their responsibility. It is useful both for those who overestimate their responsibility, as well as for those who inappropriately disavow any responsibility. It has clear applicability to adult trauma other than war, and can be used in both individual counseling or group treatment settings.

The following case study will reveal how the technique is applied. This veteran is forty-three years old and served a tour in Vietnam primarily as a truck driver delivering and unloading supplies to various military units.

> I had finished unloading a truck full of supplies to this unit; I was really tired, and was just sitting in the cab, resting . . . I happened to glance over and saw a guy in the distance by a tree; I assumed he was on perimeter (guard) duty. I also saw a second guy who was a little ways apart from the first guy and was moving in his direction. I assumed they were both Americans. All of a sudden, I heard this loud sound, a rifle shot. One guy looked like he was laying down next to a tree; the other guy was running away. I found out that the second guy must have been a VC (Viet Cong), and he had killed the American . . . and I had just *sat* there in my truck and had *assumed* he was an American! My God, I could have checked closer, or I could have yelled out, or done *something*!

Application of the steps of assigning percentages of responsibility is as follows:

Step 1 facilitates a clear explication of the event and the survivor's perception and rationale for the degree of self-responsibility assumed. The veteran is helped to verbalize the *details* of the event, preferably in the first-person as if the event were occurring now. Hazy or unclear descriptions *must* be clarified or it must be determined that a remembrance actually *is* hazy or unclear. Then the veteran must verbalize exactly *how much* of the responsibility he has assumed, in this case for the death of the American who was shot by the VC.

Therapist: Let me clarify something right away; are you feeling *totally* responsible for this guy's death?

Veteran: Yes . . . well, almost totally.

Therapist: Let's give a percentage to it. If we can assume that there is a total of 100 percent responsibility for this guy's death, what percentage have you blamed yourself for? You don't have to be *exact*, just give an approximation.

Veteran: About 95 percent.

Therapist: Are you sure that your responsibility is about 95 percent? Is it maybe *more* than that, or *less* than that?

This therapeutic interaction is to stimulate new thinking by the veteran regarding the percentage of responsibility that he has assumed responsibility for. The veteran is then challenged to *convince* the clinician (group) how it was that he *deserves* to be 95 percent responsible. The clinician (group) does *not* rescue at this point in order to force the veteran to *fully acknowledge "publicly"* that which he has already decided and been persecuting himself about all these years. It is critical for the veteran to indicate *how* and *what* he has been remembering and saying to himself to remain convinced of his (exaggerated) sense of responsibility.

Step 2 challenges the survivor's exclusion or minimization of the role of others who were at the immediate scene of the trauma.

Veteran: I would give the other 5 percent of the responsibility for the death to the vet himself; I guess if he had been a little more careful maybe the VC wouldn't have gotten that close to him.

Therapist: Wait a minute. Let's look closer at this guy's responsibility. *Were you responsible for sentry duty that night?*

Veteran: No, actually I think the guy killed was one of the guys pulling sentry duty.

Therapist: And so, he is only *5 percent* responsible for allowing that VC to get that close to him that night, and he was on sentry duty, and somehow you are 95 *percent* responsible for his death? Does that make sense to you?

Veteran: Well, no, now that you put it that way, maybe he was 15 percent or 20 percent responsible.

Therapist: Really? Are you sure that is a fair percentage to assign to him? Should he get more or less than 15 to 20 percent? (Once the veteran arrives at what appears to be a more realistic percentage of responsibility that might be assigned to the most obvious other person who bears some responsibility, the veteran is further challenged to consider how responsible he is for that other person *even being there* that night.)

By the way, did you have any responsibility for that veteran being in Vietnam? (And: Being in that unit, being there that night, being on guard duty, that he obeyed somebody's order to stand guard, for him being in-country or for being in the Army . . . If the veteran claims that indeed he *did* have some influence over the other person's being in the actual situation that occurred, he then is challenged to convince the clinician group how that person himself had *absolutely no responsibility for being there*, and how the veteran had *totally "forced"* or caused the other person to be there.)

The above strategy is also systematically applied *to all other persons who were present* at the actual scene of the trauma:

- the other veterans who were on sentry duty that night
- whoever *assigned* that deceased American to be on sentry duty
- whoever was responsible for the selection of the site where the unit was located (would this event have occurred if the unit had been elsewhere?)
- any other Americans who were in the area, and do *any* of them have *any* responsibility for what happened that night?
- the Viet Cong who actually shot the American

Therapist: Let's talk for a moment about the "enemy." *Were the VC any good at what they did? You* tell *us* how good the VC were at infiltrating behind perimeter lines.

Veteran: Well, of course, they were good, they were *damned* good.

Therapist: And if the men in that unit all were doing their jobs to the best of their abilities that night, does that mean that the VC would never have been able to kill anyone? Let's get real: DOES NOT THAT VC DESERVE SOME OF THE RESPONSIBILITY FOR THE DEATH OF THAT AMERICAN?!

Veteran: Well, yes: maybe about 30 or 40 percent.

Therapist: Wait a moment; isn't that *too much* to give someone whom you hadn't given *any* responsibility to all these years? Make sure that you are now giving what *you* consider to be a fair and realistic percentage to the enemy, no more and no less.

Thus, the veteran *comes to his own conclusion* that, indeed, his perception and remembrance of the event and delegation of blame have been extremely constricted. It may now be timely to bring to the veteran's attention that *the percentages of responsibility that the veteran has assigned to various people, including his own—now total well over 100 percent!*

Therapist: By the way, you have now assigned well over 100 percent responsibility for the American who was killed. That is impossible; that total can only equal 100 percent. Do you think that you need to recalculate some or all of the percentages you have assigned? Is yours still 95 percent, which means that all of these other people split up the remaining 5 percent?

The veteran is not specifically directed to precisely recalculate the percentages at this time. (Usually the clinician or a volunteer from the group will write down what percentages have been assigned to whom by the veteran during the group session to give to the veteran after the session is over.)

Step 3 challenges the survivor's exclusion or minimization of the indirect responsibility of others who were not at the immediate scene of the trauma. To not expand the circle of responsibility beyond individuals actually at the trauma site promotes continuation of an exaggerated responsibility for individual acts or nonacts that occur in the war zone. This is "society victim-bashing" of our war veterans, that is, blaming our veterans for licensing them to be agents of death and maiming. We allow them to carry their own *and everybody else's share* of the consequences of our nation's war policy.

Thus, the veteran is now asked to consider *if senior military officials* in the war zone deserve any share of responsibility for the various traumas that occur. In other words, did the military strategies facilitate the most likely positive (military) outcome, was the minimization of loss of U.S. casualties a primary concern, and did their strategies and policies contribute to "unnecessary" loss of life and destruction among the veteran and/or civilian population in the war zone? Ultimately, does not the military command structure at its higher levels in the theater of operations deserve to receive a piece of the responsibility?

Next, the veteran considers *the war itself.* The therapist may ask, "Would any of you even have been in-country that night, if the U.S. were not fighting in Vietnam?" What percentage of responsibility for the Vietnam war should be assigned to our political leaders, and to all the civilians who sat around and watched the latest Vietnam casualty reports on television and then proceeded with their lives, irrespective of what was happening in Vietnam? (This author contends that *when a nation goes to war, every adult in that nation bears a piece of the responsibility for every single traumatic result that occurs.*)

Step 4 rechallenges the veteran's sense of his own percentage of responsibility for behaviors and consequences in the war zone.

Therapist: Now, let us return to *you* and what *you* did and did not do, and how much responsibility you had for being in the military, for being in the war zone, for being there that night, and for what you did and did not do that night. Because you *were* there that night, you *did* sit in that truck, you *did not* say anything, and an American *was* blown away. We are not here to try and help you to explain away *any* of whatever percentage of responsibility you truly believe and feel that *you* deserve for what happened that night—once you have fully considered *all* the others who deserve some responsibility, too. And so, considering all other factors, what piece of the responsibility for that American's death do you now believe is yours? (Once the veteran has been re-oriented on this issue, the clinician moves to the next step.)

Step 5 challenges the veteran to consider if he has been "punished" enough for his personal share of the responsibility for what happened.

Therapist: Now, tell us how much you have suffered and punished yourself all these years over the *95 percent* or so of the responsibility that you had blamed on yourself for this American's death. In other words, take into account *all* the times you have suffered pain from remembering and agonizing over what happened, criticizing yourself, feeling guilty, etc. How much?

Veteran: A lot; I mean a whole lot: Not a week goes by these twenty-three years that I haven't relived that event.

The clinician/group and veteran then discuss the degree of responsibility that the veteran has now assigned internally, and how this percentage compares with the self-punishment suffered (which has been based on a much higher assumption of responsibility). The veteran must make a clear statement to the clinician (all the group members), and decide if he has engaged in (self-punishment) "enough," "not enough," or "more than enough" in comparison to his *newly assigned* percentage of responsibility. (It is often helpful for the veteran to repeat this statement to *several* individual veterans in the group.)

The above procedures are also utilized to address responsibility issues of veterans who seem to significantly deny that they had any responsibility whatsoever for particular experiences that occurred.

Step 6 explicates a non-self-destructive plan to provide additional "payback" for one's share of the responsibility. If the veteran concludes that he still has not suffered enough for this, his conclusion can, of course, be confronted by both the clinician/group. However, if the veteran can live with this reframed, less rigid percentage of responsibility, the therapist and group may now facilitate the implementation of a non-self-destructive plan. This plan provides additional payback through its positive, life-sustaining, proactive stance, rather than through a self-destructive, reactive stance. The significant reframing process will require considerable readjusting of cognitions, feelings, and memories.

Step 7 is a homework assignment, which permits the veteran some time to reflect and reframe; to refine and recalculate the set of percentages of responsibility that add up to 100 percent and truly take into account the full circle of persons and circumstances involved; and to develop an initial longer-range plan to provide additional payback, if any, that the survivor feels and believes he still must provide. The veteran provides at least a brief account to the clinician/group of the results of this homework assignment to allow for group sanction or lack of sanction. Establishing specific steps to undertake the positive, life-promoting payback plan is important, as are follow-up activities to ensure that movement has occurred.

SUMMARY OF STEPS

Let's briefly summarize the steps in the percentage of responsibilities exercise.

1. Verbalize the details of the event in the first person.

2. Ask, "What percent are you responsible for? Are you sure? Is it possible that the percentage is *more* than that; or less?"

3. Convince the listener(s) that you deserve to be _____ percent responsible. Indicate how and what you've been remembering.

4. Challenge. Who else shared responsibility? What is their fair share of the percentage?
   - Was there a perpetrator who shares responsibility?
   - Who else was involved? Other individuals at the scene? People distant from the scene? Societal influences? Please convince the listener(s) how you forced them to be responsible?

5. Recalculate responsibility so that the total is 100 percent, and accurately focus on what you did and did not do.

6. Describe how much you have suffered for the responsibility you have assigned yourself.

7. Indicate if your suffering is enough, not enough, or more than enough in comparison to your actual percentage of responsibility.

8. Establish specific life-promoting steps to promote payback, if appropriate, and commit to productive living rather than being stuck in the punishment mode.

ADDITIONAL APPROACHES TO RESOLVING GUILT

Once appropriate responsibility has been assessed, the following steps continue the process of grief resolution:

1. *Feel your feelings but distinguish between concern and guilt.* You feel very deep sadness and compassion for someone who was injured and whose car was damaged in a car accident that you are in. Upon reflection, however, you realize that you were not responsible for the accident. So you realize that your feelings reflect appropriate concern, not immobilizing guilt.

2. *Attack any remaining distortions.* You might isolate distortions that still trouble you. Write each down on a separate sheet of paper and list the advantages and disadvantages of believing it. List the positive consequences of disbelieving it, and then list as many alternatives as you can.

3. *Accept your limits.* Say out loud, repeatedly, "I am imperfect. I was imperfect then; I am imperfect now. I accept my fair share of responsibility and commit to improve." Why do humans make mistakes? Because we are imperfect. It has always been this way.

4. *Surround the survivor and the experience with acceptance and understanding.* For a year, a teenager kept the fact that she was raped secret from her parents for fear they would reject her. After she could hold it in no longer, she told her father, who embraced her and said, "I wish you had told me sooner. This must have been so hard for you to bear alone." An emaciated soldier returned to the U.S. after a year in Vietnam. The customs agent looked kindly upon the young man and said, "Do you have any contraband?" The soldier replied that he had none. The agent then said, "Welcome home, son."[144] How much more healing is kindness than condemnation. Yet we see that victims are often more self-critical than self-supporting. It is easier to be kinder to ourselves when we clearly

understand what has happened and why we reacted the way we did. Let's consider how accurate reflection leads to understanding.

- A college student was raped by her boyfriend. Shocked, she went to see him the next night, when he raped her again. She felt guilty for letting it happen not once, but twice. With counseling she learned that her behavior was very understandable. In acquaintance rape, women are not prepared to use force to stop someone they trust. They are usually so stunned that they simply hope that their stronger offender will come to his senses and stop. Stunned, confused, hurt, the student returned hoping for an apology. She had so many confused feelings and was very vulnerable. Now, after recovery, she describes the event with justifiable anger for the crime it was, and has released the guilt. She says, "I was vulnerable then. I am stronger now."
- A woman stayed in a relationship with a batterer and thought, "I must be sick to tolerate this." A relationship with a batterer is very complex. It starts with a relationship between two people who deeply need each other. The insecure batterer begins to isolate his partner. He brainwashes her into thinking that she is helpless and dependent on him. Since he can easily hurt her, she starts to feel she owes her life to him, and becomes thankful for his protection, affection, and financial support. If she married young, she will likely feel insecure about her job skills. She will likely fear retaliation against herself and/or the children if she leaves. He may also have threatened suicide.[145,146] In a similar fashion, a child is totally dependent upon adults for basic needs. The child may learn to comply with an abuser for protection and to be seductive for acceptance.[147]

5. *Understand normal decision making under extreme stress.* By definition, a traumatic event is overwhelming. That is, it overwhelms our present abilities to cope. We are not prepared for it by virtue of insufficient experience, practice, training, knowledge, or resources. Decisions are made under duress. This means that extreme emotion exists which interferes with logical processing. There is too little time to figure out the best way to cope and examine the consequences of your options.

In traumatic events, there are usually no apparent "right" decisions, nor truly good solutions. All options place us in "double binds"[148] where you are "damned if you do and damned if you don't." Thus, a woman ordered into a car by an armed man is not completely sure if complying, scream-ing, trying to talk the offender out of the crime, attacking him, or trying to run is the best course of action. All approaches pose grave dangers. No matter what she does, each option risks safety, life, health, values and/or property. Thus, indecision is to be expected.

The stress response leads a person to fight, flee, or freeze, all of which are normal, instinctual ways to survive. Especially in extreme stress, flee-ing or freezing is to be expected. Do not feel guilty for that inborn desire. During traumatic stress, most people instinctively think of survival first, and not initially about protecting others. Caring for others typically returns later—sometimes later in the event, sometimes later in life. Perhaps if a similar crisis occurs you might learn better ways to respond to the needs of others; but go easy on yourself about your survival instinct.

As Simpson[149] observes, to expect one's best in times of crisis is often un-reasonable (e.g., think of a person being tortured). Hostile environments create fear and poor choices. Might this help to explain why athletic teams usually have better records at home? We don't perform at our best when overwhelmed, terrified, out of control, and unable to see the big picture. At the time of the trauma, you were in life training. You hadn't learned all of life's lessons. You hadn't learned yet to channel such strong emotions, and trauma creates a horrible learning environment. Lessons learned from trauma usually become apparent only later in life.

The following sequence of questions can greatly help to place your re-actions in perspective:

1. Were you thinking coolly at the time?
2. Were you aware of *all* your options?
3. What were your choices?
4. Were any of them good ones?
5. Had you ever been in that situation before?
6. Was there any way of knowing for certain what was the best option?
7. Were you clearly aware of all the outcomes of the options?
8. What would have been the outcome for each choice?
9. Were any of the choices *clearly* the right one? Best one? Were any choices without a cost? Were you aware of all of this at the time?
10. Were any of your options taken away?

11. Did you lack certain information that would have helped you make a wiser choice?

12. Did you have time to fully weigh your choices; to see all the angles?

13. Were there mitigating factors (fatigue, hunger, drugs, chaos and confusion, no support from family or friends, no one to ask for advice)?

14. Was the outcome what you intended? Did you deliberately try to harm someone? Was it an honest mistake?

15. What was a reasonable expectation given the situation?[150] Rather than asking, "Did I make the *right* decision," ask, "Did I make a *reasonable* one under the circumstances?"[151]

16. Did you accomplish your initial objectives? Will there be other opportunities to do better?

17. How could you have coped worse? (Are you maybe stronger than you thought?)

18. Did your imperfect actions avert a worse disaster? In what ways?

19. How might you have responded better to create more of a sense of mastery and control? Did you know how to do that then? Was it reasonable to expect that then? Can you imagine yourself doing that now? (Try imagining your ideal response.)

20. If this were your daughter, son, or best friend who reacted as you did, how would you feel? What would you tell them? Could you understand their actions? Would you forgive them? How would you comfort them?

6. *Separate guilt from shame.* Both feel unpleasant and are easily confused. Remember, guilt is feeling bad for what you *did* (or didn't do), while shame is feeling bad for who you *are*. Guilt focuses on behavior, which is readily changeable. Shame focuses on character, which is slower to change. With shame, character feels polluted by the behavior. We ask, what kind of person would act that way? The answer is, "A bad one." This unfruitful thought keeps you bound to the past, while modifying behavior allows you to move ahead to the future. If you were truly as bad as you think, you would not be suffering as you are now. So rate behavior, not your core worth. Think, "I don't like what I did and would hope to do better now. But I am worthwhile, even though I reacted imperfectly."[152]

If you were victimized, it is natural to feel shame, but not necessary. What *happened* to you was wrong, bad—*you* are not. Alternatively, you might think, "Something *is* fundamentally wrong with *all* people. It is called fallibility, a universal aspect of the human condition. Fallible does not equal bad or worthless, though. You might think, "I am not bad. I was afraid, having my problems, pressured, trying to get out of a crummy situation. Maybe I had a bad choice then, but I can choose a good life now."

7. *Gestalt chair technique.* The process involves an interchange between yourself and an imaginary understanding friend. You play both roles, one at a time, switching chairs as is appropriate. The technique allows feelings, thoughts, and sensations to be expressed and processed at an experiential level, rather than just at an intellectual level.

- Set up two chairs facing each other, one for you and one for an understanding friend.
- Sit in the friend's chair and assume the friend's role. Ask the victim in the other chair to describe the traumatic experience, including the victim's role, responsibility, and feelings.
- Change seats and respond to the questions, this time assuming the role of the victim. When you are finished, sit quietly and allow yourself to feel the feelings. Notice what your body is sensing. Then switch seats.
- As the understanding friend, try to feel what the victim is feeling. Offer support, encouragement, advice. Ask if anything else is needed.
- Switch seats and respond.

A variation is to let the intellectual self speak to the feeling self (that finds it hard to express emotions). In a similar exercise,[153] imagine that you are two distinct people. The first person is kind, forgiving, comforting—a friend who you can count on to listen to you with understanding and empathy. The second person is the part of you in pain—the part that feels hurt, guilty, or misunderstood. Inhale slowly and deeply. As you do so, imagine that the first person lovingly takes in the damaging, hurtful feelings of the second. Now exhale. As you do so, the second person, in response to the love and acceptance of the first, releases the pain, guilt, or frustration that has been causing pain. Inhaling, imagine the second person receiving strong feelings of love, joy, and acceptance from the first. As you exhale, the distinction between the two persons dissolves, leaving you whole, complete, and healed.

8. *Consider transition.* For the present, just *consider,* but do not act upon these yet:

   - What did I learn from this experience that could:
     - prevent the traumatic event from recurring or better prepare me should it happen again?
     - make me a better person?
     - lead me to make world a little better place?
   - Where could I go from here—what's the next step?

9. *Utilize spiritual resources,* if this is right for you. Most religions teach ways to heal from legitimate guilt and reconcile with deity. A sensitive clergy person or pastoral counselor might be of help. The peaceful Tibetan Buddhists teach this exercise for feeling forgiveness. It can be adapted to one's religious orientation.[154]

   - Visualize in the sky before you a figure who, for you, embodies truth, wisdom, forgiveness, and compassion—this can be God or perhaps a figure you revere.
   - Focus on the figure in front of you. Ask that figure to cleanse you of all your negative, destructive, harmful feelings and emotions. Ask to feel yourself forgiven.
   - Visualize the figure smiling on you and your request with warm and personal affection. From the figure, visualize a stream of light flowing out and into your heart, and from your heart into your entire body, bringing you a feeling of complete peace, forgiveness, and joy.
   - Visualize the light filling you until you feel yourself made up entirely of that light. You soar up into the sky and are united with the figure. Relax and enjoy the bliss of that oneness for as long as possible.[155]

CHAPTER 23

Thought Field Therapy*

Noted PTSD researcher Professor Charles R. Figley, Ph.D., Director of the Traumatology Institute, Florida State University, has systematically investigated four treatment approaches that appear to hold therapeutic promise: thought field therapy (TFT), traumatic incident reduction (TIR), visual kinesthetic dissociation,[156] and eye movement desensitization and reprocessing (EMDR). All four of these techniques share many aspects in common. Each attempts to recover traumatic material, hasten processing, and neutralize strong negative emotions. They can all be very effective when used as part of a comprehensive treatment plan, and they are particularly useful for those individuals who are significantly and regularly distressed by other treatment approaches. He notes:

> All four of the approaches we investigated generated impressive results. But TFT stood out from all other approaches of which I am aware because of (these) reasons:
>
> 1. It is extraordinarily powerful, in that clients receive nearly immediate relief from their suffering and the treatment appears to be permanent.
> 2. It can be taught to nearly anyone so that clients cannot only treat themselves, but treat others affected.
> 3. It appears to do no harm.
> 4. It does not require the client to talk about their troubles, something that often causes more emotional pain and discourages many from seeking treatment.
> 5. It is extremely efficient (fast and long-lasting).

---

*This chapter is adapted slightly with permission from correspondence from Dr. Charles R. Figley to colleagues in traumatic stress 27 June 1995. Also referenced is Callahan, R. J. and J. Callahan. 1997. Thought Field Therapy: Aiding the Bereavement Process in C. R. Figley, B. E. Bride, and N. Mazza, eds. *Death & Trauma: The Traumatology of Grieving*. Washington, D.C.: Taylor & Francis, 249–67. This excellent chapter provides rich background and additional algorithms for anger and guilt.

Although Dr. Figley cautions that much research is still needed, he presents the steps in order to permit individuals and therapists to try it as follows:

1. *Think about the problem.* Think of the causes of your anxiety (we all have them from time to time), including the traumatic experience, and work up as much discomfort as you can. However, do not spend more than a few moments on this phase.

2. *Rate discomfort.* At a point where you feel your anxiety is at its peak, choose a number between 1 and 10 that best represents the intensity of your discomfort, with 10 being the highest and 1 being the lowest. Thus, circle a number below:

    1 . . . 2 . . . 3 . . . 4 . . . 5 . . . 6 . . . 7 . . . 8 . . . 9 . . . 10

3. *Tap the beginning of the eyebrow.* After you have circled a number, using your two fingertips tap solidly five times while thinking about the anxiety (but not too hard to cause bruising or pain) just above the bridge of your nose, approximately where either eyebrow begins.

4. *Tap under the eye.* Then tap five times approximately one inch below the bottom of either eye (again, not too hard).

5. *Tap the body.* Next, tap five times on the side of your body, approximately four inches below the pit of the arm.

6. *Tap under the collarbone.* Then tap five times on your chest just below the collarbone, approximately one inch on either side of the center of your chest.

7. *Rate discomfort.* Now take a deep breath and measure your anxiety again: Choose a number between 1 and 10 that best represents the intensity of your anxiety right now. Thus, circle a number below:

    1 . . . 2 . . . 3 . . . 4 . . . 5 . . . 6 . . . 7 . . . 8 . . . 9 . . . 10

8. *Decide.* If the intensity of your anxiety is now at least two numbers lower than it was initially, go to Step 9. However, if it is not, follow this procedure:

    Tap the little-finger side of either hand (on the fleshy part midway between the wrist and base of the little finger, where you would do a karate chop), while saying the following: "I accept myself, even though I still have this kind of anxiety." Repeat this statement three times while thinking about the problem and continuing to tap. Then, repeat Steps 3 through 7.

9. *Tap back of hand.* Next is a sequence of nine activities that are done while tapping at a spot on the back of either hand. The spot is just below and between the knuckle of the little finger and the knuckle of the next finger. (Find this spot by making a fist. Place the index finger of the tapping hand in the gap between the knuckles of the little finger and the ring finger. Slide the index finger an inch back toward the wrist.) With the hand flat, tap this spot continually while doing the following activities (about five taps for each of the nine activities):

- eyes open
- eyes closed
- eyes open, look down and to the left (head still)
- eyes look down and to the right
- roll eyes in a circle
- roll eyes in a circle in the opposite direction
- hum a few bars of some tune with more than one note
- count to five
- hum some tune again

10. *Follow Steps 3 through 6.*

11. *Rate.* As you did before, take a deep breath and measure your anxiety again. Choose a number between 1 and 10 that best represents the intensity of your anxiety right now. Thus, circle a number below:

    1 . . . 2 . . . 3 . . . 4 . . . 5 . . . 6 . . . 7 . . . 8 . . . 9 . . . 10

12. *Repeat.* Follow the above procedure at least four times to give the procedure a fair test. If your anxiety rating has fallen at least two units, TFT might be a helpful skill for you to practice. You might also try it at a time when your anxiety is higher and the cause is very clear to you. You may come up with all kinds of explanations for why your anxiety level came down. Experiment with your explanations.

SOLIDIFYING THE GAINS

If your anxiety rating has fallen to a 2 or 1, do the following. Hold your head level. Begin tapping the same spot on the back of the hand that you tapped in Step 9. As you tap, look down at the floor, then steadily raise your eyes all the way up toward the ceiling, taking six to seven seconds to do so.

CHAPTER 24

The Rewind Technique[*]

The rewind technique[157] is another special integrative technique that has been reported to be very effective for specific traumas of finite duration in adults, usually within three to four treatment sessions.[158] According to its originator, Dr. David Muss, the Rewind Technique will allow people with PTSD to get rid of:[159]

> the various involuntary, unwanted, memories of the event, such as the nightmares, the flashbacks and the dreams. As a result of this you will no longer succumb to the emotional distress which these bring about. The technique does not cancel your voluntary recall of the event. You will always be able to remember the event if you choose to. However, when you choose to recall the event, you know you will be mostly in control of your emotions and not overpowered by them as you are now when the event is unexpectedly recalled by a chance remark from a friend or a sudden news flash on the TV or radio. You will no longer be imprisoned in the trauma trap—you will be released from it.

The instructions follow. It is recommended that you first try this in a safe setting, with your therapist, after you are stabilized and a therapeutic alliance has been formed.

THE REWIND TECHNIQUE

1. *Time*. Choose a time when you will be undisturbed.
2. *Place*. Find somewhere comfortable to sit for about fifteen minutes. You may feel more comfortable with your feet up and your hands unclasped.

---

*This chapter is adapted with permission from Muss, D. 1991. *The Trauma Trap*. London: Doubleday. Copyright © 1991, David Muss. Dr. Muss is director of the PTSD Unit, Birmingham Nuffield Hospital, Birmingham, U.K.

3. *Relaxation.* Close your eyes and start to relax each muscle group of your body from your feet all the way up to your head by first tensing and then relaxing. You will find that a feeling of calmness will come over you as you slowly and systematically relax all these muscle groups. Indulge in this pleasant feeling of calmness for awhile (you might also wish to use imagery of your safe place or a pleasant scene to increase pleasant, relaxed feelings). When you are feeling truly calm, continue.

4. *Background.* The rewind technique consists of watching a film of your traumatic event, in the exact way that it haunts you, first forward and then backward. However, it is not quite as simple as that and it is very important that you follow precisely all the steps described below. Some of the things I am going to ask you to do may seem a little odd, so let's pretend that I am introducing you to a new game. As with all new games, you need to understand the rules and the setting before you play. So before you start the treatment, learn the rules with me.

5. *Floating.* First, learn to float out of yourself. Another way of saying this is: learn how to *watch yourself.* Have you been on a boat or car journey and felt terribly sick? Or have you been on a roller-coaster and felt frightened? Stop and think about this for a moment. Have you remembered what it felt like? You probably didn't enjoy that memory, did you? This is because you didn't detach yourself.

   Try now to look at the same event in a detached way. Float out of the boat, leaving your body in it, and watch yourself from the shore. Do you feel as bad as you did when you saw yourself before? I hope the answer is no. This is because you are watching yourself and not reliving the event as it (actually) happened.

6. *The setting.* You will be watching two films in a cinema. Let's assume that you have a completely empty cinema hired just for you. Imagine that you are sitting in the center with the big screen in front and the projection room behind you. Now I would like you to float out of your body and go to the projection room to *watch yourself* watching the film from there. From the projection room you will be able to see the whole cinema, the empty chairs with just your head, and perhaps shoulders sitting in the center seat, and the screen in front of you, as in Figure 24.1. (Do not proceed until you can clearly see yourself in the projection room watching yourself watching the film.) Now let's consider the two films.

7. *The first film.* The first film is a replay of the traumatic event as you experienced it or as you remember it in your nightmares, dreams, or flashbacks. In this film you will see yourself on the screen—just as if someone had unexpectedly taken a video on the day and is now showing it to you.

Run the film forward at its normal pace and stop when your memory begins to fade (or to a time when you realized you would survive). You will find it very helpful if you can start the film a little before the point where your memory of the traumatic event begins. In other words, if you were involved in a car accident with a truck, begin the film by seeing yourself driving along happily, as in Figure 24.2. You will see the truck appear (see Figure 24.3), and finally the accident (see Figure 24.4). I call Figure 24.2 the "new starting-point." It is the peaceful point you return to when you rewind the film.

So, for the forward film: remember first where you are sitting and where you are watching the film from. Then begin from the "new starting-point." Next, see yourself on the screen. Finally, let the film run along until your memory fades.

8. *The rewind.* The second film is called the rewind. You do not exactly watch the rewind. You are actually in it, *experiencing* it *in* the screen, seeing everything as if it were happening to you now, and experiencing the sounds,

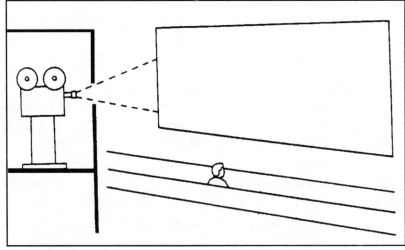

Figure 24.1

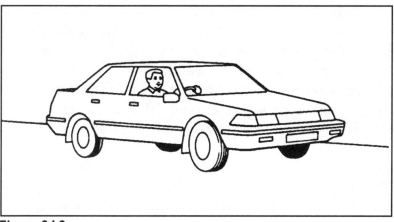

Figure 24.2

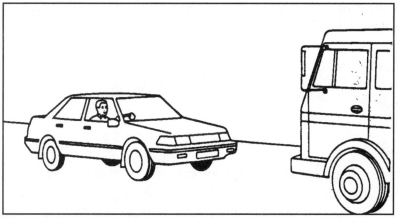

Figure 24.3

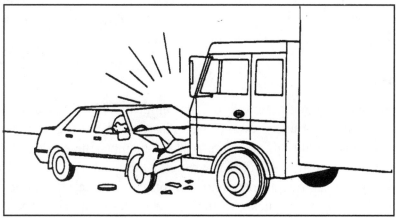

Figure 24.4

smells, feels, taste, and touch sensations. The really odd thing is that you see and feel everything happening *backward*. Thus, in the case of the car accident, first you are *in* the car after the impact (see Figure 24.5). Then you feel the car pulling away from the truck. You see the front of your car returning to its normal shape, as does the truck (see Figure 24.6). The vehicles pull farther and farther apart until the truck disappears and you finally end up with the "new starting-point," as in Figure 24.7 —you *see yourself* driving along in your car as you did at the beginning of the forward film.

Remember, in the rewind you are actually in the film, re-experiencing the event—which is now, however, all happening in reverse. The rewind must be done rapidly. You may find this difficult at first. If so, practice it slowly at the start. Once you've got it right, run it through straight after the forward film.

To give you an idea of the speed of the rewind, if the forward film takes one minute the rewind should take ten to fifteen seconds at most. You should end the rewind at your "new starting-point," which represents a good image.

SUMMARY

To sum up, with the forward film you are sitting in the center of the cinema, leaving your body there and floating in the projection room, from where you will watch the forward film. See yourself on the screen. Begin with your new starting-point. Run the first film until it fades. At this point get into the film. You are no longer watching the film, but re-experiencing the traumatic event in reverse. Rewind the event rapidly. End with your new starting-point.

CAUTION

I must warn you that going through the first film can be painful and may cause you to become pale, sweaty, or even tearful. Please don't be upset or put off. Remember that this should be the last time you remember the event in this way. After this treatment you will find that whenever the memory is sparked off the rewind will rapidly come into play, and will, on its way back, scramble the sequence, leading you very quickly to the new starting-point. The new starting-point is a good image and that is the memory you will be left with. This process

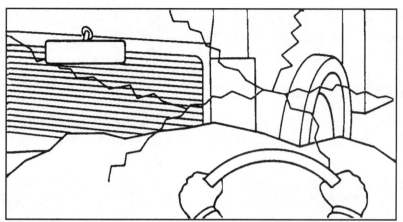

Figure 24.5

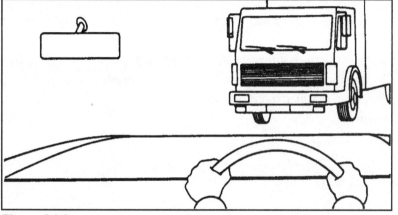

Figure 24.6

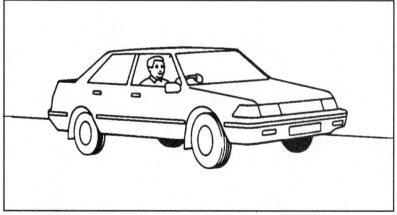

Figure 24.7

will happen faster and faster as every day goes by. As a result of this treatment, you will find that you are now able to resume all the activities which you haven't been able to do for a long time.

TROUBLESHOOTING

1. Some people find rewinding difficult and slow at first. Don't be discouraged; practice the rewind on its own until you get it right. Then go through the complete sequence without hesitating or stopping.

2. If you gloss over the really frightening or ugly part, and do not look at the film in its full detail, you will find that your PTSD symptoms will not disappear completely. You will therefore have to go back and deal with that particular section again.

3. You may be deeply shocked to find that, once you have got rid of a major haunting memory, another one appears. This shouldn't surprise you. Quite often we suppress several disturbing images and, once the major one has been removed, the next most disturbing one rises to take its place. If a deeper, concealed memory surfaces, just deal with it in the same way—rewind it.

CHAPTER 25

Traumatic Incident
Reduction (TIR)*

According to its originator, traumatic incident reduction (TIR) is a brief, one-on-one, nonhypnotic, person-centered, simple, and highly structured method for permanently eliminating the negative effects of past traumas. It involves repeated viewing of a traumatic memory under conditions designed to enhance safety and minimize distractions. The individual does all the work; the therapist or counselor offers no interpretations or evaluations but gives only appropriate instructions to the client to have him view a traumatic incident thoroughly from beginning to end. Hence, we use the term "viewer" to describe the client and "facilitator" to describe the person who is helping the client through the procedure by keeping the structure of the session intact and giving the viewer something definite to do at all times. The facilitator confines herself simply to giving a series of set instructions to the viewer, offering no advice, interpretations, evaluations, or assurances.

The viewer locates a specific trauma that he is interested in working on—one with a specific, finite duration. Then he treats the incident like a "videotape." First, he "rewinds" it to the beginning, then "plays" it through to the end—without talking about it while he is viewing it. After he has viewed it, the facilitator then asks him what happened, and he can then describe the event or his reactions to having gone through it.

---

*This chapter is adapted with permission from Traumatic Incident Reduction Association (TIRA) webpage (www.tir.org), "Traumatic Incident Reduction (TIR) FAQ." TIR's originator is Frank A. Gerbode, M.D.

After the viewer has completed one review (and one description), the facilitator has him "rewind the videotape" to the beginning and run through it again in the same fashion. The facilitator does not prescribe the degree of detail, sensory modalities, or content the viewer is to get during each run-through. The viewer will see as much as he is relatively comfortable viewing. After several run-throughs, most viewers will become more courageous, contacting the emotion and uncomfortable details more and more thoroughly. Typically, the viewer will reach an emotional peak after a few run-throughs and then, on successive run-throughs, the amount of negative emotion will diminish, until the viewer reaches a point of having no negative emotion about the incident. Instead, he becomes rather thoughtful and contemplative, and usually comes up with one or more insights—often major insights concerning the trauma, life, or himself. He displays positive emotion, often smiling or laughing, but at least manifesting calm and serenity. At this point, the viewer has reached an "end point" and the facilitator stops the TIR procedure.

In use since 1984, TIR is especially useful when:

1. A person has a specific trauma or set of traumas that she feels has adversely affected her, whether or not she carries a formal definition of PTSD.

2. A person reacts inappropriately or overreacts in certain situations; it is thought some past trauma might have something to do with it.

3. A person experiences unaccountable or inappropriate negative emotions either chronically or in response to certain experiential triggers.

In addition to eliminating PTSD symptoms, TIR often provides valuable insights which the viewer arrives at quite spontaneously, without any prompting from the facilitator and hence can "own" entirely as his own. By providing a means for completely confronting a painful incident, TIR can and does deliver the positive gain a person would have had if he had been able to fully confront the trauma at the time it occurred.

CONTRAINDICATIONS

TIR is not recommended for use with clients who:

1. *Are psychotic or nearly so.* TIR is most definitely an "uncovering" technique and hence is not appropriate for such clients.

2. *Are currently abusing drugs or alcohol.* A client should be stable and off drugs or alcohol entirely for two months before starting TIR.

3. *Are not making a self-determined choice to do TIR. For TIR to work, the client has to really want to do it.* If the client is under duress (e.g., under a court order) or trying to please someone, TIR will not work, although a reluctant client might be "sold" on the idea of doing it.

4. *Are in life situations that are too painful or threatening to permit them to concentrate on anything else, such as a TIR session.* If the client is afraid of being murdered, or is preoccupied about the possibility of having cancer, or engaged in constant fighting with her spouse, such issues/situations would have to be addressed first, by real-life coping methods or other means, before the client will be ready to undergo TIR.

Since the TIR technique is completely client controlled and unforced, clients will protect themselves if they are getting in too deeply by simply discontinuing the procedure. Hence there are no known cases of negative effects from properly facilitated TIR. A cardinal rule is never to force the client and always follow the client's interest.

WHY DOES TIR WORK?

A trauma, by definition, is an incident that is so painful, emotionally or physically, that one tends to flinch away from it. (We say that one pushes it away, blots it out, represses or otherwise does not permit oneself to be aware of it.) It is the flinch and not the "objective" description of the incident that makes it a trauma, for the flinch does not allow one to "stay with" and master the trauma. A trauma contains one or more intentions: such as the intention to blot it out, to fight back, get revenge, run away, or make sure that nothing like this incident ever happens again. As long as one has a trauma-related intention, then that person does not complete the business of trauma; one remains bound to the period of time when the trauma was experienced.

There are only two ways to end an intention:

1. *Fulfill the intention.* You can't keep intending to win a race after you have won it.

2. *Unmaking the intention by deciding not to have that intention anymore and causing it to end.* This requires a conscious decision. You have to be aware of the intention and why you formed it.

When one consciously confronts the trauma, then one sees what intentions were formed at the time of the incident, and why they were formed. Only then can condition 2 be satisfied. In other words, flinching does not work because of memory intrusions. The attempt only keeps one remaining in the past. So we form a new intention that can be completed: the intention to view fully, until it has ended. That is, all negative emotions are processed so that positive emotions can emerge. At this new endpoint, the viewer frequently understands what the intention was at the time of the incident. Usually, the end point is reached in a single session. Should an earlier or similar incident be triggered, TIR can trace back to these incidents in a single session.

When the client suffers from unaccountable uncomfortable feelings, emotions, sensations, psychosomatic pains, and unwanted attitudes, but there are no obvious major traumas in evidence that could be addressed, a type of TIR called "Thematic TIR" can be used to trace these "themes" back to the incidents they came from and eliminate them, also in a single session. For more information, or referrals to trained TIR clinicians contact the Traumatic Incident Reduction Association (TIRA) listed in the Resources, Appendix 10.

CHAPTER 26

Eye Movement Desensitization and Reprocessing (EMDR)[160]

A growing number of systematic studies have indicated that eye movement desensitization and Reprocessing (EMDR) can be very effective in the treatment of PTSD.[161] Dr. Bessel van der Kolk, a Boston University and Harvard psychiatrist and leading PTSD authority, has observed that encouraging studies indicate that EMDR "seems to be capable of producing powerful therapeutic effects in some patients with PTSD."[162]

EMDR was originated by Dr. Francine Shapiro in 1987, and was initially employed for survivors of rape, molestation, and war. Since then it has been applied to survivors of diverse traumatic experiences across a wide range of ages. Therapists consistently report that EMDR lessens negative images, thoughts, and feelings, while increasing positive images, thoughts, and feelings.

WHAT IS EMDR?

EMDR is a comprehensive treatment plan involving eight phases. A unique and central component of EMDR is that the client holds upsetting memory material in mind while following a rhythmic set of eye movements, which are thought to accelerate the processing of that material.[163] Dr. Shapiro stresses that EMDR should only be done by a licensed, EMDR-trained mental health professional; laypeople should not try it on their own except as instructed by such a clinician. Here is a general overview of the eight phases of EMDR.

1. *Client history and treatment planning.* A thorough history identifies people for whom EMDR might not be appropriate. For example, people with cardiac or respiratory problems or who are pregnant should consult doctors

because EMDR may at times bring up intense arousal (this is usually brief and occurs in about 10 to 15 percent of people). The history also helps to make a treatment plan that targets obvious traumatic events from the past that need to be reprocessed, as well as disturbing events from the past that might be related to the trauma (e.g., times of feeling out of control). Clients are often asked to identify the ten most disturbing experiences from their life. Symptoms (nightmares, flashbacks) or triggers might also be targeted for processing. Coping skills that need to be learned also become part of the treatment plan.

2. *Preparation.* A relationship with the therapist marked by trust and ease must be developed so that clients can be free to report disturbance and progress accurately—information that is essential to the clinician. EMDR theory, procedures, and expectations are explained. Clients are taught ways to relax, comfort, and calm themselves as ways to cope with distressing arousal. Then they're taught to maintain awareness during eye movements of disturbing material, knowing that they are now safe (e.g., they're taught to imagine themselves in a safe train that is speeding by upsetting scenery).

3. *Assessment.* The client and clinician identify aspects of the target to process that best represents the traumatic memory. The client then identifies a negative belief about herself that is associated with the event. For example, negative beliefs that are locked in the traumatic memory might include: "I'm no good; I'm bad; I'm incompetent, or I'm unlovable." Then the client chooses a positive preferred statement (e.g., "I'm in control, I'm safe now, I can succeed, I did the best I could, or I now have choices"). The clients also identify negative emotions and physical sensations, such as a tight chest, constriction in the throat, or a heavy feeling in the stomach. The client rates the strength of the negative and positive cognitions, as well as the degree of disturbance of the negative emotion and physical sensations. These ratings will help the clinician know how the treatment is progressing.

4. *Desensitization.* Clients are instructed to think of the targeted material (an image might be part of this, although the image is not necessary), the negative belief, and disturbing feelings/sensations. While holding all this in mind, the client is asked to do a set of eye movements by following two fingers on the therapist's hand, held about twelve inches away and moved rhythmically back and forth across the field of vision. The head is held still

as the eye movements are performed. Processing begins and new mental material typically emerges with each set. After each set of eye movements, the client is instructed to blank it out and take a deep breath. The therapist asks what the client "gets now." The client often feels the image or feelings change somewhat, or helpful insights might emerge. An associated memory or chain of memories that need to be processed also might emerge. The client is asked to "stay with that" as she follows additional sets of eye movements. Eventually all disturbing aspects linked to a disturbing memory are "cleaned out," or processed.[164]

5. *Installing and strengthening the positive cognition.* When distress has been sufficiently reduced, the preferred, or positive, cognition is repeated. The therapist might say, "As you think about the original incident, how do the words 'I did my best' (or other previously identified positive cognition) feel now?" That positive cognition is reinforced with additional sets of eye movements until it feels sufficiently valid to the client. Anything that blocks the positive cognition from feeling sufficiently valid to the client is processed.

6. *Body scan.* To further ensure that all aspects of a traumatic memory have been processed, the client is then asked to notice if any disturbing physical sensations remain as she brings up the target. If so, that sensation is targeted for reprocessing with additional eye movements.

7. *Closure.* The therapist helps the client leave the session feeling safe and comforted, even if processing is not complete. Self-calming strategies are done and the client is advised that processing will likely continue between sessions. (Even new disturbing material that comes up suggests the need for processing, and is thus a positive sign.) She is instructed to use a journal to record that processing and calming techniques to contain arousal.

8. *Re-evaluation.* At the beginning of the next session, the clinician ascertains if positive results have been maintained from the last session. New targets are identified or old targets that still need processing are identified—and processed.

When processing seems stuck, the cognitive interweave can be tried to prime the processing pump. The therapist poses a question to stimulate the connection of an appropriate positive cognition to the target network. For example, the therapist might ask, "Can a little child cause a rape?" The client thinks of that as a set of eye movements is done. Perhaps guilt changes to anger as the survivor realizes she wasn't to blame. The EMDR-trained clinician can also make a number of other adjustments to facilitate processing that is stuck.

STRENGTHS OF EMDR

As the above discussion suggests, EMDR possesses a number of unique advantages:

- *EMDR often leads to rapid improvements.* Up to 90 percent of survivors with single-incident traumatic events show significant relief in only three sessions. EMDR can also accelerate the treatment of multiple incidents although such treatment often takes longer.

- *EMDR processes various aspects of traumatic memories together: cognitions (thoughts/images), feelings, physical sensations and behaviors related to the troubling memories.* Thus, integration of the different aspects of memory is facilitated.

- *Control remains with the client.* Aspects that need to be processed arise naturally in the course of treatment. The therapist does not tell the client what to think. Clients can also stop processing at any time. For example, if processing becomes too uncomfortable, the client can signal the therapist to stop eye movements by raising a hand or turning away.

- *EMDR defuses and clears out all aspects of memory networks that might be related to a traumatic memory.* Thus, processing a recent traumatic memory with EMDR might lead a client to process a childhood memory of feeling similarly out of control.

- *The benefits of processing one type of memory may generalize to other similar memories.* For multiple or repeated trauma, similar traumas may be grouped together. Processing a representative incident from each group is often sufficient to neutralize the other incidents in that group. Thus, all traumatic events may not need to be processed.

- *Traumatic memories need not be discussed in detail if the client doesn't wish to.*

WHY EMDR WORKS

Although the mechanisms are uncertain, Shapiro offers what she thinks might explain EMDR's effectiveness. Just as a bone will heal naturally once it has been set, dissociated memories will heal naturally once processing is stimulated. EMDR helps people to confront—not avoid—disturbing memories, in small doses in a controlled and safe way. This helps pair the memory to less fearful emotions.

It is possible that moving the eyes rapidly stimulates electrical connections between parts of the brain that process memories. Theorists have noted that rapid eye movements during dreams appear to help the brain process, while high levels of affect seems to freeze eye movements and stop processing. Similarly, people with PTSD sometimes have frozen eye movements (e.g., the "1,000-yard stare" of shell-shocked soldiers). Thus, moving the eyes (or doing similar rhythmic movements) might accelerate the integration of traumatic memory with adaptive cognitions that are stored elsewhere in the brain. It is possible that the gentle processing biochemically alters the brain so that it becomes desensitized.

Clients are asked to notice memory material, by visualizing that they are a passenger on a train safely speeding by the memory. This teaches them that they can step outside the memory and observe it with safety and detachment—similar to the way meditation teaches one to view experience with detachment. Thus, the memories are paired with neutral or comforting emotions, not fear. They then are told to dismiss the memory, teaching them another way to gain a sense of control and mastery over the material. Concentrating on the eye movements provides somewhat of a distraction from the pain of distressing memories while processing occurs.

Paying attention to physical responses and relating them to emotions allows the client to break down the various aspects of a traumatic memory and see it as less overwhelming. Finally, the structure of EMDR helps to prevent overanalysis and endless ruminating, and reminds clients that they are bigger than the trauma.

WHAT EMDR CAN TREAT

- PTSD
- Grief reactions that were avoided during the trauma
- Disturbing memories that are not always identified as traumatic (death of loved one or excessive grief from other causes, abandonment, rejection, feeling powerless)
- Mental disorders that can be traced to earlier troubling events in life (e.g., a trauma-related depression; certain anxiety disorders, low self-esteem, or addictions that are connected to childhood abandonment)
- Self-defeating, ingrained beliefs whose origins are unknown (e.g., "I'm not

worthwhile" or " I can't control my life" might come from an upsetting but not traumatic event)

- Future events that are anticipated to be stressful. Desirable coping strategies can also be reinforced with EMDR.
- Fear of deciding upon a distressing medical experience (e.g., cancer treatment might be overwhelming for a person who previously had an unresolved negative experience with chemotherapy)

WHAT MIGHT BE TARGETED?

- a single trauma from adulthood.
- a single trauma from childhood.
- multiple traumas—targeting a representative incident for each group of related traumas is usually sufficient.
- triggers.
- symptoms such as dreams, nightmares, or startle response. (Processing a nightmare can lead to identification of an earlier disturbing real-life experience that can then be processed.)
- negative thoughts (e.g., the present thought "I'm powerless" often is connected to a disturbing memory).
- symptoms of walled-off memories such as memory lapses, dissociations, or the ability to access only negative material. Such symptoms might exist without a memory of a traumatic event.
- a recent experience that is not traumatic yet inexplicably distressing (e.g., an authority figure might be unconsciously triggering memories of an adult molester; a failed business reminds you of abandonment). Processing often uncovers a root memory. If not, coping skills can be taught.
- memories of people who contributed to low self-esteem.
- secondary gains.

CHAPTER 27

The Counting Method*

The last of the newer therapeutic techniques is the counting method. It has been employed by its originator, Dr. Frank M. Ochberg, Department of Psychiatry, Michigan State University, and others since 1989 with several dozen clients in an outpatient setting. In this approach, a client recalls a troubling memory while the therapist counts to 100 within a two-minute interval. In most cases, clients reported reduction in the frequency and intensity of troubling intrusive recollections. No clients reported negative consequences, and approximately 80 percent reported improvements. The following explanation is given:

> Counting affords you the relatively short interval (100 seconds), with a beginning, middle, and end, in which to deliberately recall an intrusive recollection. Thus your exposure to the memory will be titrated and you will gain a feeling of more control over the recollection. Aspects of the Counting Method include:
>
> 1. *Silent recall allows privacy.*
> 2. *Hearing the therapist's voice links the painful past to the relatively secure present and the safe, dignified partnership of therapy.*
> 3. *Feelings of terror, horror, and helplessness may recur during counting, but they will be time limited and, most likely, modulated by connection to the therapist.* Thus you will see that you can control the increase and decrease of those feelings and related thoughts, giving you a greater sense of mastery over them.
> 4. *The traumatic memory itself may be modified.* That, after all, is the ultimate objective. If and when the memory emerges spontaneously at some future time,

*Adapted from Ochberg, F. M. 1996. "The Counting Method for Ameliorating Traumatic Memories." *Journal of Traumatic Stress* 9 (4): 873–80.

it may be attenuated by the experience of the Counting Method. You will associate the dignity and security of therapy with the intrusive recollection.

Generally, memories evoked during counting will be no worse than spontaneous re-experiencing (however, occasional exceptions occur when forgotten images return). If flashbacks have been recent, vivid, and overwhelming, a companion to drive you home is advisable.

The method is different from flooding or extinction therapy for anxiety,[165] in that once you experience some mastery over the memory there may be no need for further counting sessions. The experience of connecting one significant portion of a bank of traumatic memories to the therapist's voice may generalize to all traumatic memories. Often, two or three sessions is sufficient.

THE COUNTING METHOD PROCEDURES

1. *Schedule this technique when you and your therapist feel the timing is appropriate.* The normal guidelines of safety, a sound therapeutic alliance, apply here.

2. *Schedule a session when extra time is available for closure.* The counting should be done early in the session.

3. *Identify which traumatic event you wish to work on* (if you have experienced more than one).

4. *You'll recall a memory without speaking while the therapist counts to 100.* Try to fill the 100 seconds with that memory, letting the worst feeling crest as the counting goes through the 40s, 50s, and 60s, then coming out of the past and into the present as the counting proceeds through the 90s.

5. *Get very comfortable.* You can gaze off, and you don't need to look at the therapist.

6. *The therapist begins counting: "Let's begin. 1 . . . 2 . . . 3 . . ."* (The therapist counts in a clear, friendly, natural voice. She keeps an eye on the clock to maintain a steady rhythm of approximately one number per second. Precision is not necessary, but a steady tempo is good.)

7. *At 93 or 94 the therapist can say, "Back here," to assist your return to current reality if you need a reminder.*

8. *After the counting, if you have been able to recollect a trauma, you might appear dazed, moved, or transformed.* It is okay not to speak for awhile.

You may feel some sense of accomplishment, some relief, or some residual terror from the original event. You may have recalled aspects of the trauma that were forgotten. You might be excited by the chance to share a revelation, or perhaps a bit embarrassed. If you do not speak for awhile the therapist asks, "Can you describe what you just remembered?" If the recollection is too intense for retelling, the therapist can assist by asking, "What did you recall when I was counting in the 20s and 30s?" Further probing about what happened during other parts of the counting can help elicit the fragments. The therapist takes verbatim notes to facilitate future processing.

9. *Reflection and closure.* You and the therapist discuss what has just occurred.

   - The most important goal is to end on a positive note, with you feeling composed and secure enough to leave the session. A reminder such as, "You did well. You remembered, and were able to turn on the memory tape and turn it off." Or the therapist might turn to discussing the process to lessen strong feelings ("Did 100 seem like enough time? Too much time? Did my counting help or distract?").
   - Processing of memory material that emerged may be done, if tolerable. Discuss with the therapist, reframe, and digest the traumatic memory and the way the memory was changed during counting.
   - The therapist might leave a reminder, "In the future, when you recall that awful day/night, you can remember how you turned off the tape at 94, how you heard the counting, how we revisited the scene together."

10. *If the method fails to elicit any emotions or if it does not permit you to recall the memory, discuss this with your therapist to determine jointly if you might wish to return to the method at another time or abandon it.*

11. *Further sessions.* Allow time to digest what happened after the first session. At a future time, discuss if you wish to apply the method to other aspects of the trauma. If you received partial relief, you might want to revisit the same memory and process different aspects to gain greater control of that memory. You might prefer several consecutive sessions to process these aspects. If there are other traumas, you might wish to space the method several months apart if needed. Some clients find it helpful to imagine how they wished the scene would have ended or find some creative solutions for it (such as turning the tables on the assailant).

CHAPTER 28

Dream Management and Processing

All things one has forgotten scream
for help in dreams.

—Elias Canetti

This chapter begins an exploration of other commonly used approaches to healing (chapters 28–39). You'll be wise to remain aware of the opportunities these approaches present.

Post-traumatic nightmares so frequently become a terrifying aspect of PTSD. They can jolt people awake in a cold sweat, and feel so petrifying that sleep is avoided for fear of having another. Because sleep is troubled, the victim becomes fatigued, which makes them more prone to intrusions.

Nightmares can be demystified by viewing them as simply the normal intrusion of dissociated material. They are just the brain's attempts to process walled-off memory material. The obvious difference is that these intrusions appear during sleep, often in more creative ways than the intrusions in waking life. Think of nightmares as an ally to recovery. Accessing them, rather than avoiding them, facilitates the recovery process.

Dreams are a fairly accurate barometer of recovery. Dr. Deidre Barrett, a Harvard psychologist and president of the Association for the Study of Dreams, has written:[166]

> Several studies have delineated a pattern of post-traumatic nightmares in which
> the initial dreams are fairly close to a literal reenactment of the trauma (i.e., an

almost exact replay), sometimes with the twist that an additional horror, averted in real life, is added to the dream reenactment. Then, as time passes, and especially for those whose PTSD is gradually improving, the dream content begins to make the trauma more symbolic and to interweave it with concerns from the dreamer's daily life.

The more severe the trauma, the more likely nightmares are to occur, although dreams might not occur or be remembered until after the processing of some aspects of the trauma. Barrett and her colleagues have identified several common themes and symbols in PTSD nightmares:[167]

- monsters
- danger
- being chased
- rescues
- dying
- revenge
- being threatened again by an assailant or other traumatic event
- being punished or isolated
- being trapped; powerlessness
- sexual abuse (dreams might include shadowy figures, snakes going in holes, worms, blood, good and bad sex, injury, being trapped, paralyzed, shame, guilt, anger, violence, or death)
- filth, excrement, and garbage (can symbolize evil, lack of purpose or dignity, disgust or shame)
- physical injury (losing teeth is fairly common, which might symbolize losing control, being powerless or unattractive, or being wounded emotionally)
- being visited by the deceased

Just as dissociated material can get stuck in waking life, so too can nightmares get stuck, so that we replay and rehash the same nightmares with little change. Nightmares typically remit as memory material is processed in waking life. Now we'll discuss different ways that dream material can be directly processed.

1. *Confide your dreams*. Sometimes all that is needed to diminish the intensity of nightmares is to share your dreams verbally with a supportive person or by writing in a journal. Verbalizing in a supportive environment helps to neutralize the intense emotions, and integrate the memory fragments.
    - Relax and describe your dream in detail. Break it down into the following specifics:
        - What is the setting?
        - Who are the characters?
        - What is happening?
        - What are you doing? Feeling? Thinking? What are your physical sensations?
        - What are the symbols?
        - What are the symbols saying?
    - Create a system to recall your dreams. You might keep a dream journal for such details. You might keep a pad of paper and a pen, or a tape recorder, beside your bed.

2. *Imagine that you see yourself at a specific, intense point in the dream carrying out a simple task such as looking at your hands, and saying in the dream, "This is just a dream."* Practice this before you go to sleep to serve as a cue to remind yourself that this is just a dream, should the dream, in fact, recur.[168]

3. *Confront the nightmare and find appropriate ways to modify it.*
    - Confront the monster chasing you and ask in a direct and friendly way, "What is it you want—what are you trying to tell me?"
        - One person confronted the monster and discovered that it represented himself and his guilt. He assessed his guilt and made some growth-promoting changes.
        - See if you can make the monster laugh, smile, or get it to dance.
    - Create a new ending. For example, see the assailant being caught. See yourself coping. A veteran from the Gulf War sees his buddy, "now with God." You might simply visualize yourself saying, "I am safe now, I survived," or any other positive cognition.
    - Write out or talk out what you did above.
    - Use art to draw the nightmare and then the more positive ending. Consider all the positive choices you have now.[169]

Remember, dreams—like walled-off memories—change as we learn to cope and better process dissociated material. You might dream about positive outcomes. Dreams of the deceased might include assurances that they are now well off or opportunities to say good-bye. As your recovery proceeds pay attention to the quality of your dreams. King and Sheehan have written:[170]

Dreams of growth and understanding excite both the survivor and the therapist. In them, the dreamer behaves or feels differently, sees things from a different point of view, attends to some element of the situation that she has ignored in the past, sees new possibilities emerging. The affective tone of the dreams becomes more positive. The dreamer may come to realize for the first time that she did the best she could at the time of the (traumatic event), or that she had no viable options. She may see more clearly the role of significant others, then and now.

CHAPTER 29

Healing Imagery

Health is the movement towards wholeness.
Imagery is the movement towards wholeness
made visible.

—*Rachel Naomi Remen, M.D.*

Embedded in traumatic memories are images that powerfully affect our moods, behavior, and health. Mental images even affect our immune systems. While changing our verbal thoughts can neutralize strong negative emotions, changing our mental pictures can sometimes bring about even more positive changes.[171]

In imagery, we can create mental pictures that are profoundly soothing. You have already used imagery to create a safe place and a light stream. In this chapter we will explore ways that can directly promote healing of the inner emotional wounds. Unlike the chaotic and overwhelming experience of your traumatic event, healing imagery will be conducted in a safe, accepting setting. You will have the chance to infuse your memories with dignity, respect, and control. In this chapter you'll find a number of imagery exercises to try with your therapist.

REPLACING PAIN WITH ACCEPTANCE

This imagery exercise is simple yet profound. The minimal use of words helps to discourage overanalysis while the powerful image elicits strong healing emotions. If your therapist is guiding this exercise with gentle, soothing instructions, you can signal with a raised finger when each step is accomplished.

1. *Sit or lie down in a comfortable and safe place.* Deeply relax your body from head to toe.

2. *Take two easy, deep breaths, saying a calming word or phrase such as "relax" as you breathe in and as you breathe out.*

3. *Just think of your traumatic event.* Notice what it causes you to feel.

4. *Locate those feelings in your body.* Give them a boundary and a color.

5. *Push the feelings away in front of you.* As you do, give those feelings a shape, a color, and boundaries. Think of your feelings forming a barrier.

6. *See yourself walk around the barrier.* And as you get around it you are welcomed by a most loving figure with open arms (perhaps a loving family member, Deity, or an imagined figure). You hesitate for a moment, but the peaceful loving expression beckons you and invites you forward. You move forward and embrace and are embraced by this loving figure. And you just feel that loving acceptance.

7. *Perhaps no words need to be said.* Perhaps you hear that loving figure say words like: "You are safe and secure now. You have suffered enough. Let my love surround and heal you."

   When you have fully experienced the feelings of this imagery, gently return to the present and open your eyes. Tears might appear, but they are usually warm tears, tears of relief, and healing.

TIME TRIPPING[172]

1. *Find a quiet place where you can be undisturbed for about thirty minutes.* Again get very relaxed, and take two easy deep breaths, using your calming word or phrase.

2. *Identify an event in your life that is still painful.*

3. *Call the person who experienced this difficult time your younger self.*

4. *Call your present self—who possesses greater experience, wisdom, and love—the wiser self.*

5. *Imagine that you, the wiser self, travel back in time to the difficult event, and you approach your younger self.* Your younger self looks up and sees you. Your eyes meet and there is an affinity and trust; your younger self is willing to listen to you.

6. *You enter into a dialogue with your younger self.* You ask the younger self, "What is troubling you?" The younger self expresses the facts *and* feelings of the event. You listen with great empathy and understanding.

7. *You ask, "What would help?"* You listen intently with your ears and heart for what is expressed verbally and silently. You perceive and provide for needs such as the need for:

- Understanding.
- Instruction. Perhaps you can teach coping skills that you have recently learned, or help the younger self to correct distortions.
- Support and encouragement (e.g., "Considering your experience and training, you're doing well!"; "It *will* get better!"; "You'll make it through this. I know that you will"; etc.).
- Physical help or protection.
- Advice. Think together. Use the experiences and wisdom of both to brainstorm solutions such as:
  - Perhaps you could coach the child who was abused to say, "That's no way to treat a child. I am trying so hard." The wiser self stands alongside the child for protection and support.
  - The adult might help the child say to a critical parent, "I see your point. I'd like you to help me. I think I'll develop faster if you point out the positives, too."
  - If the younger self made a bad decision, the older might say, "I see why that made sense then. Here's a better way." Imagine helping the younger self improve.
- Above all, communicate love in any or all of the forms that are needed:
  - a loving, gentle, accepting look where eyes meet eyes
  - loving words (e.g., "I love you")
  - a hug/embrace
  - a soothing touch
  - a token to remind the younger self of the wiser self's love

8. *The wiser self now returns to the future.* See the wiser and younger selves fused, strong, solid, and whole.

THE EXPERIENCE OF MATTERING

Ideally, parents will provide children with a safe, secure environment where the children feel loved, accepted, worthwhile, and safe to explore. The children from such homes tend to feel resilient. If people lacked this kind of environment as children, they will likely feel insecure, vulnerable, and defective to the core. They may need to learn how to be loving and protective to themselves. This imagery exercise provides that feeling of security and acceptance. It is especially useful for people who cannot remember pleasant times prior to their traumatic event(s). The instructions for a corrective experience are adapted from the works of John Bradshaw and Pam Levin.[173]

1. *Write down the names of your most cherished friends, family, and/or loved ones; people you felt good to be with; people who made you feel warm, safe, accepted, loved.* First identify couples, then individuals (including friends, colleagues, teachers).

2. *Find a place to sit quietly and comfortably where you won't be disturbed for about fifteen minutes.*

3. *Relax your entire body.* Take two very deep breaths, saying the word "relax" as you breathe in and as you breathe out.

4. *Imagine yourself an infant surrounded by loving people.* These can be a circle of the loving people you identified . . . or two warm, loving grown-ups—one a male and one a female—parents as you would like to imagine parents ideally . . . perhaps composite figures of people you have known and loved, who made you feel like a somebody.

5. *As an infant you needed to hear these words.* Imagine yourself hearing these alternately from a male voice and a female voice:

We're so glad you're here . . . Welcome to the world . . . Welcome to our family and home . . . I'm so glad you're a boy or a girl . . . You're beautiful . . . All our children are beautiful . . . We want to be near you, to hold you and love you . . . Sometimes you'll feel joy and laughter . . . Sometimes sadness and pain and anger and worry. . . These feelings are all okay with us. We'll be there for you . . . We'll give you all the time you need to get your needs met . . . It's okay to wander and separate and explore and experiment . . . We won't leave you . . ."

Imagine them cradling you . . . loving you . . . gently gazing upon you with eyes of love . . . and you respond to these feelings.

HEALING LOVED ONES

Imagine a loved one has been killed in an auto accident and you didn't have the chance to say good-bye. Talking about the event and your feelings has helped, but you still are having very distressing intrusions about the accident. Dr. Mary S. Cerney of the Menninger Clinic has taught this technique.[174] The client was a teenage girl who lost her sister in an accident. Her belief is that her sister is safe in heaven, yet she cannot get over the gruesome image of her sister's injury, which in this case was an amputated arm.

1. Get very relaxed from head to toe. Again, use your calming word or phrase as you breathe in and as you breathe out.

2. Can you imagine seeing your loved one now, after the accident? And what do you notice? (Perhaps she is smiling and well, but the injury persists.)

3. Can you now reach out and heal your loved one? Anything is possible in imagery. (Perhaps you reach out and restore the lost body part or otherwise heal the injury.)

4. And what does that feel like? And is there anything else that you want to do? (Perhaps you want to tell your loved one that you love them and then say good-bye.)

COPING IMAGERY

See yourself in the present confronting a trigger. See the memory of the original trauma intruding while you become very distressed. Now see yourself becoming very calm and peaceful. You feel in control. See yourself telling yourself:

- I'm safe and in control now.
- That's just past stuff—just old memories. I'm safely in the present now.
- I've survived. I'm not defeated.

CHAPTER 30

Healing Rituals

Following the Gulf War, American troops marched proudly as their country welcomed them home. Many a Vietnam veteran shed a tear and found the ceremonies vicariously healing.[175] A family holds a memorial service for a man whose body was never recovered from a flood. His little granddaughter launches a balloon heavenward with a love note saying good-bye.

Rituals are structured activities that help us heal. They help us focus our thoughts and feelings, experience them, and process them. They help us consider the meaning of what has happened, grieve losses, receive support, develop helpful new ways to view ourselves, and move ahead. Some rituals are formally structured; others can be quite simple. This chapter will explore the nature of rituals and give suggestions for developing healing rituals.

PTSD authority Dr. Don Catherall has suggested that most rituals generally contain seven parts.[176] Think of a funeral and you can easily identify them:

1. *A location* might be a gravesite, a sacred religious structure, a place where someone experienced a traumatic event, or a beloved spot in nature.

2. *A symbol.* A gravestone, for example, helps us to experience our feelings. The Vietnam Veterans Memorial is a powerful symbol. The visitor descends into what feels like a dark valley of death, pauses to pay sacred respect to the fallen individuals, then walks upward toward life and light again. A family at the grave symbolizes a new family—not diminished but unified.

3. *Props.* These include flowers, candles, photos, or written speeches.

4. *Personal support.* People verbalize love and support, and communicate it nonverbally through hugs, touch, or caring expressions. Grief is shared as people communicate their sorrow. People help survivors prepare food or

perform other helpful tasks. Comments such as, "I'll see you again," remind survivors that they are part of the community.

5. *Healing words.*
   - Remembrances help to put traumatic events and individuals' lives in perspective. For example, a eulogy by someone who knows the family can recall both the strengths and quirks of the deceased and reminisce in a loving, and even at times, humorous way. A woman nursed her husband for three years before he died from a fall. She was feeling ashamed for the times that she had gotten frustrated and impatient with him. A minister in the eulogy correctly reminded her of her extraordinary saintly patience at a time when she was open to hearing that. Informal reminiscing recalls cherished memories that may be otherwise lost.
   - Meaningful poems, songs, or music and invoking divine comfort can also promote healing.
   - Expressions of hope for the future and enduring commitment to relationships helps survivors see beyond the traumatic event.

6. *A knowledgeable, trusted guide or director.* This might be a recognized leader, a funeral director, clergy person, or one who has gone through similar difficult times and rituals before. Sometimes it is simply a family member or friend who is perceived as trusted and caring. Sometimes you might choose to lead your own ritual.

7. *Farewells.* Tossing a rose into the grave communicates acceptance of a person's passing, the wish to preserve loving memories, and the reality of moving into the future. One community drew pictures of feelings they wished to release, tore them up, and placed them in an inexpensive rocket which together they watched fly into the night.

Catherall continues that the preparation of a ritual contributes to the meaning of it. Individuals can plan how to dress appropriately, create poems, pick flowers, walk down the aisle, and make other plans. It is good to invite all people who are involved to participate—even children. A good time to hold a ritual might be at the anniversary of the trauma. The season will tend to trigger strong emotions anyway, and a ritual could provide great support to the survivors. Other significant dates might also be meaningful. For example, at class reunions the service academies hold chapel services where a roll call of deceased classmates honors their memory and gives survivors further opportunity to reminisce and grieve. The citizens of Oklahoma City gather annually on the anniversary date at the site of the bombing.

Designing your own ritual will usually make it most meaningful. Consider how your family has conducted rituals over the years. This might suggest what might be most meaningful. Catherall suggests:

1. Specify the trauma(s).

2. Identify who has been affected and how.

3. Develop symbols for life before the trauma, the trauma, and transition and transformation. The loss of illusions of security might be symbolized by an unlocked door, a picture of a child confidently leaping into a parent's arms, or a photo of an infant sleeping peacefully. A rape survivor wears one closed rose to symbolize the rape and one open rose to symbolize becoming open again to life. Religious symbols of hope and resurrection can comfort.

Again, rituals can be quite formal or relatively simple. A pilgrimage to a place that you remember with fondness and safety can symbolize a sense of security that was lost. Catherall relates another creative ritual. A young four-and-a-half-year-old girl was molested at school but was not considered a credible witness at the trial. Although the older children testified, young Catherine did not and had difficulty moving beyond the trauma. So her mother set up a pretend trial, with the policeman who had been talking to Catherine serving as the judge, and the social worker and therapist also participating. Catherine prepared by learning about how trials work, discussing the roles of the various participants, and preparing her own testimony. During the actual "trial," Catherine gave her testimony and the "judge" sentenced the perpetrator. Catherine asked for and received assurance that the "bad man" would no longer hurt her.

Let's explore certain rituals that have been used in the treatment of combat veterans. These rituals might suggest other ideas for your own healing rituals.

THE NATIVE AMERICAN SWEAT LODGE AND PURIFICATION RITUAL

This ritual is richly symbolic. According to Wilson and Colodzin,[177] war is considered abnormal and to return to the culture, individuals must be transformed and restored to balance. Thus, the returning warriors are ceremoniously cleansed before entering a dark, circular lodge. The warriors sit close together, cross-legged in a circle surrounding a pit of extremely hot rocks. They are guided to their places by a medicine man, who speaks in a soothing, calm voice of welcome, hope, healing, and transition back to the community. Water is ladled over the hot rocks, producing steam, as the medicine man pronounces a song of prayer which participants repeat together. Each participant offers a personal prayer, beginning with thanksgiving and ending with an expression of unity with all others. The medicine man speaks additional words of wisdom and guidance. After about an hour or longer, the warriors leave the lodge and smoke the sacred pipe to close the ritual.

Now let's consider the symbolism. The ritual itself honors the warriors contributions and demonstrates the desire to bring them back into the community. The medicine man, or shaman, represents healing and is a role model of spiritual strength. His guiding the warriors to their places in the dark symbolizes trust, goodness, and security, and opening the door flap periodically lets in wisdom and guidance. The circle symbolizes unity and shared suffering. In the total darkness, one confronts oneself and a sense of inner strength emerges. The sweat literally and symbolically cleanses, and the emerging into the light and fresh air of nature symbolizes transition back to the community and rebirth. If the lodge is next to a running stream, this too symbolizes cleansing.

REVISITING THE SITE OF THE TRAUMA

This special type of ritual permits one to confront the trauma from a perspective of experience and safety. Sometimes the survivor gains insights that were not afforded during the heat of the traumatic event. One of the most moving examples of this type of ritual is "Full Cycle," a University of Massachusetts project for Vietnam veterans who had been unsuccessfully treated for PTSD by conventional means.[178] Twelve veterans were taken by bus to Mylai, where American soldiers had massacred more than a hundred South Vietnamese civilians. One veteran related extreme fear as the bus approached, anticipating that the villagers would drag the veterans out of the bus and parade them as war criminals. As they walked through the peaceful village to the visitors' center, children smiled. They learned that five hundred and four civilians had been massacred, not a hundred, and many of these were pregnant women. A guide at the visitors' center greeted them graciously and asked them to sign a visitors' book. One veteran wrote, "Please forgive us." And then a healing miracle occurred. A woman serving tea said, "The past is past. We know the American people did not want this to happen. It is time to forget and become friends." A veteran wept, "Here the South hasn't forgiven the North for something that happened a hundred years ago, and these people forgive us for something that happened twenty years ago."

In the same project, two nurses with PTSD returned to a hospital, a scene of gore which intruded repeatedly into their consciousness. They assumed that they would encounter hatred. Instead graciousness and love was shown by local citizens. One nurse went to the hospital and found that the citizens had dedicated a room to the nurses who had ministered to civilians, in fact the very room where her bed had been.

Another veteran placed a marigold from Mylai on a Vietnam war memorial atop a hill as a sign of respect for the enemy he had killed. He cried, prayed for forgiveness, and released years of pain. Still another visited a battle site where he had been wounded to "return" to his comrades who had been killed after he'd been evacuated. He shed a few tears and made peace with them. Each of these individuals found a meaningful way to come to terms with his or her trauma.

Healing rituals surround the event and the survivors with healing emotions as the facts and feelings of the traumatic event are acknowledged, confronted, and honored. In this sense, healing rituals are much like healing imagery. Notice the degree of closure that has taken place following a ritual. Do not be surprised, however, if additional processing is still needed.

CHAPTER 31

Grieving Losses

We grieve what we value; we grieve in proportion to our affection.[179]

All the many complex issues involved in PTSD must be disentangled for recovery to proceed. Grief is one such issue. All events that are significant enough to cause PTSD involve loss, yet grief often gets buried in the struggle for survival. Perhaps you were too numbed to grieve. Perhaps you were too busy or were discouraged from grieving. Perhaps some aspects of the trauma still feel so overwhelming that you have avoided them. These reactions are all normal. However, continually avoiding the normal, healthy feelings of grief keeps unresolved memories of loss in active memory, emotionally charged, and likely to intrude.

Grief memories are processed much like other aspects of traumatic memories: at your own pace and when you are ready. Losses are confronted and processed so that meaningful adjustments and adaptations can be made in our lives. Of course, adjustments can only be made if we clearly acknowledge the nature of our losses. We can't adapt and find new ways to satisfy the void if losses are not confronted. Losses that are buried—not explored, experienced, and expressed—can erupt at inopportune times, resulting in a host of physical and emotional symptoms.[180] The more we fear facing the pain of loss, the more we remain in bondage to the past. So it is important to process our losses.

WHAT ARE GRIEF AND MOURNING?

Grief is the suffering associated with loss. People typically think of grief as intense feelings of sadness and sorrow. However, the experience of grief can also include bodily changes (such as fatigue and troubled sleep), and behavioral changes (such as keeping busy or using drugs to escape the pain).

Mourning refers to the process by which we explore, experience, express, and integrate our grief, and adjust to a world with the loss. Mourning derives from the Indo-European base *mer,* meaning to remember or think of. Mourning and grieving are often used interchangeably.

WHAT WE GRIEVE

In trauma, we don't only lose *something,* we also lose our way. Hard-earned gains and dreams for the future seem irrevocably lost. Development is seriously impaired. Grieving is about finding our way again. So by grieving we try to name and understand our losses. We attempt to see clearly where we presently are in regard to where we were before the loss, and where we wish to be.[181] Losses resulting from traumatic events might be tangible,[182] such as the loss of a loved one. However, there are also many intangible aspects of loss that typically need to be grieved. Thus, the death of a spouse means more than just the tangible loss of a body, which may itself have given great comfort and pleasure. Intangible losses include the deceased spouse's roles as helper, friend, adviser, protector, parent, or emotional supporter. Losing the status of being married, the surviving spouse might also find themselves isolated from old social groups comprised solely of couples. Lost too are dreams for the future, perhaps involving creating a family, traveling, or sharing hobbies. Secondary losses—consequent to the initial loss—might include having to move from a cherished home and community due to loss of the spouse's income. Having to work causes the spouse to abandon for a time their dream of writing a book. Sometimes when we grieve we discover a sense of loss for things that never were. For example, an adult survivor of incest realized that she never had a healthy, normal, loving relationship with her father. When we clearly *see* our losses, several outcomes are possible. We might:

- identify the need to mourn and find constructive ways to heal
- find ways to cherish precious memories
- accept what can't be replaced, while finding alternative ways to meet our needs
- discover or affirm inner strengths
- discover or affirm what is really important to our lives
- begin again to develop in areas that were frozen at the time of the trauma

None of these positive outcomes can occur if we simply try to flee our pain. Conversely, when our losses become clear we can take steps to get back on course. So there is a greater purpose to grieving than simply discharging sadness. When overwhelmed, we might naturally try to escape the pain. As we begin to break down the trauma and understand our losses, we are then in a better position to find our way. Specific, tangible losses might be irreplaceable but many intangibles—what they mean—are recoverable, at least in part. Traumatic events understandably involve a sense of loss. Your trauma might include the loss of:

- Life (e.g., of a loved one, colleague, or fetal child)
- Home
- Property
- Pets
- Health status: physical capacities, body parts, appearance
- Lifestyle
- Community
- Job, income, promotions (might be due to inability to concentrate or interact with coworkers, absence, medical illness, etc.)
- Memories: mementos/keepsakes (photos, baby books)
- Dreams, opportunities, hopes ("I was learning to be such a good parent and spouse; now I feel useless to my family.")
- Normal, trusting relationships (e.g., a relationship with an abusive parent that never developed, a disrupted relationship with a loved one or friend, incest that causes the removal of a parent from the home, loss of ability to connect with people)
- Innocence, a normal childhood (sense of play, spontaneity, joyful memories, discovery, warmth, zest, creativity)
- Virginity, ability to choose first sexual partner, sense of control of body
- Sexual confidence, feelings of sacredness of body and wholesomeness of sexuality, ability to enjoy sensual experiences
- Trust in others or self
- Sense of safety, goodness, beauty, humor, self-confidence, enjoyment, peace, fairness

- Previous self-concept (e.g., "I can no longer consider myself wise, prudent, a good protector, moral, etc.")
- Self-respect
- Reputation
- Spirituality (e.g., feelings of peace with God, sense of being protected and valued)
- Faith in institutions (police, doctors, military, legal profession)

UNCOMPLICATED GRIEVING

Normal, uncomplicated mourning typically follows the six "R" processes of mourning outlined by renowned grief authority Dr. Therese Rando.[183] You might think of the death of a parent who died expectedly after a long, satisfying life, although the six "R's" apply to other types of losses with obvious adjustments. The six "R's" are:

1. *Recognize the loss.* We intellectually acknowledge the loss and understand the reasons and circumstances. For example, we listen to the medical report, view the body, and participate in the funeral. All aspects of the loss, including intangible and secondary losses are identified.

2. *React emotionally.* We experience and express all emotions surrounding the loss, positive and negative. Respites and distractions from the pain are normal but eventually the hurt will be experienced.

3. *Recollect and re-experience the deceased and the relationship.* Here we review and remember realistically *all* aspects of the deceased to gain an accurate composite of the deceased. We cherish the good qualities while accepting the flaws of the loved one. Unfinished business with the deceased is recognized and completed.

4. *Relinquish old attachments to the deceased and to assumptions that no longer work.* Here we accept that the deceased will not return so we no longer expect her for dinner or expect him to call. We give up the notion that nothing bad will ever happen and accept the fact that the world is not perfect. This step does not mean that we forget the deceased; only that we accept the reality of her passing.

5. *Readjust to the world without forgetting the deceased.* We accept that our loved one will not be able to take care of us, and realize that we will need

to make some changes in order to continue living a satisfying life. We figure out ways to retain healthy connections to the deceased while accepting their passing. We might identify ways to memorialize the deceased, or remember their teachings or perspectives on decisions. We might find a support group to help us transition to our new world, learn new skills to meet needs that the deceased used to take care of, or accept life without certain needs being met.

6. *Reinvest in life—love, work, and play.* We find ways to redirect our emotional energy that will yield satisfying returns. We might find new hobbies, causes, or relationships. Cherished memories can furnish energy for these pursuits.

Rando notes that mourning does not usually progress smoothly through these six steps. Often it is two steps forward and one back. Mourning usually takes longer than we expect, as well. It helps to realize that even in uncomplicated mourning a full range of emotional, physical, and behavioral symptoms are common:[184]

- Initially shock, numbness, bewilderment, disbelief, and even denial can occur. Sometimes people can accept the loss intellectually but not emotionally. The denial can help the person get through the first few days. Denial might take the form of: "This can't be happening—it feels like a dream"; "It is happening, but it isn't that bad"; "Others are worse off than I am." Taking care of others, appearing strong, trying to reverse the loss, or keeping busy are other ways to temporarily avoid confronting painful feelings.
- After days, numbness turns to intense suffering as the loss is acknowledged:
  - Emptiness
  - Repeatedly being reminded of the deceased
  - Waves of crying and/or sadness sweep over the survivor with each reminder
  - Longing
  - Preoccupation with the deceased's memory
  - Dreams and apparent visitations
  - Physical changes include insomnia, loss of appetite, loss of sex drive

- Despair follows as the loss is accepted. Dominant feelings are sadness and the inability to feel pleasure. A tense, restless anxiety may alternate with lethargy and fatigue. Common physical symptoms include weakness, sleep disturbances, loss of appetite, headaches, back pain, indigestion, shortness of breath, throat tightness, heart palpitations, dizziness, and nausea. Sadness can be mixed with anger at the deceased for leaving or for other disappointments, relief at not having to care for the deceased any longer, or gratitude for being alive. Some people seek company while others withdraw. People might alternate between avoiding reminders and cultivating memories. Many wish they had treated the deceased better, and a significant minority (about 40 percent) think they are losing their minds.

- Sadness and emotional swings may last for years. Even after recovery, waves of grief may return on anniversaries or other significant dates (grief spasms).

COMPLICATED MOURNING

Rando defines complicated mourning as a response to loss that does not progress normally through the six "Rs." That is, there is a problem or "sticking point" at one or more of the processes of grieving. Many forms of complicated mourning involve trauma. Complicated grief symptoms are similar to those of uncomplicated grief, except that they are more prolonged and intense. In addition, clinical depression, anxiety disorders, compulsive gambling, low self-esteem, guilt, fear of relationships, chronic grieving as attempts to keep the loved one alive, and other symptoms associated with PTSD are common.

The following is a list of factors that can complicate the mourning process:

1. Denial is excessive and persistent:
   - An incest survivor thinks, "I can't believe my father would do that to me—he loves me."
   - A mother of a son who died in an automobile accident says, "I don't want to know what really happened. Don't tell me the details or show me the accident report."
2. Preoccupation with anger and rage might prevent one from acknowledging the underlying grief.
3. Ambivalent feelings toward the deceased are not acknowledged.

- A woman only recalls her father as loving when he was sober, and can't permit herself to feel anger for his violence when drunk. Thus, she does not complete her business with him by processing her anger.
- Anger is displaced from the deceased person to others such as doctors or relatives, as a way to avoid the primary source of anger. For example, a woman could not acknowledge her anger at her usually careful husband who died in a careless industrial accident. Instead she raged at his managers for not preventing the accident.

4. Unresolved guilt ("If only I had . . . ") blocks processing of grief.

5. The traumatic events were too sudden and overwhelming to confront. Often multiple losses seem impossible to break down and grieve singly. Perhaps you were too preoccupied with survival or too numb to grieve.

6. Other people discourage grieving or are unavailable to support the bereaved.
   - Most cultures routinely sanction funeral rites for the deceased. However, most cultures do not routinely provide ways to grieve miscarriage, abortion, suicide, sexual abuse, rape, domestic violence, or family dysfunction from alcoholism.
   - When a child dies, spouses may be unable to support each other because of their own grief.

7. People may learn a variety of myths that discourage grieving (see page 243).

TIPS FOR GRIEVING

1. *Go as slowly as you need to.*

2. *Look for all emotions.*

3. *Use pre-trauma photos to help identify "losses."* As someone once said, "the child you once were you still are." Although trauma seems to bury the beautiful qualities of an individual those qualities still exist and may again be cultivated.

4. *Memorialize the loss.* Memorials like the Vietnam Veterans Memorial help to contain grief. It gives grief a place to reside, wrapped in dignity, respect, and love, and gives us a way to stay connected. It says, "I love you, I

MYTHS THAT COMPLICATE MOURNING

1. *Grief is a weakness.*
Grief is a normal, understandable human experience that happens because we deeply value what has been lost. Grief is part of what makes us human, but like guilt, it is not meant to last forever at an intensely painful level. The grieving process allows us to feel the pain, express it, then move on with fewer long-term negative effects.

2. *If I start to grieve I will lose control and cry forever.*
According to the research, losing control is unlikely. You will more likely feel sad for a time, but you will recover. Should you lose control and cry for awhile, so what? This is a normal way to express pain so that we can recover sooner and retain our humanity.

3. *If I stop to grieve, I will lose the gains I have made in life.*
As a rule, the sooner one resolves grief, the more productive one is able to be. Conversely, unresolved grief will detract from performance and enjoyment. Grieving does not mean that life's progress will stop. Grief work does take time but it is an investment of some time, not all of one's time.

4. *If I recover and feel joy, I will show that I don't care.*
Some combat veterans think they must continually grieve as a memorial to their fallen comrades, and feel disloyal if they stop feeling intense pain. We might ask, "Are there better memorials to the deceased than prolonged pain? Are there better ways to stay close to them? Do you think they want you to go on grieving and stop living? Might they prefer that you memorialize them with happy memories and a fruitful life?"

Others think that no longer feeling intense pain over their mistakes indicates betrayal of their values. We might ask, "Can we commit to living well without being emotionally distraught? Can we motivate ourselves with a carrot rather than a stick?"

5. *If I stop grieving I will forget the loss.*
When memories are no longer numbed, we remember the loss more completely—but with more peace and less pain.

6. *If I give up the loss I give up a part of self.*
Is it really prolonged anguish that we wish to preserve or cherished memories and a satisfying life course?

7. *The deceased (or offender) is a saint or a sinner. I must either love or hate him.*
This idea makes it impossible to process normal ambivalent feelings. Every mortal is somewhere between the extremes of perfect saint or complete sinner. So it is normal for a child to grieve a parent who was loving at times, yet have great anger for the criminal things the parent did. Conversely, to be angry at a generally decent deceased person does not make the survivor a bad person or mean that they didn't love the deceased.

8. *Grief shows a lack of spiritual faith.*
Faith may help people keep going, but it does not insulate one from human sadness. Certainly Job was no stranger to grief, while Jesus wept.

always will; this gives me a way to remember you while continuing on with my life. I will not forget you."

5. *View upsurges in grief as opportunities to resolve grief and heal emotionally.* Look for grief from previous losses that might make you more vulnerable to more recent losses.

6. *Be willing to give up guilt, shame, the desire to judge or punish yourself, and the hope to change the past.*

7. *Consider how loss might lead to gains:*
   - increased empathy and capacity to help others
   - clearer understanding of what really matters; greater wisdom
   - constructive changes; commitment to use time and life energies wisely
   - the knowledge that you can survive anything; recognition of inner strengths
   - gratitude and appreciation for what you still have
   - awareness of personal vulnerabilities
   - recognition of the need to develop new skills to strengthen yourself

8. *Consider thoughts that might help you better deal with the losses. For example:*
   - "My baby is safe with God."
   - "My deceased loved one is in a better place."[185]
   - "I'm a good person who went through a bad experience."

9. *Consider the possibility of forgiving loved ones or others who disappointed you.* This difficult process will be discussed in chapter 37.

   You might find the journey of grief exercise that follows very helpful.

THE JOURNEY OF GRIEF EXERCISE

Once we have confronted our pain, there is nothing left to fear. The journey of grief is like a voyage into darkness and sadness. We keep traveling into the darkness and sadness until eventually the darkness gives way to light and gladness. Then we have seen the whole picture and no longer need to run from the dark.

We will not lose ground if we pause to grieve. Grieving is like restful sleep. Sleeping takes time, but we awake refreshed for the next day's journey. In the same way, grieving allows us ultimately to progress further.

Begin your journey of grief with a sense of discovery and the nonjudgmental attitude of a scientist. That is, do not judge your feelings or reactions as good or bad. Just allow them to be and observe them.

Below are a series of questions to respond to. It is suggested that you place each question at the top of a separate blank sheet of paper. Number the sheets and questions and answer each question in turn. Keep a fairly steady pace. You can go as slowly or as fast as you want. For major traumas or traumas that were prolonged you'll probably be wise to advance in small doses. Return to questions as often as you like until you feel that you have completed your journey.

The journey of grief exercise consists of three parts: damage assessment, broadening the perspective, and readjusting and reinventing.

Damage Assessment

A military commander receives a casualty report. This permits the commander to see where the unit is in terms of capabilities and needs, and how best to proceed. At times the commander might determine that time is needed to regroup and re-train. At other times, the commander will know that the unit is ready to advance with confidence. In the Journey of Grief Exercise you, of course, are both the unit and the commander, gathering accurate information in order to determine how best to proceed.

1. Briefly describe what happened. That is, list the traumatic event(s) and when it/they happened?

2. What did I seem to lose? (Consider the obvious tangible losses, as well as intangible and secondary losses. Ask yourself, "How am I different since the trauma?; What does the loss mean to me?; What gains had I made that were reversed?")

3. What negative impacts have the losses had on me? What painful feelings have resulted?

4. Do the losses following the trauma remind me of earlier losses such as death, abandonment, or neglect? What did those earlier losses cause me to feel?

5. What factors have prevented me from grieving my losses?

Broadening the Perspective

Here we view the loss in its complete, realistic context. As we have noted previously, there is a tendency in PTSD to see only the negative aspects of our experience.

6. What hasn't been lost? (What do I still have such as abilities, capacities, relationships, other tangibles, and intangibles?)

7. What has been gained from the loss?

8. What have I learned?

9. What positive benefits can still be derived?

10. What has helped me to cope and survive? Has there been some goodness in the world that has assisted me?

11. What inner strengths have emerged or have I discovered in myself? (What personal qualities got me through the loss? What beautiful aspects are still there? What did I do well to survive? What have I done since the trauma that is honorable or noteworthy?)

12. What do I still value?

13. What could have made things worse for me? For others?

14. What do I miss most about the losses?

15. What memories do I still cherish that perhaps were buried by the trauma?

16. What won't I miss about the losses?

17. What can I still enjoy?

Readjusting and Reinvesting

The purpose of grief is not to remain in a hole of sadness but to find ways to go on living fruitfully.

18. What would I wish to say to the people involved in the losses, including myself, to help complete unfinished business?

19. What thoughts might help me to deal with the loss?

20. What do I still need?

21. What would help me heal?

22. What losses are replaceable? (Are my tangible losses irrevocable? If so, how else might I fill my needs?)

23. What will help me set a good life course? (How can I transition to a more satisfying way of life and go on without the things I've lost?)

24. Imagine yourself a year or two from now. You think of the loss and remember it, but the intense pain has ended. What has happened to enable you to do this?

CHAPTER 32

Making Sense of Trauma
Coming to Terms with Suffering

We ask, "Why? Why?! Why!!" Why did it have to happen? Why to such a good person? Why to my loved ones? Why to me? Why is there so much evil? Why did God let this happen?

Without resolution these questions keep us stuck and powerless. On the other hand, responding to these questions can be very empowering and liberating, even if the answers are not totally satisfying. Some counselors feel it is best to not ask the questions since one cannot fully answer them. They correctly point out that those who continuously ask why are more likely to be depressed. Or angry demands for answers might deflect one from accepting losses and moving on. So they think it wise to accept that bad things happen, and move on. This is one option.

Another approach is to more fully address the questions, answer them as completely and as quickly as possible, accept the limitations to our understanding, and then move on.

When we ask why, we are really asking "Why do we suffer?," a question that has plagued philosophers throughout history. Let's tackle this question and resolve it as satisfactorily as we can. In short, we suffer because the world and its people are imperfect. More specifically, we suffer for four reasons:

1. *We sometimes suffer as a result of our own imperfections.* If we drive loved ones away because of our anger, it is good to recognize our shortcoming and make adjustments. A traumatic event might catch us unprepared, unskilled, unable to function at our best under duress, or careless—in short, imperfect. If we accurately accept responsibility for our flaws and try our best to improve without self-condemnation, then suffering is not in vain.

2. *We sometimes suffer as a result of the imperfections of others.* We live in a world where each individual has free choice. Mother Teresa wisely observed, "Even God will not force us to do good. We must choose to do good." A world of free choice permits individuals to rise to the very noblest of heights. As the humanitarian Albert Schweitzer observed, "Man is fallible, but infinitely perfectible." History is full of noble individuals and we need not look too hard to find people like Schweitzer, Mother Teresa, Abraham Lincoln, Arthur Ashe, or the kind neighbor down the block. On the other hand, a world of free choice permits people to choose evil. It is difficult to comprehend why a person would choose evil over good, or know for certain what factors are operative in an individual's life. But we can consider and understand the possibilities.

- People tend to reenact what they see and learn. If a child grows up in a violent home, he is more likely to become a victimizer than one who grows up in a loving home. The encouraging news is that the majority of abused children do not grow up to be abusers. However, the bad news is that the vast majority of prison inmates have a history of abuse. Sometimes victimizers have been numbed to all feelings of conscience, guilt, and compassion by a history of brutality. Sometimes they have not learned to interact in loving ways and lash out in frustration and pain.

- Brain damage has been observed in victimizers to a greater degree than would be expected by chance. Shaking or battering a child can damage areas of the brain that help to regulate emotions. This might help to explain explosive, uncontrollable anger and/or lack of remorse in some victimizers.

- Certain biological abnormalities can lead to mental or medical illnesses that are sometimes associated with victimizing behavior. These include certain forms of epilepsy, schizophrenia, or bipolar disorder (manic-depression). Similarly, brain tumors, viral infections such as encephalitis or rabies, strokes, multiple sclerosis, Huntington's chorea, some forms of mental retardation, and substance abuse might interfere with affect regulation.[186]

- The Chinese philosopher Lao Tsu observed that bad and good coexist in each individual. We each grow up in environments that can favor the cultivation of one or the other. Beyond the influence of family, risk factors for victimizing include media violence and/or media sexual exploitation. Feeling incompetent or insecure, some people attach to hate groups made up of like-minded individuals who seek to control others.

3. *Sometimes we suffer as a result of chance.* Rabbi Harold Kushner[187] writes of a woman who lost her loved one in a plane crash and cries out, "What did I do to deserve this?" He responds that bad things sometimes happen randomly to good people. Not all bad things happen because we are bad and deserve them.

4. *Sometimes we suffer so that growth becomes possible.* Orthodox Judaism's most illustrious philosopher, Rabbi Joseph B. Soloveitchik, stated, "God left an area of evil and chaos in the world so that man might make it good."[188] Thus, suffering confronts us with the possibility of elevating ourselves and others. We cannot control others or force them to choose good, but we can choose for ourselves what course to follow and perhaps influence others. Perhaps more important than why a traumatic event happened is what we will do to make the suffering meaningful.

A young widow, Whitman[189] writes of the loneliness she felt following her husband's death. In gratitude she sees more clearly what a loving, complex, often tormented person he was and wonders how she might have listened more and tried to understand him better instead of being so petty. She realizes through her grief that she was overcoming her fear of being alone. She gained compassion as she realized she could no longer condemn the alcoholic who tried to escape his pain. In short she realized that her suffering was more than pain, it was the shaping of her soul. Similarly, through his anguish, Vanauken[190] came to view the loss of his beloved wife as "a severe mercy" because of his soul's enlargement that ensued.

Understanding suffering as clearly as possible and taking responsibility only for that which we can control can help us to come to terms with suffering.[191] We accept that the world is imperfect and that very bad things can happen. Accepting does not mean that we like or allow bad things to happen. It only means that we acknowledge that they do and move on with as little bitterness and cynicism as possible.

CHAPTER 33

Hypnosis

Because survivors of trauma have already learned how to dissociate, many therapists will enlist this skill as an aid to recovery. Hypnosis is one strategy that uses dissociation in a comfortable way. There is nothing mysterious or magical about this effective strategy. As we discuss it, you will realize that you are already familiar with many of its aspects from previous strategies we have discussed.

In hypnosis, one deeply relaxes and opens the mind to possibilities. We voluntarily loosen our grip on the way things normally are and redirect our minds in productive, often creative ways.

As we relax we sharpen our concentration, perhaps focusing attention on:[192]

- Forgotten details. For example, a firefighter remembered only the cries of the person he could not save. Watching the fire from an imaginary safe place under hypnosis, he recalls the people he did save and all that he did to save them. As a result his guilt was reduced.

- Solutions or a better future ("What would the solution look like, sound like, feel like?").

- Positive feelings, beliefs, or self-images ("Was there a time when you felt safe, etc.?").

- Ways to value previously dissociated parts of the self.

- Lessons learned from the trauma.

- Healing suggestions that are agreeable to you ("You'll most likely find yourself worrying less and focusing more on the enjoyable aspects of situations.").

- Pain management ("Give the pain a color, temperature, and shape; see the color changing and cooling.").

The American Psychological Association has stated:[193] "Contrary to some depictions of hypnosis in books, movies, or on television, people who have been hypnotized do not lose control over their behavior. They typically remain aware of who they are and where they are, and unless amnesia has been specifically suggested, they usually remember what transpired during hypnosis. Hypnosis makes it easier for people to experience suggestions, but it does not force them to have these experiences."

Peaceful imagery or other forms of induction are often used to obtain a relaxed state. In a soothing, rhythmic voice the therapist might say, "Imagine walking slowly down stairs"; "Imagine that your limbs are warm and heavy"; or "Imagine resting in your favorite sofa, pleasantly fatigued, perhaps after taking a walk on a spring day." Induction usually takes ten to twenty minutes or more, but with practice might be accomplished within seconds. Hypnosis ends with a simple suggestion.

The case below is adapted from Schwarz,[194] and will give you an idea of how hypnosis might be used to help a person integrate trauma material. Bill remembers his image in a photograph taken shortly after his traumatic event. In it he looks sad, anxious, and numb. Thoughts of this image, along with the negative feelings, often intrude into his awareness. He dislikes this image of himself and tries to put the memory out of his mind—a way of dissociating parts of the self.

Therapist (T): What would be the opposite of sad, anxious, and numb?

Bill (B): Safe and happy, I guess.

T: (After induction): Think of a time when you *strongly* felt safe and happy.

B: I remember being in high school with my friends. We felt so safe and secure then . . . and happy.

T: Good. Go there fully. Be in that place feeling strongly safe and happy. Recall what your face looked like and all the senses that you experienced then. Say the words *safe and happy* with feeling, with every fiber of your being. Good. I'm going to touch you lightly on your wrist for a few seconds as a cue to recall this resource state. (Hereafter, the word CUE will indicate the therapist's touching Bill's wrist to cue the resource state of safe and happy. If being touched is uncomfortable, then the therapist could simply say the words safe and happy as the cue.)

The therapist goes through the following steps:

1. Imagine that you are sitting in a movie theater before a blank movie screen. On the screen is a still image of yourself before the trauma. Bring back the resource state to where you are sitting in the theater and keep that state with you as you watch. (CUE)

2. And you float out of your body to the projection room such that you can look down on yourself watching the screen. Imagine that the safe and happy feelings come strongly to you there as well. Keep these feelings with you in the projection room. (CUE)

3. Let the still image on the screen run to the point where the trauma is over and you are no longer in danger—a point where you knew you'd survive. Perhaps as you continue watching with me, watching yourself from the projection booth watch the movie, you gain new understanding and perspective. You know, of course, that you can make the movie stop or get smaller if you wish to. Remember not to associate with the movie but to watch from a distance, keeping in your resource state. Please raise an index finger when the movie has run through.

T: Good. Imagine that you leave the projection room and go into the screen to visit your younger self, the survivor who is not yet recovered. What does that younger self need?

B: To know that he's not a bad person.

T: Yes. And what might the older self say to comfort the younger self?

B: You made the choice that made the most sense at the time.

T: And what else?

B: It was a difficult situation. I still value you. You'll continue to survive and heal. (CUE)

T: Bring your younger self off the screen and sit together in the here and now. (CUE) Pondering that photograph . . . from experience you have learned to infuse unhappy feelings with acceptance, compassion, love, safety . . . and you notice that photo changing. (CUE) I'll count to five now as you return safely and comfortably to the present.

The jettison technique[195] can be used at the end of a therapy session or for relief from difficult memory work.

1. Make a fist and you have all your fears and problems clasped there in your fist.

2. On the count of three you will open your fist and all your anxieties will disappear, and you will feel happy, confident, and calm.

CAUTIONS

- If you decide to use hypnosis, it is important that you feel safe and in control. You might first practice using it to increase calmness and self-esteem before experimenting with it for other uses. Discuss with your therapist how hypnosis will proceed and be sure that you are comfortable with the plan. Agree upon a signal to stop if the process becomes too distressing, such as a raised hand.

- In many states, memories recovered under hypnosis are not allowed in court. Discuss this with your therapist before using hypnosis if litigation is planned. While most people will not create a memory that is suggested, the possibility exists that some might. Others might have a vague uncertainty as to whether or not a suggested memory occurred. Thus, it is crucial that the therapist not try to influence one's memory. Again, the principle is that hypnosis should remain under the control of the client, with the therapist acting only as a collaborator and guide.

- Hypnosis is a procedure that can be useful within a broad treatment plan. It should only be used by therapists who are trained in its use and who also have sufficient training and experience in the treatment of PTSD.

- Some people are more prone to experience intrusive memories when they become very relaxed. So be sure that you and your therapist have worked on skills to cope with intrusions before trying hypnosis.

CHAPTER 34

Expressive Art Therapies

Because experiencing and expressing trauma material is so important to recovery, the expressive arts are being increasingly incorporated into PTSD treatment plans. The expressive arts help unlock rigidly held memory material in ways that normal conversation or thinking might not, especially those memory aspects that are nonverbal. Once expressed, the material can be processed and healing proceeds. The expressive arts are particularly appealing for a number of reasons. Some people find it difficult to talk directly about their traumatic experiences. Perhaps the trauma happened to preverbal children or to children who were told by the perpetrator never to talk about the trauma. For some, the feelings seem simply too complex for words. Some self-conscious people find it difficult to talk directly about their feelings. The expressive arts shift the focus to the project. It becomes easier to describe the feelings *it* expresses.

The types of expressive arts include visual arts (drawing, painting, sculpture, collages); movement/dance; music; language arts (storytelling, essays, poetry); drama; and play/sand-tray therapy.

We shall briefly explore and sample some forms of the expressive arts—enough to gain a general understanding and appreciation for what they can bring to the recovery process. As you will see, the expressive arts do more than access traumatic memories. They put us in touch with who we really are, the parts of us that reside beyond the intellect. They also can tap wisdom and healing powers in ways that normal conversation might not.

Some mental health professionals have specialized training in art therapy. Sometimes art therapists will be part of a treatment team. They may work with individuals or groups.

VISUAL ARTS THERAPY

As Spring[196] notes, in the process of creating art, history and feelings surface in symbolic language. Once formed and expressed, art can be interpreted, processed, and transformed. Since we can handle art, we can gain a greater sense of control over inner states depicted by the art. And the simple act of creating rekindles the inner forces of hope and healing. For example, a person might depict:

- Safe places; places to contain painful emotions such as a big freezer for painful memories
- Life or self before the trauma to find "lost" characteristics to recover
- Nightmares[197] and new endings to them
- What happened
- The worst moment or event
- The moment of survival
- Separate pictures of self and the event (moving them around helps to show that the two are not the same)
- Positive and negative feelings about a victimizer
- Strengths shown during the traumatic event
- Where I am now, how I have improved since the trauma (e.g., draw a picture of self before treatment and now[198])
- Feelings (that were numbed or lost, that I'd like to have, that I have after creating the art)
- What I'd like to become in the future
- A collage of positive and negative outcomes including what I've learned and strengths I've gained
- A memorial to honor losses
- How to be safer in the future
- Coping in the future
- Comforting a friend or a pet who survived the trauma or one similar to it
- Beauty for enjoyment's sake

An art therapist who specializes in PTSD typically assembles the art materials and assists the person throughout the creative process. The art therapist will emphasize that the value of art therapy is in the expressive process. Artistic talent and the quality of the product are not important. If possible, the creator will discuss the various aspects of the project with the art therapist since verbalizing helps integrate the various components of disintegrated memories.

MOVEMENT/DANCE THERAPY

The mind and body are connected. The body accurately reflects what is going on in the mind and emotions, even if the intellect disguises this. As Roth observes, "The body is a reflection of all that is being felt and held inside."[199] In this regard, our bodies are rather like art which can express, reveal, and teach. Conversely, even subtle bodily movements can exert positive effect on the mind. Movement and dance therapists are trained to use the mind/body relationships in the recovery process in a variety of ways:

- *Movement activities relax and strengthen the body.* Simple exercises like stretching and breathing can discharge tension while more vigorous activity both strengthens and relaxes. As a result, the mind is also relaxed and strengthened. This helps to lift the mood and stabilize the sensitized nervous system.

- *If we pay attention to the body we can learn if we are frightened or tense.* We notice areas of discomfort; we observe movements that are restrained or full of strong emotion. We gradually gain comfort with those emotions as we just notice them in a nonjudging manner.

- *Circle dances, ball tosses, or other group activities help to build a sense of community and counter feelings of isolation.* We can sometimes connect more readily with people on a physical level than a verbal level. Unspoken trust can build as people in groups synchronize movements to each other. A therapist might nonverbally mirror one's physical movements through dance to communicate empathy and trust.

- *Memories might contain rigidly stored emotions and physical aspects that might only be unlocked through movement.* Movement might allow the person to safely express anger and defensiveness. Once this is accomplished, the way might be cleared to allow other strong but hidden emotions to be expressed, such as inadequacy, guilt, shame, sadness, and loss.[200] Once unspeakable memories are unlocked they can be released, processed, and eventually verbalized.

- *Abused persons may be disconnected from their bodies because they contain pain.* Movement can help to release that pain and detect emotional issues underlying the physical discomfort. The person can then learn to use physical discomfort as cues to comfort one's self emotionally and physically. Eventually, through the joy of movement, the body becomes associated with pleasant sensations.

- *A person might be able to physically act out complex or confusing feelings that cannot be verbalized.* This not only permits discharge of strong feelings but also provides a sense of control and an opportunity to better understand and integrate those feelings.

- *Movement can activate self-protection and expression.* A person might have bodily memories of freezing during a traumatic event. Now, through movement, the person can unfreeze that memory and create a new bodily memory. She can symbolically push away an offender or enact other nonverbal ways of protecting herself. She might also symbolically enact ways to say yes to healthy situations. A firefighter might recreate a desired rescue response now that there is less danger and fear.

- *Movement/dance can be used for nurture and comfort.* For instance, cradling or rocking provides support. Bowing to people communicates respect.

- *In a safe setting, movement helps one experience joy and personal empowerment.*

- *Since body movement reflects personality, fluid body movements can help the mind function in a less fragmented, more integrated way.*

- *Like meditation, movement helps us simply to be ourselves.* Words are not so important.

- *Games like Red Light/Green Light teach impulse control.*

- *Physical activity raises endorphin levels, improving moods and lessening pain.*

The many uses of movement/dance has prompted Roth to observe, "If you just set people in motion, they will heal themselves."[201] Sessions begin with an explanation of activities and boundaries. They end with a discussion of what happened to maximize processing and integration. Like art, the purpose of the therapy is not to perform but to learn through the process. So there is no requirement to be a good dancer nor is there pressure to perform in any set manner.

MUSIC THERAPY

Like dance/movement, music helps us pass intellectual barriers to processing. Combined with relaxation, music can stimulate images, emotions, memories, and body sensations. Afterward, the stimulated material can be processed verbally as one explores the meaning of the stimulated material.[202]

Depending on the type, music can evoke a wide range of moods from anger or loss to calm, tenderness, and love. One type of music might elicit negative memories. Shifting to a different type of music might elicit long buried feelings of empowerment and hope that can help to transform negative memories.[203] As noted music expert H. L. Bonny observes, music can stimulate changes in mood and memory perceptions by its innate "tension/release mechanisms . . . instrumental color, melodic line, (or) cadences."[204] Soothing music at the end of a session might facilitate a feeling of safety.

Off has described how drumming can be used to help overcome feelings of powerlessness and anger and develop assertiveness in a victim of abuse. The client and music therapist each have a drum. The client begins to drum but the therapist must ask permission to start playing. The client sometimes says "yes" and sometimes "no," and may tell the therapist to stop at any time. The therapist will sometimes support the beat and sometimes interfere. Afterward they discuss what it felt like for the client to be supported or disrupted, to have a say in whether the therapist began or stopped, or to say nothing. Anger is described in imagery in order to understand gradations. The client explores the idea of saying "Stop" as soon as she wants something to stop, and is encouraged to stop the therapist's drumming on subsequent rounds with increasing comfort.[205]

LANGUAGE ARTS THERAPY

Poetry therapy uses the written or spoken media in the healing and growth process. Poetry therapy uses not only poetry as a tool, but also stories, autobiographies, literature, journals, letters, essays, and song lyrics. In this type of therapy, you might create, read, and discuss your own written pieces or study the creations of others. Written or spoken media provide a safe place to contain strong emotions—we can control and understand what we put into words.

The process of speaking or writing our own stories begins to stir our inner creative and problem-solving forces. As we examine what we have created, we become more aware and appreciative of who we are inside. We gain confidence over our emotions and a sense of competence.

As we read or listen to the stories of others we gain a sense of connection, a realization that we are not alone, that others understand and share our burden. We can gain distraction from our own problems and inspiration as we learn from others. The discussion that is stimulated can lead to insights and greater understanding of our experience.

According to Alston, stories help give order to chaos. That is, they help us understand what can be confusing and complex. Notice how Homer's myth can be useful to war veterans:[206]

> Homer's *Odyssey* is the story of a warrior who returned home after being gone for twenty years. The battle for Troy lasted ten years and his return home took ten years. His wife Penelope struggled to keep her suitors from taking over the bed and home of her husband Odysseus, the warrior. The journey home was perhaps more costly than the long battle. Odysseus faced the perils of sea monsters, the alluring invitations of the Sirens who offered him knowledge, and the temptations of the Lotus Eaters who offered him mind-erasing drugs. When he wandered into their home, at first, Penelope didn't recognize him. Here we find parallels to the story of the Vietnam veterans, some of whom are still on the way home after more than twenty years. Like Odysseus, they have been facing demons in the psyche that are as threatening and alluring as the fantastic creatures in the ancient Greek story.
>
> When Odysseus finally returned, his wife Penelope thought he was yet another impostor trying to trick her. Finally she tested him by casually mentioning that she had moved their great bed. This would have been an impossible task because the bed that Odysseus had made for her was built around a great tree: it could not have been moved without destroying the tree. When she saw his outrage, she recognized him. She actually saw his great love for her in his anger at the apparent destruction of their beautiful marriage bed. Along with his father, son, and larger family, she bade him enter his own home and return to the life of the hearth and community. Such a story of war, alienation, and return is timeless and finds echoes in the stories of Vietnam veterans and their families.

Alston also relates Campell's[207] story of a woman who cannot relate to her traumatized and numbed husband, and asks a healer for a potion to cure her husband. The healer instructs her to bring a whisker plucked from the face of a tiger. After six months of bringing a tiger food, gradually getting closer and closer, she tenderly snips a whisker as the tiger nestles its head in her lap. However, the healer tosses the whisker in the fire, explaining that a woman who can accomplish such a feat needs no potion. With little or no interpretation, the listener realizes the need to discover inner strength when magical cures do not exist. However, groups might also discuss various aspects of the story. For example, what might the wife have felt at various points of the story? The husband? The tiger? There are no "correct" answers; this approach allows one to develop a broader range of feelings.

Stories can be told randomly, around a fire, or after supper. Stories of heroes who coped or blessed your life create a hopeful tone and a sense of safety. Fanciful stories, such as Dr. Seuss's *Oh the Places You'll Go*, contain uplifting themes about coping. Any personal or entertaining story helps to create a sense of community. Stories can also memorialize the deceased or affirm that your experience mattered.

If poems are created, they need not rhyme. They just need to express your honest feelings. Some find the rhythm and pattern of poetry soothing. The ideal poem will relate to your negative feelings but also communicate hope. An uplifting poem can break the inertia of depression and anxiety, soothe, and heal. *Fear,* by J. Ruth Gendler,[208] is an excellent example of this type of poem.

Some find writing letters to other survivors quite healing and comforting. Letters to the deceased can also help maintain a healthy connection or sense of closure.

Registered poetry therapists are trained in literature and psychotherapy. They can be very effective helpers in the healing process.

DRAMA THERAPY[209]

Drama therapy uses drama/theater processes to let clients tell their stories. In the process they express feelings safely and appropriately, gain new understanding and perspective, solve problems, and set goals. Integration is facilitated because the drama balances verbal with nonverbal processes. Dramas can range from improvised and informal reenactments to scripted theatrical productions with props, masks, and costumes.

In one form of drama, psychodrama, individuals reenact a traumatic event to gain insight and control. Group members take assigned roles. Action is slowed to facilitate processing. New reactions or endings can be tried. The group might devise ways to protect the survivor. The individual might assume different roles to gain new perspectives. Afterward the drama is processed for insights and understanding.

PLAY/SAND-TRAY THERAPY

Play can be a very useful part of treatment for both adults and children. For example, Helen found it very difficult to talk about the abuse she experienced as a child. However, using a doll house to recount that experience, she could slow down the events and found it easier to talk about her thoughts and feelings. The doll house became a form of art that contained and gave distance to her distressing feelings. She could move the doll house closer or farther away or she could move figures in the house around to gain mastery—just as one does with visual art. Eventually, the gradual exposure of play permitted Helen to talk directly about her experiences. She was then able to progress to other treatment strategies described in this book. However, it was nonthreatening play that started her progress.

Dr. Wendy Miller, cofounder of Create Therapy Institute in Bethesda, Maryland,[210] explains that listening to a person's language during play will often reveal the form of art that is best to try. For example, an adult is asked to express his story or the world he experiences on a sand tray containing sand, water, and miniature people, structures, and animals. A person who says, "I am sitting under a gray cloud" might resonate with visual arts, while one who says, "I'm running around," might be suited to movement/dance therapy.

The sand tray also becomes another form of art, allowing the individual to explore and further integrate his experience. Dr. Miller writes, for example, that:

> One child who kept trying to build a dam that would hold everything back was, in the therapist's mind, attempting to create a metaphor of absolute strength, an image of something that would unfailingly hold back his anger. After watching many failed attempts, the therapist guided the child toward a dam that let the water through in a steady, regulated way, allowing both flow *and* control. This child needed to see that rather than completely binding his anger, he could find a way to live with the anger by expressing it in nondestructive, controlled ways.

In this case, the metaphoric play helped the child explore a new way to deal with feelings.

BLENDING THERAPIES

The expressive arts might be blended in various ways depending upon the creativity and skill of the therapist and the receptivity of the client. For example, music is readily blended with movement/dance or with visual arts. A therapist might direct your attention to your posture while you are creating art or discussing what you created. If the feelings that your body is communicating can't be verbalized, the therapist might ask you to use a form of movement to express them. The skillful therapist will also blend art therapy with other forms of treatment thus forming a complete treatment plan.

CHAPTER 35

Life Review

We have observed that traumatic events are so intense that they capture more than their fair share of our attention. In the life review strategy we recall our entire lives, not just the traumatic events. A number of positive outcomes occur from this strategy:

- *We gain perspective on our lives and ourselves.* We see more clearly that there is more to our lives than the traumatic event, and more to us than what we did during the traumatic event. One elderly survivor chuckled sagely, "Well, I survived the war and lots of years since then. Surely that counts for something!"

- *We contradict core beliefs that were acquired in early life or from the traumatic event.* For example, we might identify evidence that challenges our belief that we are worthless, have never contributed to life, or have never experienced love or happiness.

- *We can put our lives in better balance.* Assessing our lives realistically, we might rediscover what is really important and how we want to live the rest of our lives. Paying attention to their lives, many say, makes their lives richer and renews cherished ideals.

- *We make better sense of our lives.* In examining our lives we better understand why we are who we are. When we "get it all off our chest," we not only discharge emotions but gain a chance to make sense of the memories.

- *We find memory gaps, sometimes indicating dissociated material.*

- *We gain acceptance of ourselves and our shortcomings.* In reminiscing about her life, one woman gave herself a diagnosis of "extenuating circumstances" in crediting herself for doing her best and surviving, even if imperfectly. When done in a group, we also gain a "comfortable acceptance of the life cycle," as we see that all people go through ups and downs in their short lives.[211]

- *Reminiscing has been associated with less depression, psychological well-being, and seeing one's life as meaningful and satisfying.*[212] One cannot help but look at a scrapbook of an individual's life to realize that all lives have meaning.

Life review is simply reminiscing about one's life. It can be done by making an oral or written history. Some prefer talking into a tape recorder. Some prefer writing an autobiography and, perhaps, making a scrapbook of mementos. The point is to see one's life in its entirety.

An excellent structured approach to the life review has been developed by Dr. Benjamin Colodzin. His instructions follow.[213]

THE LIFE REVIEW

The goal is to learn more about who you truly are. You will be looking for information that can help you develop "anchors" to help you weather stormy moments in your life. You will look for strengths that have gotten you through thus far. You will be reconnoitering for the available choices that can bring acceptance and peace more powerfully into your life. These choices will be found inside yourself. As you search, you will ask important questions that have meaning to you. How can you find your place in this world? How can you obtain a measure of peace in your life? Is it possible to make sense out of the ugly things that have happened? Such questions are more important than paying attention to what's wrong with you or the world.

There is more to us than we habitually notice. We are more than a worker or a survivor of a traumatic event. The purpose here is to reconnoiter the path of your life—the experiences you have lived through—to take a look at the happenings that helped form you into the person that lives here-and-now, and to see if perhaps you can relocate some parts of yourself that you may have lost touch with over time. Some are parts that will be painful to remember; these are the places where you lost your balance, where you were knocked down somehow by life. Other parts will be very nourishing to recall; these are likely the places where you learned some of what you know about holding your balance.

It's important to begin with the basic rule that this reconnaissance is something you do for yourself and no one else. As you proceed you will need to write down your recollections, which means you will create a written record that is just for you. It helps to be honest if we are not worried about the judgments of others. If you wish to share something that comes up, that is fine. But it is also fine not to.

Your mission is to pay attention to the terrain and report what you see accurately. Only in this case, the terrain is your life and the only one you will report to is yourself. To begin, you will look through what has happened in your life, using a particular method I will explain shortly, scanning for the different important experiences that have happened. The reason for doing this is to help fill in missing pieces in the story of who you are.

The things that have happened that occupy your thoughts most often are not the whole story. If you are old enough to read this book, you've been alive a long time and have been through many experiences of different varieties. You have not only lived thorough some traumatic event(s), you've also been through a lot of other experiences as well. *In paying attention to what you have known, you can become more clear about what you need to know.* Many survivors have stated that in the here-and-now of their lives they do not know how to relax or to reach a place of peace. And because repeated exposure to this way of experiencing leads such individuals to tell themselves the story: "that is who I am," you may tell yourself you cannot experience these things, that the experience of peace is not included in "who I am."

What I am going to request that you do here is to take a time out from holding so tightly to the story you have been telling yourself; time out to make sure you've got the whole story about who you are; time out to go through your life with an open mind; time out to explore. The chances are that somewhere in your life you have been happy (if only for a short while). Somewhere in your life you've felt confident and proud of who you are. There was a tendril of strength. Somewhere in your life you've felt some kind of fear and found a way beyond it. There was a victory. Somewhere in your life you have played and been relaxed. Somewhere you have tasted a good taste and found a drink that quenched your thirst. It will be helpful to find where these places are. Not so you can share them with anybody else or so anyone else can judge you, but because it is helpful for you to remember that you already know that there is more to you than the story you've let yourself see. The experiences you have had point to the skills that you have used, skills that you may not yet recognize as something useful for your life now. *It's easier to relearn something you once knew, than to learn something that you have never done before.*

One purpose of this exploration is to reclaim some of the territory of yourself that you may not be using now—to remember that it is also part of your identity—so that when you consider this idea of "me," you can tell yourself a bigger story than you were remembering before. Although I won't ask you to accept this just because I say so, I will tell you what I have observed again and again: as the story you tell yourself about who you are gets more and more filled in, you become able to make more choices about how you want to live now. Your job at this point is neither to accept or reject this statement, only to try it and see for yourself if it is helpful.

Searching Inside Yourself: A Basic Method

The writing method I will now describe can help you to regain pieces of your story. It is not a game; it is a serious psychological tool of considerable power. You are not ready to use it unless you are willing to listen to what you have to say.

In working with this kind of technique, you will have to use your imagination. You don't have to have a particularly good imagination: you just need at a minimum to know what a road looks like. Do you know what a road looks like? As long as you've got that one figured out you can start using this method.

The first step is to imagine your life—made up of all your experiences—as if it were a road. First, you're born; that's the beginning of the road for you here on planet Earth. Each place you've been and each event you've known exists along the road you have traveled. There's more of the road, untraveled as yet, but we will not look that way now. You were born, and the road started there. It stretches all the way to right now. Your reconnaissance assignments will be along this stretch of the road.

You're going to look at some of the things that have happened along the road. It would be best if you got a paper and pencil ready at this point, because you will be writing down some information about what you observe along the road. You won't want to write down too much. When you observe some important scenery along the road, you'll want to write down just enough so that you'll have a record of it. Here's how it works:

> First, imagine yourself sitting up in the distant hills, overlooking the road. The road of your life. You will not be on the road; you are removed from it, looking down at this road from higher ground. You will be looking along the road,

checking the scenery, looking at the things that have happened in your life. At first, you will look for the things that really made a difference in shaping you as you are.

Before you begin, I will explain how you write down your observations on this reconnaissance.

Imagine, for example, that you suffered a serious loss when you were six years old—such as the loss of a family member. This might well be an important event in your life, something that made a difference. When you scan along your road, it might be a piece of the scenery that you would notice. Another possibility might be that when you were six years old, you met another child who became your friend and taught you important things. This could perhaps also be something that made a difference in your life.

When it is your life, it is for you to decide. These important events can happen at any age in your life. You do not need to follow any particular formula. You are requested here to give your mind free rein, to follow the scenery along the road, looking for the things that made a difference. As you tell yourself about your own story and re-encounter some of your important scenery, you make a record of what you observe. You just need to write enough so that the key word or words that you write down will remind you of the scenery you are seeing on that piece of the road.

Going back to the examples, the road watcher who lost some family member when he was six might simply write "family"; he knows what experience that refers to. The one who made an important friend when he was six might write "friend" or the friend's name. *Write just enough so you'll know what you're talking about when you refer back to it later.* Since you're not writing this for anyone else, there is no need to be detailed.

Here's how to use this method. In your mind's eye, imagine a picture of the road. You are not on the road; you are up in the hills or other high ground, and the road appears in the distance. The road starts where you were born and stretches through all the territory up until now. You are not on any part of the road; you are reconnoitering it from a distance. You may see a flat and straight road or it may be very curvy. It may have peaks, valleys, or just about anything.

To start your reconnaissance, you will lift your imaginary binoculars to the start of the road from your vantage point on high ground. At the same time, you say to yourself, "I was born there." Then begin to sweep along the road with your binoculars as you say to yourself, "and after that . . . " Look for whatever shows up along the road of your life that made a difference. Do not attempt to structure your thoughts; just look at what comes up. Do not force your thoughts, worrying, "I should probably include this or that." Just imagine yourself scanning along the road while you hold this thought about the important things that made a difference in shaping you as you are and see what shows up in your field of view.

Repeat this procedure along your entire road up to now. Try to limit yourself to ten key items or so on this first reconnaissance. This will help you focus on some really important events. Take twenty or thirty minutes and see what you come up with. One of the curious things about this reconnaissance is that even though you are looking in just one direction along the road—from the past toward the present—you do not always remember the things that made a difference in the order they happened. When you have read these instructions to this point, you have the information necessary to take your first scan. When you are ready, give it a try.

When you have finished, look at your key words: Do you identify some with positive feelings and beautiful scenery along your road? Do you identify some with negative feelings and ugly scenery along your road? Which ones recall experiences where you felt good about who you are? Which recall experiences where you felt the opposite?

The answers to these questions contain clues about what these experiences mean to you inside. As you have recorded these experiences, you see, you have been reclaiming parts of you, experiences that you are intimately familiar with because you were there. So as you look back and remember the friend that made a difference, or enemy, or loved one, or idea—or whatever else you came up with—you can ask yourself: "Do I want more of that in my life now? Do I want less?"

You might see if the keywords you have identified form a mixture of experiences that you would judge from your present vantage point as "good" and "bad," "positive" and "negative," "beautiful" and "ugly." If they appear heavily weighted in one direction, you have gained information that the story you are telling yourself about your life is focused in that direction. This means it is possible that your individual "life tree," in adapting to your life circumstances, may have once needed to reach away from certain aspects of your story, aspects you may now be ready to reclaim. This type of scanning can give you clues about where you are paying attention and where you are not.

Your answers are a beginning. They are a way to start telling yourself what you are looking for and what you do not want to look at. If you have spent a great deal of your time with your attention focused on scenery that you don't want to look at, it is easy to feel like you have no control. As you begin to get some information and some insight about the kind of experiences you want more of now, you will be better able to steer your life in that direction toward the things you need to maintain balance. As you do that, you gain more control.

Unfinished business.   As you make your scans and find events that made a difference, you may notice that some of them have a particular quality associated with them that can be termed "unfinished business." Events that are related to "unfinished business" can stimulate some inner reaction that is unbalancing when you turn your attention their way. You may have listed many events that had a major impact on your life. If, when you remember them, it is easy to look, observe, and put those memories "back on the shelf" in your mind, chances are good that those events do not contain "unfinished business," and that you have made peace with whatever happened and have laid it to rest. Events related to "unfinished business," though, tend to evoke some kinds of reaction: anger, fear, love, sadness, or some other feeling. Places where you locate this "unfinished business" can be very important clues as to where to direct your future peace-making activities.

Searching for Inner Peace (twenty to thirty minutes)

In this next reconnaissance exercise, you will again imagine yourself on high ground, looking at the road of your life. However, instead of looking for everything that happened that made a difference, you will be looking for a specific type of scenery that made a difference.

During this reconnaissance, I'd like you to scan for the places in your life where you have felt natural and at peace—places you were doing what you felt you were supposed to be doing, where your balance felt most firm and made a difference in who you are. You will be looking for those experiences that held some quality of nourishment, connectedness, or sacredness as you lived them.

Perhaps, for example, you may observe yourself at three years of age playing with your favorite toy. If it truly made a difference, write it down. Nothing should be judged as too silly, too trivial, or too anything else. You alone will use this record; if you are engaged on this mission then you have chosen to learn just what kind of story you are telling yourself about you. Any experiences that pop up while you are scanning along the road are part of the story. So if you find your scan hovering on an idyllic fishing vacation, a positive sexual experience, a good idea, work on some project, a flower in your garden, whatever—write it down. Again, take twenty to thirty minutes and try to limit yourself to items of particular strength.

When you have completed this exercise, you will remember that there have been moments in your life—even if they were a long time ago—when you felt good. If you came up with a blank sheet (i.e., nothing has ever felt good), then you have gained some basic information about the story you have been telling yourself, namely, that life never feels good. In this special case, you may need to do some special work to remember the best in your life. Try this exercise again— only instead of looking for high "peaks" or wonderful moments, just look for the time where there was the most calm and the least discomfort in your life. This can be a starting point in helping you find the places in your experience where you were most comfortable with yourself. For those who are experiencing post-traumatic distress, it can be very difficult to locate the places in one's experience that held nourishment, peace, or positive spiritual resonances. One person who tried this exercise remarked that their road looked like a concrete airport runway and nothing else. I asked that attention be turned to looking for any places where there might be cracks in the concrete, and a blade of grass had sprung up. If one's life has been filled with "nonpeace," look for the places along the road where the "nonpeace" was a little less and made a difference.

If you did come up with some observations on this scan, take a moment to consider what is on your list. The chances are good that you would like to have these sorts of experiences in your life now. Even if they happened a long time ago, you see, you are telling yourself the story of the experiences you appreciate now. So the person who is doing the appreciating, the one who has chosen these particular memories out of all that has happened, is the you that is alive in the present.

You are beginning to get some clues about the sort of experiences that might bring more meaning to your life. This does not mean that you need to try to relive the past. That is not possible. It simply means that you have located some experiences in your past that tell you what makes it feel good to be alive. As you remember those experiences, they may help you face decisions about how to live now. They give you a sort of homing beacon to take readings from when you are facing the tough choices. You can ask yourself, "If I choose to go in this direction, will it move me toward those good feelings?" I like to think of these places along the road as spiritual "anchors," places that are like safe havens within our minds. They have power to help us return to balance when we are afraid or otherwise paying attention to what is "not okay" in our experience.

Because the knowledge of your innermost needs and feelings come from inside you, and not from anyone else, they are authentic, legitimate, and to be trusted as arrows pointing the way along your healing path.

Even if you have not been able to get at this knowledge for a long time, it is still there. Focusing your attention on the scenery on your road where you experienced your own balance may make it easier to make choices that help you get back there.

If you remembered a time when you felt very relaxed, for example, and you have not been able to relax for a long time, then you can help yourself relax now by imagining that you are back in the experience where you once relaxed. This is a way to make good use of your prior experience. Your body responds to the relaxing image in your brain.

Searching for Inner Wounds (twenty to thirty minutes)

For the next reconnaissance, use extra caution. Follow the same basic method as before. This time, you will be looking at some of the ugly scenery along your road, the places where painful and frightening things have happened—the places where you most seriously lost your balance.

This type of reconnaissance is the one you are most likely to avoid because it is very uncomfortable to recognize and pay attention to our fear and pain. There is no need to push yourself; when you are ready you will stop avoiding this scenery. When you are not ready it is best to be honest with yourself.

To do this reconnaissance, scan along your road and stop to write key words where you find places where pain or other ugliness happened and made a difference.

Because of the special nature of this type of scenery, you may have some strong reactions. If this occurs, make a record of what you were thinking/feeling when the reaction occurred. This is another clue about what is important to you. When you are finished with this reconnaissance, use your "internal radar" and scan your muscles for signs of tension. It is common to tense up when doing this difficult work. If you find a high tension level, take the time to breathe back to balance before you move on to something else.

If you have an extremely strong reaction as you observe this scenery along your road, break off the exercise and return to it later. Try to be honest with yourself about what you were observing on your road when the reaction happened. If this exercise is too difficult for you to complete at this time, you may consider finding some outside help in paying attention to these parts of the story. The people you trust the most and the people with similar scenery in their lives are good places to start a search for the right kind of help.

Please understand that if you have lived through "unusual experiences" that were overwhelming, it may be very difficult for you to fill in the parts of your story that can be found in this exercise. You may experience a very detailed reconnaissance, or you may feel as though you cannot see the terrain clearly. Sometimes seeing this terrain clearly takes time, similar to peeling an onion one layer at a time, little by little.

This is not an easy or comfortable job. Almost every trauma survivor I have encountered who has done this type of work agrees that "It gets harder before it gets easier."

Though we might wish it were otherwise, this is an accurate statement. I know of no way to take the hurt out of that which is painful. Yet it is also true that it does get easier. Your healing pathway can lead through being stuck with uncomfortable feelings to a more balanced position. If there are hidden dark spots inside that are very painful, they may need to see the light of day in order for healing to occur.

Searching for the Open Heart (twenty to thirty minutes)

Now for another type of reconnaissance. This time, you will be looking for the scenery where love occurred inside you. It may have turned out with a happy ending, and it may have been disastrous. How it turned out is not the central question here. Look for the places along your road where love happened and made a difference. It doesn't need to be sexual love—it could also be love of a parent, a friend, an animal, an idea, a place, or generalized compassion without an object—anything that fired up your heart in a way that really counted. Repeat the basic procedure: Start on the high ground and observe your road and scan forward in time, repeating: "I was born, and after that . . . " Sweep along the road, and find the scenery where love happened in your life and made a difference.

You may have had a terrible childhood, and perhaps you can remember no loving scenery until after you left home. Scan on. Or you may remember love as a child, but nothing since. Keep scanning. Something happened, somewhere. Even if it is not what happened along most of your road, there are places where you can find that scenery somewhere; some kind of love, or caring, that made a difference. Find those experiences and record key words. Again take twenty to thirty minutes and limit yourself to the most important items.

RECLAIMING OUR WHOLE SELVES

These exercises help people to reconnect all aspects of their lives. If you have been telling yourself that you have never known pleasant or loving moments, then perhaps this will stretch the story because you have examined for yourself your whole life story. *You are a human being with the ability to live many, many different ways.*

You may also choose to use this inward scanning method to fill in other parts of your story. Choose any subject that is important to you as the "filter" you place on your scan. If you are having a problem with anger, for example, you might want to look at the scenery along your road where anger has happened and made a difference. If you are working on a relationship, you might want to recheck the relationships along your road. You might need to take a look at what has happened along your road in relation to work, money, or your body. Your road belongs to you: you can retrieve what you need from it when you are ready.

CHAPTER 36

Building Self-Esteem

Two conclusions are apparent from the research: self-esteem helps protect people from anxiety and stress, and self-esteem is a most important predictor of happiness and life-satisfaction. So investing time in building self-esteem is most worthwhile. The tendency following a traumatic event is to feel shattered, perhaps worthless. But self-esteem can be developed, regardless of one's history or circumstances. Although space will not permit an in-depth survey of this important topic, we can note the principles and develop important foundation skills. Further reading is suggested in the Resource section, Appendix 10.

WHAT IS SELF-ESTEEM?

Self-esteem is a *realistic, appreciative* opinion of oneself. *Realistic* means accurate and honest. *Appreciative* implies positive feelings and liking. Self-esteem involves a clear view of self and a quiet gladness to be yourself.

It should be apparent that self-esteem is not destructive pride that says we are better than another as a person, or that we are more capable or self-reliant than we truly are. This would be arrogance and deception. Nor is self-esteem the shame that says one is worse as a person than another, totally incapable, and lacking in worth. Rather, people with self-esteem retain a healthy humility as they are aware of their strengths and weaknesses. Yet weaknesses are viewed as rough edges—not the totality of who they are. Deep inside at the core, they are quietly glad to be who they are. This deep satisfaction motivates them to grow and improve.

The person with self-esteem views people on a level playing field, each with different skills and talents, but no one more worthwhile as a person than any other. So a person with self-esteem will respect one in authority but not be intimidated. The person in authority has certain well-developed skills and attributes. But that makes him different, not better as a person. So the person with self-esteem is not driven to compete with another to prove his worth. He may be motivated to succeed by enjoyment and a sense of mastery, but not to prove his worth as a person.

Having self-esteem is not the same as being selfish or self-centered. I think of Mother Teresa who had a quiet inner gladness, yet was enormously altruistic.

HOW DOES SELF-ESTEEM DEVELOP?

Children are more likely to develop self-esteem if they have parents who model it and show the children that they are valued for who they are. They show interest in the children's friends and activities. They respect their opinions, although they care enough to enforce limits that are in the children's best interests. The parents' expectations are high—after all, they believe in the children. The standards are reasonable, however, and the parents give a lot of support. Rewards are favored over punishment.

The obvious question is, "Can adults who lacked this kind of parenting develop self-esteem?" The answer is "yes," provided they learn ways to satisfy these unmet needs. Can adults who lose self-esteem regain it? Yes, the principles are the same. Think of self-esteem building as a skill that requires steady practice and reinforcement.

HOW DO I BUILD SELF-ESTEEM?

To change self-esteem is to first understand the factors upon which it is built: (1) unconditional worth; (2) unconditional love; and (3) growing. (See Figure 36.1.)

While each building block is essential for development of sound self-esteem, the *sequence* is crucial. Let's briefly describe each building block.

UNCONDITIONAL WORTH

Unconditional worth means that each person has infinite, unchanging worth *as a person*. This worth comes with a person's creation, and cannot be earned nor lost by poor behavior. This is not the same as market or social worth, which clearly are earned and lost. This core worth is not comparable. So you might be a better doctor and I might be a better teacher, but worth as a person is equal. In theological terms, worth as a person is a given; each and every soul is precious. We might conceptualize this worth as follows (see Figure 36.2):

Figure 36.1
THE FOUNDATIONS OF SELF-ESTEEM

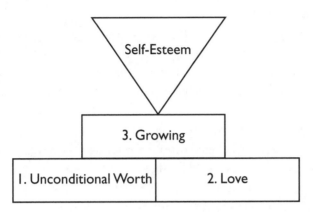

Figure 36.2
THE CORE SELF

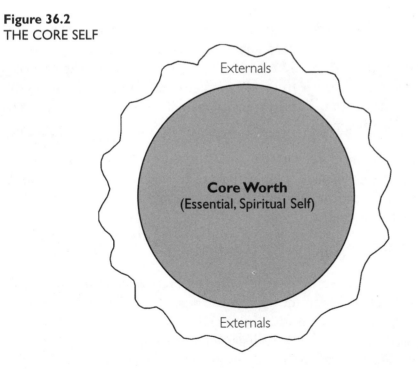

The core self is like a crystal of great worth. Each facet represents a beautiful potential or attribute in embryo. Each person is *complete* in the sense that he or she has every attribute needed (such as the seeds of love, integrity, intelligence, and talents). However, no one is *completed* or perfect, since no one has developed all attributes fully. Yet the worth of the core is infinite. People sometimes ask, "But how can I have worth if I have never accomplished or produced anything noteworthy?" And I ask them to think why parents might spend two million dollars to save a two-year-old child that has fallen into a shaft in the earth.

Some externals (e.g., respectful treatment, making wise decisions) shine up the core and help us enjoy its beauty more. Other externals (e.g., criticism, abuse, unkind behaviors) can cover or camouflage the core like a dirty film. The basic core is still there, however, unchanged in worth as a person.

The goals of strengthening this building block are:

1. *Separate core worth from externals.* Externals include performance, appearance, health/disease, condition of the body, wealth, race, social status, gender, education, how we are treated, and traumatic events that happened.

2. *See clearly one's inner strengths.* The idea is not to see each strength as completely developed, but to appreciate that the capacities are there, in embryo, to think rationally, to feel, to sacrifice, to love, to make responsible choices, to recognize truth and worth, to create, to beautify, to be gentle, patient, or firm. These capacities exist in each person, at different stages of development.

With these goals met, one is freed to find satisfaction and joy, even in poverty or fading health. This understanding permits us to experience value and worth amidst our imperfections. It gives us the perspective that there is more to us than what happened to us or what we did.

UNCONDITIONAL LOVE

Whereas unconditional worth refers to a thought process, *unconditional love* involves feelings and applies to the appreciative part of our definition of self-esteem. Many people understand with their minds that they have worth, but they do not *feel* a gladness, a joy inside. Each person has the capacity to love, although this capacity might be underdeveloped or buried at present. But love is like a seed and is capable of cultivation. Love is:

1. *A feeling* that you *experience*. Each one recognizes it and responds to it when one sees it.

2. *An attitude*. Love wants what's best for the loved one at each moment.[214]

3. *A decision* and a commitment that you make every day. Sometimes you "will it," even though this may be difficult at times.

4. *A skill* that is cultivated.

Can you recall television's Mr. Rogers telling children each day that it is *you* he likes? Not your clothes, your hairstyle, or other things that surround you, but you. This is a way of saying, "I love your core, the part that is deeper than the externals." Just as Hitler and other violent dictators learned hatred in their youth, the great lovers of the world *learned* to love. It is a skill, a talent, something that can be cultivated at any season of life. If you did not receive love from your parents, it is even more important to learn ways to provide this essential nutrient for yourself. Love is the *foundation* of growth. It is a way of feeling like a somebody of worth (i.e., not that it *gives* you worth but that it lets you *feel* it).

Self-love is similar to self-acceptance. *Accept* means to take in, to receive gladly. To self-accept, then, is to receive ourselves kindly, acknowledging our flaws and experiences.

GROWING

Growing is the process of moving toward our potential. It is a never-ending process where you develop your capacities and attributes at a pace that is suited to you, not someone else. I like many names for this factor: "coming to flower"; "elevating ourselves while we elevate others"; "love in action"; "developing"; "reaching for excellence."

We feel more satisfied with ourselves and our lives when we know that we are on a satisfying course. This building block could involve many activities including striving for competent and ethical behavior, developing talents or virtues, implementing healthy behaviors, or producing something meaningful.

Many people assume wrongly that if they can only do something noteworthy and achieve social acceptance then they will achieve inner peace and satisfaction. So they desperately and impatiently strive for quick results. This approach rarely succeeds if the first two building blocks are not in place. However, if the first two building blocks are in place, then people are free to grow because it is deeply satisfying, not to prove their worth. This produces happy achievers not driven neurotics. Again, the sequence is crucial. A person who can separate competence and confidence from worth feels secure enough to patiently try just about anything.

HOW DO I IMPLEMENT THESE PRINCIPLES?

Reasoning that self-esteem can be built systematically, I developed a college course based on the foregoing principles. Initial data indicate that the course significantly reduced anxiety and depression and raised self-esteem. The skills are described in a separate work (*Building Self-Esteem: A 125-Day Program*; see Appendix 10). Space will permit us to include some of the skill-building exercises here along with two additional exercises.

SKILL BUILDING ACTIVITY: NEVERTHELESS! (SIX DAYS)

The following is a very simple and effective skill. It reminds you of your unchanging worth amidst stressful situations that can undermine that perception. It is based on these principles:

1. Feeling bad about events, behaviors, outcomes, or some other external can be appropriate (i.e., as in appropriate guilt or disappointment). This is different from the unhealthy tendency to feel bad about the core self (this has been described as shame).
2. Saying "My skills are not quite adequate for the job yet" is quite different from saying "I'm no good *as a person.*" Feeling bad about failing is very different from "I am a failure" at the core.
3. It's okay to judge the behaviors and skills, but not the core, essential self.

In short, we want to acknowledge unpleasant external conditions without condemning the core self.

The Nevertheless Skill Concepts

People who dislike the self tend to use "*Because ... therefore*" thoughts:

> *Because* of my mistakes (my lack of training, my weight, or some other external condition), *therefore* I am no good as a person.

Obviously, this thought will erode self-esteem or keep it from developing. So we want to avoid such thoughts.

The nevertheless skill provides a realistic, upbeat, immediate response to unpleasant externals—a response that reinforces one's sense of worth by separating worth from externals. Instead of a "*Because . . . therefore*" thought, we use an "*Even though . . . Nevertheless*" thought. It looks like this:

Even though _____ , **nevertheless** _____
    (some external)   (some statement of worth)

For example: Even though *I botched that project,* nevertheless *I'm still a worthwhile person.*

Other nevertheless statements are:

- I'm still of great worth.
- I'm still an important and valuable person.
- My worth is infinite and unchangeable.

Perhaps you can think of others that you like.

Drill

Get a partner you feel very safe with. Ask your partner to say whatever negative things come to mind, be they true or false, like:

- You really blew it!
- You have a funny nose!
- You mumble when you talk!
- You bug me!
- You're a big dummy!

To each criticism, put your ego on the shelf and respond with an "*Even though . . . Nevertheless*" statement. You'll probably want to use some of your cognitive therapy skills. For example, if someone labels you "a dummy," you could respond, "Even though I behave in dumb ways sometimes, nevertheless . . ."

Steps for the Nevertheless Skill

1. For each of the next six days, select three events with the potential to erode self-esteem.
2. In response to each event, select an "*Even though . . . Nevertheless*" statement. Then record on a sheet of paper the event or situation, the statement used, and the effect on your feelings of selecting this statement and saying it to yourself. Keeping a written record reinforces the skill. Set up your record like this:

Date	Event/Situation	Statement Used	Effect

SKILL BUILDING ACTIVITY: COGNITIVE REHEARSAL (TEN DAYS)

Self-esteem can be cultivated by mindfully acknowledging what is presently "right" about one's self. For many people this is difficult because habits of negative thinking make it easier to identify what's wrong. Although there is a time and benefit to acknowledging shortcomings and weaknesses, when these become the dominant focus—to the exclusion of strengths—self-esteem suffers.

This exercise, then, is designed for practice in acknowledging and reinforcing strengths with appreciation. Doing this is a way of loving. This skill is based on the research of three Canadians—Gauthier, Pellerin, and Renaud,[215] whose method enhanced the self-esteem of subjects in just a few weeks.

To warm up, place a check if you sometimes are, or have been, reasonably:

_____ clean	_____ appreciative
_____ handy	_____ responsive to beauty
_____ literate (come on—if you've	or nature
read this far, check this)	_____ principled, ethical
_____ punctual	_____ industrious
_____ assured or self-confident	_____ responsible, reliable
_____ enthusiastic, spirited	_____ organized, orderly, or neat
_____ optimistic	_____ sharing
_____ humorous, mirthful, or amusing	_____ encouraging, complimentary
_____ friendly	_____ attractive
_____ gentle	_____ well-groomed
_____ loyal, committed	_____ physically fit
_____ trustworthy	_____ intelligent, perceptive
_____ trusting, seeing the best in others	_____ cooperative
_____ loving	_____ respectful or polite
_____ strong, powerful, forceful	_____ forgiving or able to look
_____ determined, resolute, firm	beyond "faux pas" (mistakes)
_____ conciliatory	_____ patient
_____ rational, reasonable, logical	_____ tranquil or serene
_____ intuitive or trusting of own instincts	_____ successful
_____ creative or imaginative	_____ open-minded
_____ compassionate, kind, or caring	_____ tactful
_____ disciplined	_____ spontaneous
_____ persuasive	_____ flexible or adaptable
_____ talented	_____ energetic
_____ cheerful	_____ expressive
_____ sensitive or considerate	_____ affectionate
_____ adventurous	_____ graceful, dignified

Check if you are sometimes a reasonably good:

_____ socializer	_____ follower
_____ listener	_____ mistake corrector
_____ cook	_____ smiler
_____ athlete	_____ debater
_____ cleaner	_____ mediator
_____ worker	_____ storyteller
_____ friend	_____ letter writer
_____ musician or singer	_____ thinker
_____ learner	_____ requester
_____ leader or coach	_____ example
_____ organizer	_____ mate
_____ decision maker	_____ taker of criticism
_____ counselor	_____ risk taker
_____ helper	_____ enjoyer of hobbies
_____ "cheerleader," supporter	_____ financial manager or budgeter
_____ planner	_____ family member

Perfection was not required for you to check these items, since *nobody* does any of these all of the time—much less perfectly. However, if you checked a few of these and have managed to maintain reasonable sanity in a very complex world, give yourself a pat on the back. Remember, this was just a warmup. The exercise that follows has been found to be very effective in building self-esteem.

Cognitive Rehearsal

1. *Develop a list of ten positive statements about yourself that are meaningful and realistic/true.* You may develop the statements from the list on the preceding pages, generate your own statements, or do both. Examples might be: "I am a loyal, responsible member of my_____ (family, team, club, etc.)"; "I am clean, orderly, etc."; "I am a concerned listener." If you mention a role that you perform well, try to add specific personal characteristics that explain why. For example, instead of saying that one is a good football player, one might add that he sizes up situations quickly and reacts decisively. Roles can change (e.g., after an injury or with age), but character and personality traits can be expressed across many different roles.

2. *Write the ten statements on a sheet of paper.*

3. *Find a place to relax for fifteen to twenty minutes.* Meditate upon one statement and the evidences for its accuracy for a minute or two. Repeat this for each statement.

4. *Repeat this exercise for ten days.* Add an additional statement each day.

5. *Several times each day look at an item on the list, and for about two minutes meditate on the evidence for its accuracy.*

If you prefer, you can write the statements on index cards and carry them with you. Some find the cards easier to refer to during the day.

Notice how you feel after practicing this skill which disputes the all-or-none distortion "I am no good," by substituting appreciative thoughts and feelings. Students especially enjoy this skill. Comments they have made over the years include:

- Hey! I am not so bad after all.
- I got better with practice. I didn't believe the statements at first. Then I found myself smiling on the way to school.
- I feel *motivated* to act on them.
- I felt peaceful and calm.
- I learned I have a lot more good than I give myself credit for.

A Variation of Cognitive Rehearsal

Integrating traumatic memories sometimes brings an unexpected benefit. As we clearly see the whole picture, we can often see ways in which our inner strengths were revealed, and see beyond the negatives that previously felt so all-encompassing. As you consider each traumatic event—your motives, what you felt and did during and after—what inner strengths were shown? Consider what you did to survive and cope, what you did to protect yourself or others. What have you done since to carry on or lift people? Here we are simply recognizing the truth and not minimizing our limitations. Do any of the strengths you have recognized in yourself apply lately, at least in part, to the trauma? Consider also the possibility of seeing yourself as:

- Emotionally strong, courageous, determined, unwilling to give up the fight
- Having good motives and intents: caring, concerned, willing to help and try again
- Resourceful, quick thinking, clever (e.g., just to survive)
- Principled (e.g., to be troubled by this means I have a conscience; to change course, when appropriate, indicates integrity)
- Honest (e.g., to acknowledge the damage, pain, my limitations, the need for patience in healing)
- Physically strong
- Resilient
- Stronger now in some ways
- Others?

Try putting each strength on a separate index card. Refer to one at a time, several times a day. Consider the evidence for its accuracy, drawing from not only the trauma but from the rest of your life.

SKILL BUILDING ACTIVITY: NEVERTHELESS II (SIX DAYS)

Whereas the first nevertheless skill focused on unconditional worth (a cognition), this nevertheless skill focuses on unconditional love (which involves feelings). Remember the premise that unconditional love is necessary for mental health and for growth. *Unconditional* means that we choose to love even though there are imperfections that we would wish were not there.

Let's take two people who are overweight. Jane thinks, "I am fat. I hate myself." Mary thinks, "I am really glad inside to be me. I'd feel better and enjoy life even more if I lost some of this fat." Notice the difference in emotional tones between Jane and Mary. Which one is more likely to adhere to an eating and exercise plan to lose weight? Which one is more likely to arrive at their desired weight without being emotionally distraught?

To review some of the key concepts of the first nevertheless skill:

1. We want to acknowledge unpleasant external conditions without condemning the core self.

2. People who dislike the self tend to use "*Because … therefore*" thoughts (e.g., Because I am fat, therefore I hate myself) which erode self-esteem.

3. The Nevertheless Skill provides a realistic, upbeat, immediate response to unpleasant externals—a response that reinforces one's sense of worth by separating worth from externals.

The second nevertheless skill uses this format:

Even though _____, **nevertheless** _____
               (some external)   (some statement of love/appreciation)

For example: Even though *I am overweight*, nevertheless *I love myself.*

Other Nevertheless statements are:

- I sure love myself.
- Inside I am really glad to be me.
- Deep down, I really like and appreciate me.

Perhaps you can think of other statements you like. Try the second nevertheless skill over a six-day period, recording the results just as you did for the first one. Try to say the nevertheless statement with real feeling. You might try this at times in front of a mirror, looking into your eyes, and seeing beyond the imperfections into the core with the love you would have for a good friend.

A graduate student shared with me a wonderful experience she had with the nevertheless skill. She was driving with her six-year-old son who happened to be upset with her. In response to his criticism she said, "Nevertheless I'm a worthwhile person." The boy retorted, "You're not worthwhile, Mommy." She calmly replied, "Yes, I am, and you are too, and I love you so much!" She said, "Michael looked at me so strange because he wanted to be mad at me—he was caught off guard." The anger quickly faded. I've since thought how fortunate that boy is to have seen his mother model a way to buffer criticism, and at the same time be reminded of her love for him.

LOOKING AT YOURSELF THROUGH LOVING EYES

Developed by family therapist John Childers, this strategy combines the skill of dissociation with art to experience a loving self-image.[216]

Step 1: Establish the experience of being an artist.

Each of us has within ourselves an artistic part of our personality. This artistic part is able to create new and wonderful drawings of the world around us. These drawings need not look exactly like a tree, house, or person. That is not important. What is important is your freedom to express your artistic self on paper. Imagine, for the time being, that you are an artist. In a few minutes, as an artist, you'll use crayons and paper to create a wonderful drawing. But for now, just imagine being an artist.

Step 2: Identify someone you know who loves you.

As an artist, you'll be drawing a picture of someone in your life who you know loves you (and has treated you respectfully). Take a moment to think about people in your life—perhaps Mom, Dad, Grandfather, or Grandmother; perhaps a brother or a sister, a classmate, teacher, or coach. Select one very special person. A person you know loves you.

Step 3: Describe to yourself the characteristics that make that person special.

In a minute or two you'll draw a picture of this special person but first think about how to draw this special person. For example, how does this special person look? Is he or she tall, medium, or short in height? What color of hair does this special person have? What's the color of his or her eyes? Do the eyes sparkle? Does this person have a smiling face? Is this person reaching out with his or her arms? How does this person's voice sound? Does it sound soft? Loud? Strong? Kind? If voice sounds could be colors, what colors would this person's voice be? How would you describe this special person's feelings? Continue to think about this special person's qualities for a few more minutes. Those things that make him or her so very special to you. As you think about this special person, who loves you, become aware of your own feelings. How are you feeling right now? Loving? Warm? Excited? Happy?

Step 4: Draw a picture of the person who loves you.

Now let the artist within you draw a picture of this special person—this special person who loves you. Feel free to begin drawing this person now, selecting just the right crayons to color this person as you see him or her. If you want to, you can use colors to describe this special person's voice and feelings as well. You may want to write a few words on this drawing that also describe this person. Take your time and enjoy drawing this special person who loves you. As the artist, once you have completed your picture you may want to give it a title.

Step 5: Imagine being this special person and able to see yourself through his or her loving eyes.

Now, I would like you to imagine that you are this special person. Imagine being this special person you have drawn. Float outside of yourself and imagine becoming this special person who loves you. Okay, as this special person, I would like you to think about how you see yourself. You see yourself through the eyes of someone who loves you. Look carefully at yourself through these loving eyes. In a few moments, I'll ask you to draw a picture of yourself through these loving eyes. But for now, please continue to see yourself through these loving eyes.

Step 6: Describe and draw what is loved and seen through loving eyes.

Seeing yourself through the eyes of someone who loves you, you see yourself as someone to love. Describe to yourself what you love about the person you see. Continue seeing yourself through the eyes of someone who loves you. Okay, please draw a picture of yourself as seen through the eyes of this special person who loves you. As you draw and color this picture, continue seeing yourself through loving eyes. Use colors and/or words which describe your looks, behaviors, and feelings as seen through loving eyes. Continue your drawing, seeing yourself through the eyes of someone who loves you. Your drawings may be lifelike, or abstractions or splashes of color. Whatever you choose to make them.

Step 7: Re-associate into your own body, bringing back lovable feelings.

Now, slowly come back into your own being. Looking at this picture of yourself you see yourself as someone who is lovable. Seeing yourself as lovable, say silently to yourself, "I am lovable," and notice the warm, loving feeling growing within you.

CHAPTER 37

Unfinished Business
Resolving Anger

He who pounds a pillow is in touch with
neither his anger nor the pillow.
—*Thich Nhat Hanh*[217]

Unresolved anger is a costly burden. It keeps traumatic material highly charged and in active memory. It keeps us chained to the past, in bondage to a heavy load that we carry around each day, a load that erodes peace, happiness, and eventually health. Whereas chapter 16 suggested ways to *manage* anger, this chapter will explore ways to *resolve* it.

Resolving anger from a serious offense or trauma is not easy. It does not usually happen quickly or all at once. Rather, it is a process that may not progress until considerable healing has taken place. The complexities of the simple term *resolving anger* suggest why the process is not simple at all and why it takes time. Resolving anger involves five processes:

1. *Re-experience and express enough anger to get in touch with your feelings.* This does not necessarily mean raging and screaming. Chronic, uncontrolled anger can reinforce anger and actually prevent processing. Conversely, those people who chronically bottle up their anger may need to let it out in order to loosen rigidly contained material. As the emotional pendulum swings, people discover a balance point, a place somewhere between detached intellectual control and uncontrolled emotions where memories can be honestly and effectively processed.

2. *Gain understanding.*

- We learn through anger to better understand ourselves. Anger following a traumatic event is usually accompanied by underlying grief, fear, disappointment, hurt, or insecurity. As we recognize these primary emotions we can touch and soothe them so that the anger can subside.

- We identify the true source of our anger and hurt. Perhaps we are upset at a loved one who died. Perhaps we are angry that loved ones did not protect us. Perhaps we are angry at ourselves. Directing our anger at the government, the media, or some other secondary source might deflect us from resolving the primary issues and putting them to rest.

- We seek to understand the offender's viewpoint. As much as possible we seek to replace hatred, revenge, and resentment[218] with understanding and compassion.

3. *We say what has needed to be said to gain a sense of closure.*

4. *We seek outcomes that can help bring the event to completion.*

- Sometimes an apology, the words "I hurt you, I was wrong, I am sorry," can be enormously healing. Sometimes to simply have one's pain respectfully acknowledged can be healing. Sometimes just knowing that the offender has gone as far as he is capable of toward recognizing the pain he caused is helpful.

- At times seeking justice will seem appropriate. For example, incarceration of an offender can protect you and others. It may do the offender no favor to permit him to hurt others without being disciplined.[219] Compensation for damages might also be needed. If you hold the offender accountable, do so for the safety of yourself and your community, not as a personal matter. Recognize that confronting a childhood abuser in court or in person can prove traumatizing all over again.

- Often we will not receive the things we wish for to set things right. Perhaps the offender is dead. People who were disturbed enough to commit serious offenses will likely be unable or unwilling to treat your pain respectfully now. The legal system often fails to find and punish offenders. So instead we discover ways to do what we can and accept these limitations.

5. *We release anger and resentment as we learn other ways to protect ourselves.*

THE GESTALT CHAIRS TECHNIQUE

This technique is very effective to help resolve unresolved anger. Gestalt chairs can be used to process unfinished business with an offender who is dangerous, unavailable, or unable or unwilling to deal with your hurt.

1. *Arrange two chairs facing each other at an angle.* Sit in one.

2. *Take two easy deep breaths.* Relax. Calm yourself as you prepare to get in touch honestly with your feelings. Remember that feelings are teachers. Exploring them in a secure environment is healthy.

3. *Imagine the offender sitting in the other chair.* Notice what it is like being with this person.

4. *Begin a dialogue.*
   - Start by saying a positive statement (e.g., "Years from now I want to have good feelings when I think about you, but right now I don't. My aim is to resolve this, not hurt you.")
   - Explain what you want (e.g., "I want you to hear and understand my hurt and not have you cut me off with 'I'm sorry' or 'I didn't mean it' before hearing me out.")
   - Tell the person what you are thinking and feeling:
     - Describe what happened.
     - Describe the impact of the offense, and especially your feelings (e.g., "I felt . . . ; Now I feel . . . ")
   - Remain seated. Think. Feel your feelings—the anger, the hurt, the sadness.

5. *Change seats.* Allow the offender to think and feel his feelings—his own hurts, disappointments, frustrations. Allow the offender to respond. Express the offender's perspective, including his view of what happened, his thoughts and feelings. Stay seated after talking. Think. Feel—as though you were the offender—all his feelings.

6. *Keep changing seats until both have fully expressed themselves.*

Look at the person who is listening. Stay with your feelings until they are fully experienced and expressed. At some point, you'll probably want to:

   - Check to ensure that what is said was understood. ("Do you understand why this was difficult for me? Are you hearing that?" Then let the other person respond. Both can pose this question.)

- Ask the offender, "I'm trying to understand—what were you feeling? Why did you do that?"

- Consider creating an opportunity for the offender to say those healing words: "I hurt you. I was wrong. I'm sorry."

- Consider if there were two angry or hurt people, or just one.

You might consider taping such a dialogue to better hear the feelings expressed and further process the dialogue. Gestalt chairs can be used for dialogues with "failed protectors," people who are deceased, or yourself. Here the older self asks the younger self questions such as, "What happened? What were you feeling? What do you need? How would you like to see things change?"

The gestalt chairs technique helps overcome avoidance. Sometimes it leads us to the questions, "What could the offender be teaching? Is it possible he is teaching me how to self-accept even when others don't?"

FORGIVING

Formerly a theological concept, forgiving has made its way into the psychological literature as an effective tool for resolving anger. To forgive is to release resentment, hatred, bitterness, and desires for revenge for offenses or wrongs done to us. It is a closing of the account book and a release of the debtor so that we don't allow him to set up camp in our homes. One rabbi who lost his family in the Holocaust said that he chose to forgive because he did not want to bring Hitler with him to America.[220] It is like opening the doors to our homes and taking out the garbage.

Forgiveness is something we choose to do whether the offender deserves it, asks for it, or apologizes. While it is *easier* to forgive when the offender acknowledges the hurt he caused and subsequently changes his ways, forgiveness is really about the offended, not the offender. We voluntarily forgive because we no longer wish to suffer, realizing that getting even does not heal.[221] We choose not to hate the offender, even though we hate what they did.

What Forgiveness Is Not

Forgiving is made more difficult by some common misconceptions. Forgiving does not mean:

- Minimizing the offense or its impact. In fact, acknowledging the hurt is usually necessary to heal and move beyond it.

- Forgetting the offense. Indeed, it is wise to remember the offense so that we can avoid being hurt in that way again. The offense, if confronted, can furnish useful experience, wisdom, and empathy. However, it is possible to remember without bitterness.

- Condoning the offense or permitting it to recur.

- Reconciling or trusting. Trust, the firm belief in one's integrity, is necessary to rebuild a healthy relationship and must be earned over time. However, even if reconciliation is not possible, forgiveness can occur at any time.

When Forgiving Is Needed

For many of us, forgiving when someone has hurt us has to be learned; it does not come naturally. Failure to forgive can lead to a wide range of symptoms, any of which might indicate the need to forgive.

- Sarcasm
- Rancor
- Anger
- Backbiting
- Criticism
- Grudges
- Suspicion
- Resentment
- Cynicism
- Mistrust of others
- Sensitivity to criticism
- Desires for revenge
- Demanding
- Anxiety
- Depression[222]
- Fatigue
- Tension
- Others are uncomfortable being around you

- You bristle when the offender's name is mentioned or you think about them
- Loss of peace, happiness
- Fear, expectation of disappointment
- Need to control others to prevent them from hurting you
- Hatred
- Mood swings
- Self-medication
- Difficulty trusting
- Difficulty tolerating flaws

Forgiving can help to lessen these symptoms, sometimes in unexpected ways. An interesting case was reported in the journal *Psychotherapy*. Tom was a critical father who could not hold a job because of his anger and sensitivity to criticism. Months of counseling unearthed the origin of his anger—an alcoholic, critical father. He acknowledged his pain, which he had buried. Tom also talked it over with his pastor. As a result, Tom visited his dad and said in effect, "Dad, I prayed for help to forgive you. I think maybe it worked. I want you to know I love you and forgive you for your alcoholism and your criticism." To his surprise, Tom's father cried and embraced him. Although his relationship with his father didn't change much, *Tom* changed. He became a loving and gentler father, less sensitive to criticism, and able to hold down a job.[223]

Is forgiving a serious offense easy? No. Can it be done? Yes. Bill is one who rose above bitterness. After six years in a WWII concentration camp, he looked surprisingly vigorous, living a life of love and forgiveness. He had watched his wife and three children be machine-gunned to death, then pleaded for his captors to take him next. They said, "No, you speak six languages. We need you." About that terrible moment in his life, he said, "I had to decide then to hate or to love."[224] Again, forgiving is an act of will which we choose because we realize that we are more than the offense and no longer wish to carry it around with us.

Ideas that Block Forgiveness

1. *That act is unforgivable. I can never forgive it.* There is a difference between a despicable act and an unforgivable one. The unforgivable act only requires our willingness to change it to a forgivable one.

2. *I should not be angry or hurt. I should be able to forgive.* These would be nice, but we are human and never perfect. We can only forgive as best as we can.

3. *The offender is all bad. He must pay.* The offender is weak, perhaps sick. Anyone who knowingly hurts others has paid, is paying, and will pay a price in terms of his own suffering. We can't fully know the painful history of others. But even the worst people can be our greatest teachers if they cause us to learn forgiveness.

4. *I must remain bitter to insure that it never happens again, until justice is secured.* Remembering and wisdom protect, not bitterness. Justice and protection can be sought with or without bitterness.

5. *Staying mad will get it out of my system.* Reliving and rehearsing anger keeps it in focus and causes us to be controlled by it.

6. *I'll betray myself or others if I drop the grudge.* We ask if there are better ways to show loyalty than infection with anger.

7. *I'll make myself so invulnerable and strong that no one can hurt me.* To be human is to love. To love is to be vulnerable. The only way to never be hurt is to avoid loving. It is possible to remain loving, but with greater wisdom regarding whom we choose to trust.

Whom to Forgive

Anger and other symptoms can be a cue and an opportunity to forgive all parties involved in your hurt. We might explore our life history and notice people along the way. It is good to start working on people responsible for traumatic offenses. Then we might work on forgiving those less directly involved such as those who failed to protect or support us. We can forgive ourselves. The skills we'll discuss can also be applied to other offenses from critical teachers to prejudiced people.

How to Forgive

1. *Ask:*
   - What percent of the offender's behavior can be explained by a desire to hurt you personally? What percent can be explained as a reflection of his own pain or frailties?
   - Am I prepared to condemn the offender's behavior but not the offender?
   - Am I open to learning ways to protect myself without bitterness?

- Could I envision releasing some of my anger and shifting my focus more to life's loveliness?
- Is it possible to relinquish some responsibility for settling the account? One person with a spiritual perspective found comfort in the suggestion that "The battle is not yours, but God's."[225]

2. *Decide to heal.* As Trout has noted, "The moment one definitely commits oneself, then Providence moves too."[226]

3. *Find constructive ways to identify and express all feelings.* The goal is not to rehearse the pain forever, but to release the infection and soothe the wound so that it can heal. Writing in journals, artistic expression, or confiding to another trusted person are some ways to do this.

4. *Rely on yourself to heal, not the offender.*

5. *Forgive as best you can.* Remember that forgiving is a difficult process that does not usually happen all at once or once and for all. Surges of negative feelings do not invalidate your progress. They may indicate the need for further healing. Do your best and go on living. Forgiveness may occur when we are not expecting it.

6. *After processing your feelings, try rituals to symbolize the release of your hurt.* For example, you might draw your pain on a balloon and release it into the sky.

7. *Discriminate.* Remember that not all offenders are unwilling or unable to respect you. Some people who hurt us are not willfully malicious. Many people will appreciate the chance to air differences and restore relationships.

Forgiveness imagery

1. *Identify a loving figure* (parent, relative, Deity, etc.)—someone who loves you and makes you feel safe, like someone important.

2. *Think of a person who has offended you.* Reflect upon the offense, assigning responsibility for the wrong they did.

3. *Express your pain in the presence of the loving figure.* Physically locate your feelings of rejection, inferiority, violated trust, anger, or other forms of hurt. Give the pain a shape and color. Imagine the love of that loving figure surrounding you and infusing the places that hurt.

4. *Imagine the offender's real life battles* (trials, challenges, difficulties). Imagine the adversity they are facing. What is it like to face it? Imagine them as a hurting child, perhaps a victim.

5. *Imagine their strong points.*

6. *Can you recall shared good times?* Joyful experiences? Ways they supported or made you feel good? This can sometimes account for part of the difficulty of letting go.

7. *Accept responsibility for taking offense.*

8. *Send your forgiveness and healing to the offender.* Imagine something nice happening to him, such as filling the gaps and needs of his childhood. Imagine wishing him well. See him filled with and behaving with loving-kindness.

9. *Scan your body for remaining hurt or heaviness.* Feel it lifting away from your body and taking shape in front of you. The loving figure pulls you through the hurt and heaviness, embraces you, and whispers kindly: "The hurting is healing. You are safe, loved, and protected now." You feel your entire body filled with peace.

Forgive in writing

1. Make a list of all the people you have not yet forgiven. For each person, complete this statement for each offense.

Dear_____,

I felt _____ when _____
    (hurt, angry, etc.)   *(describe what happened)*

because _____. I still feel _____.
    (why you felt as you did)   *(describe present feelings)*

If possible add an empathic thought that reflects the other's emotional state/view at the time, such as: "You were probably feeling pain/insecurity yourself at the time," or "I guess you thought harsh punishment was good discipline." Then, "I want to forgive you."

Signed _____

2. After completing Step 1 for each person, finish this sentence:

Dear_____,

To the best of my ability, I now choose to forgive you for all these hurts. I release my burden of ill will toward you now, and free you and me to live.

Signed _____

---

3. Some people find it useful to ritualistically burn their writings as a symbol of closure.

CHAPTER 38

Prolonged Exposure

As we have discussed, trying to avoid or forget traumatic memories does nothing to neutralize them. In fact, the more we fear and flee them, the more negative energy we give them, enabling them to remain so negatively charged. The opposite of avoidance is exposure, or fully confronting troublesome memories. Prolonged exposure is a method of inviting traumatic memories in a controlled way fully into our awareness in a safe environment.

In prolonged exposure we, bring *all* aspects of traumatic memories into awareness. When we stay with the memories we fear, we soon realize that they can't really hurt us; they are distressing but not dangerous. Confidence replaces fear and begins to neutralize the memories. When we connect those distressing memories to feelings of deep relaxation rather than more fear, the memories are neutralized further. Connecting traumatic memories to soothing emotions is called deconditioning. That is, the nervous system breaks the conditioned response of reacting to recalled memories with arousal. We are actually training our nervous system to be less sensitive to these memories, hence the process is sometimes called desensitization. Finally, exposure to all aspects of traumatic memories permit the memory material to be fully processed and integrated. Recall that intrusive memories usually do not contain all aspects of traumatic memories. If we were to permit full recall in a safe environment, the mind would have a chance to integrate these memories and place them in long-term memory. However, traumatic memories are typically avoided before integration occurs.

When we voluntarily let fears fully into awareness, some people will feel some relief right away. Some will feel troubled initially, much as Pennebaker found in those who began writing about their traumas. However, because processing is occurring, benefits might begin to become apparent fairly quickly, often within two to three weeks under certain conditions. (See cautions and considerations section, on page 301.)[227]

HOW IS PROLONGED EXPOSURE DONE[228]

1. *Prolonged exposure is done with a psychotherapist in up to fifteen exposure sessions.* Each session typically lasts sixty to a hundred and twenty minutes. Usually sessions are held once or twice a week.

2. *You start by making a hierarchy of distressing events.* Think of a ladder. At the top of the ladder is the most traumatic event that you experienced. At the bottom is the least traumatic event. Between these two endpoints are other traumatic events arranged in order. Or you might choose to break a traumatic event into parts, with the most distressing aspects at the top of the hierarchy. Assign a SUD rating to each rung (e.g., 0 = not at all distressing; 10 = most distressing).[229]

3. *Relax deeply.* Usually this is done with two easy deep breaths followed by progressive muscle relaxation. To deepen feelings of safety you might use safe place and/or pleasant memory imagery.

4. *Choose a starting point on the hierarchy.* Some wish to start at the highest rung, hoping that positive results will generalize. However, the potential for retraumatizing exists if memories flood and overwhelm awareness. Most approaches start at a rung associated with moderate levels of distress. This permits one to be challenged but not overwhelmed, while confidence is gained.

5. *Recount the selected event.* Tell what was happening before, during, and after. Use the first person and the present tense, as though it were happening now ("I'm walking to my car . . ."). Describe what you see, hear, smell, touch, and taste. Describe your body's reactions, your surroundings, weather, clothes, what you are thinking, feeling, and doing. Recall what the perpetrator or others are doing. Verbalizing seems to help integrate the material.
   - The therapist will help you set up the scene by giving some details, such as the date, and asks you to begin retelling. In the approach developed by Dr. Edna Foa, the client simply retells whatever details can be

tolerated for the first few times. Usually more details surface with re-peated tellings.

- With successive tellings, the therapist will prompt you to include more and more details. It is especially important to process the most distress-ing aspects of a memory, so-called "hot spots." Thus you will take more time with hot spots, slowing down and recalling more detail. Your ther-apist might prompt you to recall other aspects, such as feared conse-quences.
- If you finish retelling the story before time is up, go back and repeat it in even more detail. As additional details come to light, more process-ing occurs. Although this might be more distressing, eventually your nervous system will react less to the memories, a process known as habituation.
- Monitor SUDs every five to ten minutes. Your therapist will ask you to rate your discomfort quickly, without your leaving the scene. You will continue to retell the story until SUDs drop by half or to a mild to mod-erate distress level.

6. *End the exposure with relaxation.*

7. *Cognitive restructuring is done before and after exposure to eliminate dis-tortions that increase arousal* (e.g., "This shouldn't be so hard"; "The world is totally unsafe"), and to connect the memories with more adaptive thoughts (e.g., "It's okay that I need to work at this"; "The world is *some-times* unsafe."). Evidence for unproductive thoughts is tested and core be-liefs are uncovered. The amount of time spent in cognitive restructuring increases as the amount of detail retold increases.

8. *Your therapist will give you an audiotape of your recounting, and you'll lis-ten to it at least once per day for about thirty minutes.* As you listen new details might arise for processing, and you'll likely tend to get less aroused with repetition. Perform a relaxation strategy such as progressive muscle relaxation before you begin and after you listen to the tape. You might also wish to end with pleasant memory imagery. Do not listen to the tape be-fore bed because of its potential to trigger nightmares. Find a unique place to listen to the tape. You would not wish to associate negative emotions with places such as your bed, favorite sofa, or kitchen table. Instead find a neutral place, such as a chair in the corner of a room. Monitor your SUDs and notice decreases.

9. *Sometimes variations might be introduced to the exposure portion of therapy sessions.* Your therapist might ask you to project yourself into the future, imagine the worst case happening, and stay with it until even that can be tolerated (e.g., imagine that loved ones discover your secret and reject you). Exposure to feared situations can later be supplemented with role playing, where you practice coping in situations you'll likely confront to gain confidence.

10. *As soon as possible, you'll also confront in real life fearful situations that you've avoided.* You'll make a hierarchy and gradually encounter these situations, staying in them long enough to notice a drop in SUDs by at least half and/or for thirty to forty-five minutes to gain confidence. For example, rungs might include wearing clothes worn when one was traumatized and walking near the scene of the traumatic event if that is now safe to do. Before doing this real-life (in vivo) exposure work, review your coping skills. You might wish to carry flashcards with coping skills and adaptive thoughts. At first, your therapist or a skilled and trusted friend might accompany you.

11. *Remember the other strategies that you have learned thus far to feel safe, reduce arousal, and lift your mood.* Use these regularly between sessions.

CAUTIONS AND CONSIDERATIONS

1. *Prolonged exposure is somewhat controversial.*[230] If done too soon or too fast, it can retraumatize the client.[231] Because of this potential, some experts feel that it should only be tried when other approaches have not worked effectively, and only then once a strong therapeutic alliance has been formed. Other experts feel that prolonged exposure can sometimes lead to greater, more lasting improvements than some of the other strategies typically tried, suggesting its use in combination with other strategies.

2. *Prolonged exposure is contraindicated for people with current substance abuse, a history of impulsivity, risk for suicide, ongoing life crises, difficulty using imagery, uncontrolled depression, inability to tolerate intense arousal, cardiovascular risks, and psychotic or personality disorders.*

3. *Prolonged exposure is indicated for people who are motivated, who become aroused when exposed to specific memories, and who can describe concisely the traumatic event.* Before using, insure that your symptoms are stabilized,

that you have good self-esteem, and that you have developed a range of coping skills.[232]

4. *Prolonged exposure has mostly been used with combat and rape.* It is not yet demonstrated to be effective with child abuse. Possibly, it is best used for single or time-limited events, in combination with other strategies.

5. *Don't allow your SUDs to get so high that processing is blocked.* If retelling becomes too stressful:

   • Slow down the retelling.

   • Recall helpful reminders, which can be written on flash cards, such as: This is difficult, not dangerous—I can handle it; This is just a memory—the event is past; I know how to calm myself down.[233]

   • Remind yourself of the positive aspects of the traumatic event as well as the negatives. For example, you might recall what you did to survive or help others. You might recall that blood is also a sign of life and creation, not just death and hurt.[234]

   • Try to calm yourself without avoiding the thoughts.

   • If you have to distract from the process, calm down and compliment yourself for doing as much as you did.

6. *Prolonged exposure is usually not effective with unresolved guilt, anger, or sadness.* Process these first before trying it.

7. *Don't expect to not have distress after prolonged exposure, just more reasonable levels of it.*

CHAPTER 39

Complementary Approaches

ACTION-BASED PROGRAMS[235]

Contemplate the children who enter the world. They are enthused and full of adrenaline as they anticipate new adventures. They relish the world which is full of things to discover, explore, and master. They take delight in new challenges and spontaneously play with them and with others. Trauma elicits a similar kind of physical arousal but with very negative feelings. Action-based programs recreate this type of physical arousal, but this time surrounded by some of the positive feelings and experiences that we just contemplated.

Many action-based programs trace back to Outward Bound. This program includes action experiences in nature such as hiking, mastering outdoor obstacles, and working together in teams in a safe emotional climate. Such emotionally positive experiences rekindle positive emotions that exist in pre-trauma memory, or in some cases provides new positive emotional experiences. For example, an Outward Bound program for combat veterans leads small groups into the wilderness for four days where group members might engage in hiking, climbing, rappelling, negotiating rope obstacle courses, practicing survival skills, and white-water rafting. A variation might include a helicopter ride, this time with a sense of joy and safety, not fear. Throughout the experience a trained leader creates a compassionate emotional climate and sense of camaraderie, where thoughts and feelings can be safely discussed among group members. Individuals are encouraged to participate in the activities but no one is forced beyond his comfort zone. Leaders at some point might tactfully discuss participants' options, reasons for their choices, the effects of those choices, and how similar choices might affect everyday life. The program frequently results in favorable outcomes, such as:[236]

- An openness to trust others again (this follows from the strong bonds that naturally form as, for example, group members helping each other overcome physical obstacles).

- A feeling of success, accomplishment, overcoming adversity, enhanced self-esteem, and empowerment.

- A recapturing of the positive qualities of soldiering (courage, triumph, selflessness, self-confidence, dedication, determination, interdependence, compassion, responsibility, brotherhood, power, competence) without the horrors of war.

- A sense of being energized by nature, physical activity, and camaraderie.

- An awakened sense that one can grow and change their life.

Although action-based programs are not therapy or substitutes for therapy, they can be effective adjuncts to therapy. They might help to prepare some individuals for therapy or expedite the healing process.

TWELVE-STEP RECOVERY PROGRAM

Dr. Joel O. Brende, M.D., has developed a twelve-step recovery program as a support for those with a spiritual perspective. The program, in essence, invites God, as individually understood, into the recovery process. Participants explore the Twelve Spiritual Steps, which are:[237]

1. Acknowledge traumas and seek God's help.

2. Seek meaning.

3. Seek healing in order to trust.

4. Seek self understanding and openness to change.

5. Seek understanding and control of anger.

6. Seek understanding and control of fear and helplessness.

7. Seek resolution of guilt through forgiveness and love.

8. Seek healing in grief.

9. Seek to surrender self-destructive tendencies and commit to life.

10. Seek to replace revenge with justice and forgiveness.

11. Seek knowledge and direction in order to find a renewed purpose in life.

12. Seek to love.

Consistent with Alcoholics Anonymous, participants are encouraged to make meaningful changes while turning over to Deity with an attitude of acceptance that which cannot be presently changed.

Many other twelve-step groups, tracing back to the AA model, can help survivors with specific problems related to PTSD such as substance abuse, gambling, or eating disorders. See page 398 in Appendix 10 for Dr. Brende's Trauma Recovery Publications and locations and phone numbers for a variety of twelve-step program headquarters.

PART VI

Moving On

CHAPTER 40

Transitioning

The life you have led doesn't need to be the only life you have.

—Anna Quindlen[238]

Ponder what you were like before the trauma. It might help to look at a photo taken before the trauma, if you have one. What interested you? What got you excited and curious? What made you laugh? Cry? What did you consider beautiful? What was your sense of spirituality like? What were some of the qualities that you liked about yourself? What were some that you'd wished to improve?

Then consider the trauma and the ways that it understandably affected you. Perhaps much of your growth and development seemed to be put on hold.

Now ponder your future. What would you be wishing to feel more of? What would you wish to be doing and thinking? What important aspects of your life do you wish to rekindle? On what new adventures do you wish to embark?

Trauma changes people. We are never quite the same afterward. On the other hand, in many ways we are still the same people—older, wiser, able to pick ourselves up, dust ourselves off, and get back on our life's journey; able to overcome despair. Often we have learned better ways to cope in similar situations.

Trauma is but a detour over which the human spirit triumphs. As you continue to heal, the present and future will become increasingly important to you. Should distressing feelings recur, you now know that this might simply be a cue to process unprocessed material. Distressing feelings might also signal new opportunities for growth. This part of the book will explore ways to move beyond recovery. As you progress through the remaining chapters, you might consider how you will choose to recapture your dreams and/or create new ones. You might begin to create a time line from now into the future. As you read ahead, you might add goals and dreams to the time line as they occur to you. You might also consider starting a letter to a loved one, written a few years in the future, telling of the positive changes that have happened.

Interestingly, research[239] has shown that trauma cannot only be overcome, but can actually have positive effects on one's life. In fact, people who experienced traumatic events reported more growth than those who did not.[240] Such positive effects include:

- *New possibilities* (discovery of meaning, interests, life path; desire to leave a legacy for children)

- *Personal strength* (inner strength discovered and developed, improved self-esteem, self-assurance, confidence to survive that generalizes to other situations, accepting the need to protect self, replacing simplistic or naive ways of thinking with more adaptive views)

- *Spiritual change* (stronger faith, greater insights, less attachment to material things)

- *Appreciation of life* (reordered priorities, living life to the fullest, slowing down, spending more time with family, seeing everyday hassles in perspective, seeing what's really important, finding joy in the simple things)

- *Relating to others* (greater compassion and desire to lift others, appreciation for others, relationships more valued, accepting the need to trust others and disclose, accepting the need to be assertive in relationships, fewer petty quarrels)

Contemplating the positive in the traumatic experience in no way minimizes one's suffering. Neither is simplistic positive thinking implied. What is suggested is that we see accurately all aspects of the trauma, so that it might be better integrated. We deny neither negative nor positive aspects. Unfortunately, some victims see only the negatives. Scurfield[241] suggests how each negative in combat can be balanced by a positive aspect. These examples are easily adapted to other forms of trauma (see Table 40.1).

In recalling traumatic events, people are not usually glad that they occurred. But they can be glad for what they have done with their lives in the aftermath. As Sipprelle reported:[242]

Table 40.1
THE NEGATIVE AND POSITIVE ASPECTS OF COMBAT

Negative Aspect	Positive Aspect
Sense of loss, grief, hurt	The extraordinary sense of comradeship experienced in combat suggests that the veteran has already experienced deep friendship and therefore has the potential to do so again
Confusion, questioning of values and life direction	Healthy questioning and reaffirmation of one's values
Difficulties in dealing with "everyday" stresses	Knowing that one can remain committed and proficient under very trying circumstances
Fall in self-esteem due to imperfect behavior and difficulty in adjusting to post-trauma life	Appreciation of the strength it took to survive both the war and the postwar recovery years
Disturbing loss of trust and faith in the country's institutions	Healthy questioning of those institutions, realizing that when government becomes immoral, everyone suffers
Intolerance for insensitive, impersonal authority figures and institutions	Strong convictions that one deserves to be treated with respect and dignity
Isolation and alienation from others, who are assumed incapable of understanding the trauma experience	Shared bonding among veterans that would not be possible without having the combat experience[243]
Loss of belief in God, religion, or faith in humanity	Marked positive changes in outlook, expansiveness of world view, profound spiritual/religious insights; potential for religious rebirth
Dwelling on the fact that one should have died; resentment over suffering	Concept of "bonus time"—to consider survival extraordinary and to appreciate and take advantage of limited time on earth
Fear of risks or danger, or being "adrenaline junkie" who is constantly exposed to dangerous, needless risk	Appreciation of thrilling and peak experiences that did occur in the war, and the willingness to experience healthy and safe stimulation today
Bemoaning and resenting one's postwar difficulties and deprevations	Profound appreciation of freedom and the ability to persevere despite pain
Painful memories	Appreciating the ability to remember lessons
Accepting total or exaggerated degree of responsibility for war zone trauma	Realization and appreciation that situations are often complex, with diverse influences to consider

Fifty years after surviving the Bataan death march and a subsequent forty-two-month internment at slave labor in Japanese POW camps, a seventy-year-old veteran was interviewed. He stated that he would not repeat his experiences for a million dollars, but recalled them as the most enriching, ennobling experiences of his entire life.

We can ask ourselves, "What frame of mind would it take to view my trauma this way?" Some people figure out a way to change the trauma from a stumbling block to a building block.[244] Gradually, perhaps imperceptibly, a victim of trauma can transition to survivor and then thriver. A victim is one who merely undergoes a traumatic event. Surviving suggests a certain fighting spirit and determination to keep going. Thriving implies that one is living well. From the perspective of experience, thrivers have learned to appreciate themselves, others, and life. They have learned the art of being happy despite adversity. They have learned optimism. Optimism does not mean that one expects everything that happens to be wonderful. It means that one thinks, "No matter what happens, I can still find something to enjoy, to find satisfaction in." Optimists find and accept partial, imperfect solutions. Optimists, therefore, can examine negative events and accurately see their positive potential.

CONSTRUING BENEFIT IN TRAUMA

Make three columns on a blank sheet of paper. In the first column, list the negative impacts trauma has had on your life. In the second column, list the positive impacts that have occurred as a result. In the third column, list the positive things that could still occur in your life. Keep this exercise in your journal. Refer to it often to reinforce your sense of optimism.

THE ELDERLY CHILD REMEMBERS

Trauma therapist Beverly James uses this strategy to help victims of childhood trauma rehearse a happy future. This strategy, however, adapts well to survivors of any trauma. She explains that this dramatic strategy "playfully allows the (survivor) to imagine a future for herself in which she has integrated her traumatic experience into the fabric of her interesting life. It is best accomplished with a small group . . . joining the (survivor) in treatment in an individual session. It is helpful to have on hand some amount of dramatic play props for both (males and females), such as hats, masks, scarves, jewelry, dishes, building materials, make-up, etc." The strategy is explained as follows[245]:

Today we are going to imagine ourselves in a future time. You are going to be wonderful old ladies (or old guys) who are hanging out together having a good time. You have been successful in taking care of yourselves, in following your careers, and in raising your families. This is a time in your lives when you are very creative. There are many things you enjoy doing. You work part of the time and find your work interesting. Although you are old now, you have kept your bodies active and healthy. You have good friends that you enjoy spending time with, and today you are visiting with some of these good friends. You are in a restaurant [on a mountain top, fishing, on an airplane . . .] and are talking about your lives. You are going to talk about a long, long time ago when you were about [use current age] years old and feeling bad [worried, scared . . .] about the [trauma, the future . . .]. You are going to talk about how you felt way back then, how you got stronger, and then how you went on in your life to be successful. Talk about how it is for you now that you are an older person who is thinking back so long ago. And how does it feel when, as an older person, you think back to the (trauma) and remember that it was an important part, but just one part, of your very interesting life. First, let's get some props and costumes together. Should I be the waitress [friend, ranger, boat-cleaner]? Are we ready? Let's begin. Action!

CHAPTER 41

Intimacy and Sexuality

With sufficient healing, the areas of intimacy and sexuality can become increasingly meaningful in the lives of PTSD survivors. It is fitting, then, to explore these areas now.

SNAPSHOT LENS

Following a traumatic event, victims tend to see the world through a new lens. They see themselves as worthless and undeserving. Others now seem untrustworthy, and relationships dangerous, while sex is confusingly different. It is as though a snapshot has been taken through a clouded lens. A moment in time determines the view that persists. To retain the old lens is to remain a victim. To carry on despite the clouded lens is to be a survivor. To clean off the lens and take a fresh look is to thrive.

We have talked about gaining an accurate view of self when we explored self-esteem building. We'll now separate the two areas of intimacy and sexuality—two areas of conflict and confusion for PTSD survivors—so that we might see them clearly and be liberated to create new and satisfying experiences. Each new experience is an opportunity to create a new, positive memory. We want to scrub off our lenses on self, relationships, and sex—all of which interrelate. The thriver learns to view the self as capable, strong, good, worthy, and deserving of happiness. Relationships are seen as an opportunity to joyfully bond in a loving, committed, enduring relationship, and sex is seen as a beautiful aspect of a loving relationship.

INTIMACY

Intimacy means that we share what we are really like, who we really are, and what we have been through. Two people are intimate when they truly know each other and, it is suggested, like and accept one another. Sharing thoughts, feelings, values, and sometimes sexual love are ways to be intimate. In addition to making life more joyful, intimacy is important in PTSD recovery. People who actively connect with others following a traumatic event seem to fare better. For example, Holocaust survivors who made an effort to get involved with others had better mental health than those who did not. These people formed social groups with friends, family, and neighbors. They self-disclosed or confided what was happening in their lives—their pains, concerns, even finances. They used the telephone, visits, and letters to stay in touch, and provided support for their comrades. They also accepted support from others. The researchers concluded that staying isolated is bad for your health. A positive finding in this research was that survivors were more likely to help out family and friends than those who did not endure trauma.[246]

Unfortunately, PTSD survivors seem to have more relationship difficulties such as divorce and avoidance of intimacy. Some appear to marry in hopes of recreating their pre-trauma life[247] or escaping difficult circumstances before sufficient healing has taken place. For some, fear of intimacy interferes with connectedness. As one survivor said, "I heard that love casts our fear, but in my case fear cast out love." Sheehan has identified five fears that interfere with intimacy and which must be neutralized in order for intimacy to grow. Otherwise, survivors will sabotage intimacy in ways that include workaholism, picking fights, abandoning their partner, or drinking. As you'll see, these fears make perfect sense for one who has survived trauma so be understanding toward yourself. The fears are:[248]

1. *Loss of control.* In intimacy, we open ourselves up emotionally. This means that we are prone to emotional intrusions of unresolved memories. This can lead to avoidance or anger to prevent loss of control.[249] It is logical, then, to sufficiently heal so that intimacy might progress. In some cases, survivors fear being controlled by their partner. This follows logically from trauma where choice and control were taken away, especially when it was another human wresting control from the victim. The antidote is to find a trustworthy person(s) who can be viewed as an ally and teammate. In such a relationship, we gradually learn to relinquish or share some control.

2. *Abandonment.* We manifest this fear by never loving again, engaging in casual sex without emotional involvement, being distant or revengeful in relationships, or overreacting with clinging, jealous insecurity. This follows

from being left by significant people, or by their failure to protect the victim.

3. *Rejection.* To protect against this fear the survivor might not let herself be fully known, or will reject the other person first. This fear arises from the feeling of being damaged and unlovable, and by the perception that people would reject her if they knew her secret.

4. *Attack.* In close relationships, people are more vulnerable to put-downs, teasing, or other abusive acts. Such behaviors seem like a betrayal of the unspoken pledge to support and protect one's loved one. One who has become sensitized to danger will have an even greater need for safety. Because of this vulnerability, survivors are likely to feel threatened by even small disagreements. A "you are with me or against me" mindset might develop which makes communication difficult.

5. *One's own tendency to hurt others.* Survivors may not see their anger, disappointment, or hurt as normal feelings that can be constructively dealt with, or they may lack the skills to do so.

Intimacy is more likely to flourish if survivors:

1. *Accept the fears.* View them as normal, understandable consequences of trauma without judging yourself. Normalizing fears is one way to neutralize them.

2. *Replace ideas that block intimacy:*

   • *All men/women are no good.* This idea would lead one to either avoid all intimacy, or to permit someone untrustworthy to enter one's boundaries, since there is apparently no hope of finding someone decent. In truth, some people do not reject, abandon, attack, or take advantage of others weaknesses. Some people respect and honor others, even with their imperfections. This is the essence of love.

   • *Nobody has gone through the terrible things I have gone through. Nobody can relate to me.* Even among young, apparently healthy college students you will typically find a wide range of severe traumas. No matter what you have gone through, many others have experienced similar traumatic events. People exist who will relate to you with compassion. Some people have learned this compassion through the things they have suffered, while others have learned compassion by being raised in loving homes.

- *Nobody could accept me if they knew what I've been through.* Some people may not. When trusted with secrets, however, some people will accept and respect the survivor more.
- *It is demeaning to be flawed, and foolish to reveal vulnerabilities.* Everyone is flawed, and sharing our true feelings is the essence of wholesome intimacy.
- *I can't burden others with my problems.* If people care about you, they will want to know about the bad times as well as the good. People in high-quality relationships create time for humor, play, and affection. And when discussion of difficult emotions is needed, they make time for that, too.

3. *Develop communication skills.* Visit your library or talk with your counselor. There are many, many effective skills for resolving differences peacefully, expressing affection verbally and nonverbally, expressing negative feelings constructively, complimenting, and standing up for yourself. (See the books *Fighting for Your Marriage* and *Getting the Love You Want*, in Appendix 10.)

4. *Gradually risk and discern.* As wisely as possible, involve trusted people in your life. Allow them to help to meet your needs. With the right person, disclosing your true self can be pleasantly surprising. Hiding your true self creates barriers. As fears are permitted expression and are respected, trust builds. The climate of safety that develops also fosters the expression of positive emotions. It is possible to be known emotionally without disclosing details that are too uncomfortable to discuss. Test the waters and discern how the other person responds. Caution may indeed be wise if the other person is too defensive to reciprocate, is judgmental or abusive, or will not keep confidences. Heed those warnings. When you discern, however, that the other person is safe, begin to accept nurturing in the form of emotional support, listening, and compliments.

5. *Notice how conflicts are handled.* Conflict in relationships is normal and to be expected. However, it is the way conflict is handled, and not the presence of conflict, that has been found to predict marital success. Attacking verbally or physically, withdrawing, sulking, threatening, criticizing, raising the voice, manipulating, dishonesty, and jealousy are styles that create interpersonal distance. Approaches that favor intimacy include good

listening skills, sticking to issues, kind humor, patience, calmness, emotional openness, sharing control, complimenting, empathy, and willingness to tolerate differences.

6. *Consider picking up where they left off before the trauma.* This could mean building the type of healthy relationships that were enjoyed before the trauma, or cultivating better ones. Ponder the kind of relationship that you'd enjoy. Try to create a vision of what it would be like.

RESTORING WHOLESOME SENSUALITY AND SEXUALITY

Our bodies are part of the way we experience being alive, and sexuality is an important aspect of this experience. Bodies allow us to feel the wind through our hair and the joy of a warm embrace. Yet commonly, people with PTSD feel shamed emotionally. Because the mind and body are connected, they also feel physically and sexually shamed. Physical and sexual sensations that were once innocent and wonderful become conflicted and confusing. Understandably, sexual difficulties often arise.

Several studies have indicated that males and females with PTSD are more likely to experience sexual problems than those without PTSD. These problems include sexual disinterest, aversion, dissatisfaction, and performance difficulties (erectile problems, premature ejaculation, painful intercourse, impaired arousal or climax). For example, in one study 80 percent of Vietnam veterans were found to have clinically relevant sexual problems.[250] It is common for survivors to feel anxiety, disgust, shame, and a devalued body image during sex.

Sexual difficulties are certainly likely if the traumatic event involved some form of sexual abuse, although other forms of trauma produce similar difficulties. For example, survivors who were abused in any way (sexually, emotionally, physically) commonly feel shamed emotionally and sexually. Beautiful women or handsome men might not feel attractive despite positive feedback from others. If bodies were treated as objects in the past, it is difficult to see them now as beautiful. They may be driven to have a perfect body. Yet despite successful exercise and dieting they still feel ashamed, dirty, and ugly outside and in. Victims might find ways to avoid sexual relations by wearing unattractive or drab clothes, gaining weight, mutilating their bodies, or developing psychosomatic illnesses.

Following sexual assault, sex itself can become a trigger. It is now associated with humiliation, exploitation, danger, secretiveness, and shame. Even if the present partner is trusted, the smell of semen might trigger painful memories. Likewise, certain ways of being touched—even nonsexual touches—or certain positions taken by the partner during lovemaking might trigger traumatic memories. If the victim climaxed during rape, then climaxing becomes associated with shame. The victim may have dissociated from her body during the trauma, and might again dissociate when her present partner becomes aroused. She may see the face of the rapist in her husband even though the rape occurred years ago and the husband is loving and devoted. So it is understandable that the victim might avoid sex, touch, and intimacy, and find it difficult to relax and enjoy sexual relations. Others may be drawn to sex in unhealthy relationships (a futile form of repetition compulsion) in an attempt to "make sex right" again. (It doesn't work because the context is all wrong.) Some feel too shattered to resist manipulative lovers as unhealthy sex in unhealthy relationships maintains the problem.

Emotional numbing, depression, and substance abuse also help to explain why sexual difficulties can arise in all forms of trauma. As with other areas in PTSD, we can pick up where we left off in our development as regards wholesome sensuality and sexuality. The transition period is an excellent time to do this.

Understanding and Neutralizing Disgust

Along with fear, disgust is another emotion that is commonly fused with traumatic memory material. It is helpful to understand this emotion as a way to neutralize it.

Disgust is a strong emotion which, like other emotions, can serve a protective purpose—in this case, keeping something away that is harmful. With permission, we'll explore some essential concepts from William I. Miller's *Anatomy of Disgust*.[251]

Disgust conveys a "strong aversion to something perceived as dangerous because of its powers to contaminate, infect, or pollute by proximity, contact, or ingestion." Other words for disgusting are repulsive, revolting, and abhorrent. Disgust is close to sentiments of contempt, loathing, hatred, horror, even fear. Disgust is often accompanied by feelings of uneasiness, panic, or incompetence—particularly if the disgusting object caused us to feel helpless in the past. The emotion of disgust may be accompanied with physical sensations of nausea, queasiness, or sick feeling; "it makes my skin crawl" or "it gives me the creeps."

It is normal to feel disgust. Disgust rules mark the boundaries of self; they keep out what is threatening. The relaxing of these rules marks privilege, intimacy, duty, and caring. Thus, the initial disgust with body functions or parts (e.g., menstruation, odors, or hair) is overcome as a "prelude to normal sexual behavior."

Certain objects, such as decaying garbage, pose obvious threats of contamination. Their odors, sights, or tastes might be described as "fetid, foul, stink, stench, rancid, vile, revolting, nauseating, sickening."

The fear of disgust is not just that the body will be contaminated, but also that the soul will become dirty inside. Thus defects of character can seem disgusting—vulgar. Think of sexual assailants in rape. It is not just that perpetrators "mock principles we feel should be better served; it is that they impose vices on us: distrustfulness, cynicism, and paranoia." This is why it is normal to feel disgusted following rape. It is not sex per se that disgusts, but sex in the context of exploitation. Sex is used to defile, and it is natural to assume that sex could do so again. Lost perhaps is the perception that sex in a different context and setting could also lift the individual. Sex out of place, without love, is disgusting. To say it another way, sex can be uplifting, wholesome, and enjoyable when experienced in a committed, loving, and responsible relationship. It is normal to be repulsed by sex that is misused for selfish pleasure, domination, power, or ego gratification.

Disgust by association.   Like fear, disgust has a strong tendency to fuse with memories in confusing ways. For example, disgusting smells are associated with shame and immorality (e.g., "I stink"). Strong sexual smells that are disgusting in the context of rape might then also become fused with shame.

Disgust can become state-dependent. That is, any present situation that disgusts (defecation, present sex, disgusting entertainment) can trigger a full blown disgust/shame reaction. It is natural, then, that sex will be aversive and avoided. Instead of being a source of satisfaction and beauty, it brings back uncomfortable feelings. Because of the proximity of the sex organs to the anus, sex can become confused with decay and its odors so that all parts of the body in the genital region become devalued.

Another infrequently mentioned aspect of disgust is that we tend to view our bodies as we view ourselves. If people view themselves badly (i.e., disgusting), then their orifices and secretions are viewed as disgusting and likely to repulse a lover. (This fear of repulsing is challenged by engaging in a sexual relationship in the context of love, trust, and dignity.)

The positive side of disgust.   As Miller observes, disgust can benefit humans. Disgust can help us avoid what is harmful and seek what is elevating. "Morality, cleanliness, and loathing of cruelty depend on it." Indeed, we "recoil from the stench of sinful deeds." If we are disgusted by certain behaviors, it shows that we still have an appreciation of good behavior. Disgust with misused sex and bad character means we still have an appreciation for good character and sex used within a healthy context. In fact, walling off sexuality is a way to protect it until it is safe to experience in a safe context.

We note that disgust for certain things is not necessarily static. As we mentioned, initial disgust with the human body is overcome as a prelude to normal sexual behavior. Anything that was once beautiful and pure can become disgusting, and vice versa. A rose is beautiful and decaying garbage is not. But the beautiful rose eventually decays, and the decaying garbage can eventually become the soil used to grow a rose.[252] Disgust can be neutralized and modified, although the imprint of disgust might not change overnight. Miller notes that love enables people to overcome disgust.

Strategies for Rebuilding Wholesome Sensuality and Sexuality[253]

1. *Normalize the genital area.* Survivors need to relearn that the genitals are normal, matter-of-fact parts of their bodies. James approaches this process in a straightforward, playful way with her young clients. Following a discussion of appropriate names for body parts, James explains:[254]

   First of all, let's take "butts." Do you realize that everyone in the world has a butt? What good is a butt? You're right, it's good for sitting on. What would it be like if people didn't have a butt? They couldn't sit down. There'd be no chairs in the world. Everyone would lie down a lot. What would cars look like? What else is the butt good for? What comes out of the butt? If we didn't have a butt, then poop would come out somewhere else. Where could that be? What would that be like? What would bathrooms be like?

   [A similar process would continue for "vagina" and "penis." The message to be left with the child is that all humans have these things, they are efficiently designed for their unique functions, and they are neither glorious nor shameful, that is, "parts are parts."]

2. *Neutralize feelings of disgust.*

- Realize that sexual abuse temporarily contaminates the body, but not the soul, unless we take in the message, "I am only an object."

- Consider disgust normal without judging yourself. Look at disgust and objectively examine what it is saying. Is something disgusting because it is presently dangerous, or does it just trigger memories of the past? Ask, "Will this really contaminate me, or is it just an unpleasant thought?"

- Discriminate. Break down overwhelming feelings of disgust into parts to gain a sense of control over those feelings. What specifically is disgusting? Is it all aspects of sex or just certain behaviors? Is it all touch or just certain types? Distinguish disgust related to sex from disgust related to other body functions. You might try writing about this to gain a greater sense of control.

- Separate disgust with sex from shame. Remember that shame is feeling bad for who we are at the core, rather than feeling bad for what we did or for what was done to us. Feeling polluted by your own or others' behavior signals a need for cleansing and healing, not a destruction of self. Regarding shame, a survivor of rape might ask, "Am I bearing the costs for another's crime?"

- Neutralize disgust with love for self and others whom you choose to let in. Think, perhaps, of your affection for a newborn baby or a trusted lover.

- Shift your focus. Don't focus exclusively on the negative, but also see the beauty. Ask yourself, "What else is there to notice?" Look for opportunities to appreciate the beauty of the human body. Tasteful art is one way to do this. Enjoy the curves and proportions of the body; notice how beautiful they are. Also notice nonsexual aspects of people. Just appreciate the wholesome beauty of people: enjoy the countenances, colors of dress, overall appearance, or personality. Wholesome sensuality is broader than sexuality. Sensuality applies to using all the senses to enjoy the pleasures of the world. Thus, we can enjoy a sunset, a flower, or a good meal, too.

- Create a wholesome vision of sex within the context of a committed, loving relationship. What would that relationship be like? Would it be marked by mutual love, respect, trust, tenderness, laughter, admiration, and security? More simply, perhaps you just treat each other well. Imagine that you and your partner know each other not just physically, but emotionally, philosophically, and creatively as well. You might view sex as the culminating expression of a good relationship, one marked by hugs, good conversation, and play. You might envision comforting and pleasuring your mate, while receiving the same in return. If desired, you might envision sex for the purpose of creating babies who are loved, nurtured, and trained so that they grow into decent people who are good company. It might help to ponder the differences between unhealthy and healthy sexuality, as summarized in Table 41.1.

3. *Learn the paradoxes of satisfying sexuality, suggested by Engel:*[255]
   - The harder you try to make something happen sexually, the less will happen. [In other words, relax. Go slow. Allow whatever happens to happen. Have reasonable expectations. Take a moratorium on genital sex if you wish, and focus on other aspects of physical intimacy—touching, stroking, holding, hugging, kissing, fondling, and other expressions of affection that many people find just as satisfying as intercourse. This period of abstinence can allow other satisfying aspects of a relationship to grow without pressure to perform.]
   - The way to cure your sexual problem is to not try to cure it.
   - The way to be able to have sexual activity whenever you want is to learn to recognize when you do *not* want to have sex. [Recognize when sex does not feel right, and say so.]
   - The way to relax is to learn to recognize when you are anxious.
   - The way to learn to concentrate is to recognize when you are not concentrating.
   - The way to be able to please your partner is to learn what feels good to *you*.

4. *The sensate focus is useful for a wide range of sexual problems, and is especially useful for PTSD.* This technique enables partners to learn or relearn to enjoy the simple act of touch, without the expectation or pressure to perform sexually. Sensate focus is so called because the person focuses only on the sensation of touch. Because the focus is in the present and grounded in physical reality, there is less tendency to dissociate. The directions are:[256]
   - As closely as possible, you'll focus on touching your partner's skin. You will focus just on the exact point of contact between your fingertips, hand, and forearm, and your partner's skin, noticing what it is like to touch and be touched by your partner's skin.

Table 41.1
UNHEALTHY VS. HEALTHY SEXUALITY

Unhealthy Sexuality	Healthy Sexuality
feels secretive and shameful	feels good; is celebrative; adds to self-esteem
is illicit, stolen, exploitive, abusive, and/or demeaning; the victim is used, then abandoned or dominated	is healing; has no victims; loves, lifts, trusts, cares for, and protects the other person
compromises values and spirituality	deepens meaning and spirituality; adds to the feeling of closeness to God
fear provides excitement	shared vulnerability and regard provide excitement and deep satisfaction
reenacts childhood abuses	cultivates a sense of being an adult
disconnects one from oneself	adds to one's sense of self
is self-destructive and dangerous	enhances the sense of safety and security
uses conquest, control, and power; an "I-It" relationship	uses love; honors the partner; shares control in a meaningful way; an "I-Thou" relationship
pain is covered, medicated, escaped, or killed in a sterile way	pain is surrounded and infused with love and intimacy
is dishonest	is responsible to both parties; enhances integrity
becomes routine, grim, joyless	is stimulating, challenging, playful, and fun; becomes more interesting as feelings are honestly shared
requires a double life	integrates the most authentic parts of the self
demands perfection	accepts the imperfect
is separate from intimacy and a loving relationship; confuses sex with caring	exists within a loving, respectful relationship
creates distance or enmeshment/engulfment	creates comfortable intimacy
overemphasizes superficiality (looks, talents, etc.)	is more concerned with feeling comfortable with one's partner and the partner's goodness, kindness, and decency
overemphasizes fears from the past	focuses primarily on building the relationship
is selfish, focused only on self-gratification	also considers the partner's pleasure and well-being

Adapted with permission from Carnes, P., with J. M. Moriarity. 1997. Sexual Anorexia: Overcoming Sexual Self-Hatred. Center City, Minn.: Hazelden. Copyright ©1997 by Patrick Carnes.

- With tender, caring, gentle movements, caress your partner. That is, using the flat of your fingertips, the flat of the hand or fingers, palms, wrist, or even the forearm, slowly stroke your partner's skin in long, sweeping strokes. The strokes are much lighter than a massage.
- This technique is intended for your pleasure as well as your partner's, so don't worry about doing it "right." Just focus on your own feelings and assume that your partner is okay. Your partner just relaxes passively and enjoys the experience, focusing only on the point of contact.
- Go very, very slowly. Then cut the speed in half. Focus only on the point of contact.
- Relax and be silent. There is no speaking, groans or moans, or sexual movements.
- Afterward, honestly discuss what the experience was like. Honestly discussing what was enjoyable and what was not increases trust and communication.

Without pressure to perform, this technique often helps partners to feel valued for things other than being a sexual partner.

5. *Distinguish sex from love, affection, and attention.* When we see the differences clearly, we can better choose how to experience sex in the context desired.

6. *Prepare for flashbacks during sex.*[257] First, ask your partner for help. Communicate to your partner what you have experienced and how it has affected you. Teach your partner how to recognize signs of flashbacks, and to check it out if you appear to be experiencing one. Instruct him/her to gently bring you back to the present and comfort you with comments such as, "It's me, you're safe now" and to wait until flashbacks stop to respond sexually. Should a flashback occur, open your eyes and notice where you are. Notice that your partner is not the perpetrator—notice specific differences between your partner and the perpetrator and between the present surroundings and the place where the sexual assault happened. Use easy deep breaths and calming self talk to relax, or focus on a symbol of safety or security.

7. *Discuss using the rewind technique with your therapist, rewinding to a point where sex was viewed positively.* Sex, here, could simply mean viewing someone as attractive or beautiful.

8. *Create a collage of wholesome sexuality and sensuality.* You might include images that remind you of your pretrauma views, as well as images of what you wish to create. You might include pictures of a loving parent with child, the opposite sex with a kind face, a person at home in nature, or beautiful art which celebrates the beauty of the body.

9. *Use eye movements to integrate the past and present.* Create a wholesome vision of sexuality—where sex is seen within the context of love. You might, for example, imagine a couple embracing warmly as they watch a sunset. Perhaps you'll use an image from your collage. Then pick or create a wholesome image of sexuality from a time before the trauma. Think of the first image, then think of the image from the past. Then do a set of eye movements to reinforce the connection.

10. *Somatic trauma therapy is useful for someone who froze during some form of sexual assault.* An actual safe place with an actual safe person is imagined. Then the person lies down and pummels a mattress with feet and arms, and visualizes running to the safe place. This tends to loosen the traumatic freezing and infuses the memory with a feeling of contact rather than isolation.[258]

11. *When women experience painful intercourse, practicing Kegel exercises, which strengthen the pelvic floor muscles, are often helpful.* The pubococcygeal muscle tightens when the vagina and rectum are contracted, as when stopping the flow of urine or when going up in an elevator. The feeling of relaxing this muscle is similar to an elevator going down. Ten repetitions done two to three times daily over at least six weeks is recommended to increase muscle strength. During intercourse it may be best if the female is on top of her partner in order to maintain the ability to stop if intercourse becomes painful. The female tenses those muscles and feels the sensation of contraction, as she says to herself, "Up the elevator." She says to herself, "Down the elevator" as tension is released. A side benefit of the Kegel exercises is that they help to prevent incontinence with aging or pregnancy.[259]

12. *Consider trying healing sexual imagery or stories.* One imagery approach utilizes the assumption that confronting painful memories dissipates their control over the victim. This approach involves four steps:
    a. Recall negative sexual experiences and their results.

b. String these negative experiences together and form an image that represents them.

c. Stay with the image. Let it settle. Go into it.

d. Notice what comes into your awareness.

For example, one survivor's negative sexual memories included experiences of abuse, being used and rejected by lovers, and seeking empty sexual liaisons to escape her pain of loneliness. The image that represented these experiences was a sense of darkness that enveloped her and settled over her. As she allowed the darkness to settle around her and went into the darkness, she noticed that her fear subsided. She felt at peace. In the midst of the darkness she noticed an ember, a flame of brightness. To her the light symbolized the love that she was seeking and had once experienced in the presence of her grandparents. She realized that it was *love* she wanted to cultivate and preserve. As she became aware of love, she no longer made choices in her relationships that were contrary to love.

Healing stories are another type of imagery. In a very relaxed state, simply imagine seeking the ear of a trusted, wise adult. You relate the negative experience to this adult who listens with great love and compassion, then offers a soothing antidote. For example, a woman who was raped as a teenager, hears, "I'm sorry that your first sexual experience wasn't a beautiful and tender one. That must have been so difficult for you. I want you to remember, though, that sex with someone you truly love and who truly loves you is beautiful and tender. You're smart. You'll find a relationship where there's love and commitment. And then sex will be wholesome and right." The people in the story give each other a warm hug, the young girl thanks the adult, and that ends the story.[260]

CHAPTER 42

Meaning and Purpose

My legs you will chain—yes, but not my will—
no, not even Zeus can conquer that.

—*Epictetus*

In this century the famous psychotherapists Carl Jung, Rollo May, and Viktor Frankl have described an anxiety that is associated with a lack of meaning and purpose. Perhaps the most profound thoughts on this subject have been written by Viktor Frankl. Frankl survived the horror of the World War II concentration camps. He noticed that those who had goals, a reason for living, and meaning and purpose in their lives withstood the suffering better. He marveled that some people in the most dire straits found joy in serving their comrades. He himself transcended the meaningless, miserable world of a concentration camp by envisioning his beloved wife's love, and seeing himself at some future time lecturing to others on the lessons of the concentration camp. He also realized that one could take consummate pleasure in something as simple as watching the sunrise through the barbed wire. He reaffirmed that one might imprison your body, but no one can take away the last freedom, one's attitude toward suffering. He developed the school of psychotherapy called *logotherapy*, which helps people find meaning in their lives, and found great meaning in his own life by helping others find meaning and purpose. He has said, "What man actually needs is not a tensionless state but rather the striving and struggling for a worthwhile (freely chosen) goal."[261]

A psychological scale has been developed based on Frankl's work. Research with the purpose-in-life scale has shown that those with meaning and purpose are happier, less anxious, and freer of psychopathology in general. Scurfield poignantly exhorts survivors to give up vengeance as their purpose for living, and replace it with love, peace, and joy again.[262]

REDISCOVERING THE MEANING AND PURPOSE WITHIN

All individuals already have within them the seeds of great meaning and purpose which can be nourished and cultivated. Take a few moments to ponder and respond to these questions as a way to get in touch with these seeds:

- Why did you survive? For what purpose?
- Why didn't you commit suicide?
- Why have you kept going?
- What is it that makes my life worth living?[263]

Perhaps this exercise helped you get in touch with:

- a realization of what life has invested in you
- hopes and dreams; anticipation of experiencing life's loveliness (one survivor said, "Life still holds adventure.")
- a realization of to whom you matter
- faith in the future ("I had faith that my suffering would resolve.")
- expectations of being useful (because of what you have learned, and because of who you are)
- hopes in and for others ("As bad as I feel, perhaps someone will help me find greater joy"; "I've seen others get through this—so can I.")
- trust in your sense of discovery ("I believe I'll find greater meaning and more enjoyment.")
- inner resources, sense of worth ("Deep down, I know I am worth something; I am not a quitter; I believe in myself; There's more to me than this trauma; I've been to the depths and now I know I can survive anything.")

FURTHER CULTIVATING MEANING AND PURPOSE

We might categorize methods of finding meaning and purpose into three groups.

1. Giving something meaningful to the world.
2. Experiencing and enjoying the world's wholesome, beautiful pleasures.

Giving something meaningful to the world. Contributing in ways that make the world a better place:

——————— establishing or joining a social or political cause (family, politics, science, church or synagogue, Mothers Against Drunk Driving, Parents of Murdered Children, etc.)

——————— creating art, poetry, writing; other creative expression that makes something new, beautiful, or useful

——————— giving money or material support to a worthy cause

——————— altruistic service, self-transcendence, building up or helping others

——————— giving in small ways (it needn't be grandiose) that are useful to others, like picking up trash by the road, beautifying your yard for your neighbor's benefit—not yours, giving a coworker, spouse, or neighbor a hand unexpectedly, lifting anyone in any small way (a smile, thank you, listening ear, etc.)

——————— committing to doing your best at your job today

——————— simply observe what you do to meet others' needs

——————— sharing with others what you have discovered to reduce your own suffering

Experiencing and enjoying life's pleasures/beauties. Enjoy:

——————— nature (e.g., get up early and watch the sunrise; gaze at the constellations at night)

——————— intimate love

——————— friends

——————— connecting with neighbors

——————— entertainment

——————— exercising your body

——————— notice what you appreciate in others; tell them

——————— cathedrals; majestic or beautiful buildings

——————— faces

——————— teamwork

Developing personal strengths and attitudes:

——————— peace of mind

——————— personal growth; holiness, goodness of character, self-actualization

——————— courage, taking responsibility for my own life. (The "I can't" often means "I won't take responsibility for my own life," a form of avoidance.[264])

——————— refraining from criticizing, complaining, whining, backbiting, and other negatives.

——————— improving the mind

——————— understanding, empathy, patience, compassion

——————— loyalty and honesty (survivors will not betray others as they were)

3. Developing personal strengths and attitudes.

The existential psychotherapist Irvin Yalom writes, "One begins with oneself in order to forget oneself and to immerse oneself into the world; one comprehends oneself in order not to be preoccupied with oneself."[265] In other words, self development is a means to engage further in the world in a meaningful way. Describing the most fulfilled people, psychologist Abraham Maslow said that "Self-actualizing people are, without one single exception, involved in a cause outside their own skin, in something outside of themselves . . . and which they love."[266] Echoing this thought in *On the Meaning of Life*, historian Will Durrant said, "Join a whole, work for it with all your body and mind. The meaning of life lies in the chance it gives us to produce, or to contribute to something greater than ourselves. It need not be a family (although that is the direct and broadest road which nature in her blind wisdom has provided for even the simplest soul); it can be any group that can call out all the latent nobility of the individual and give him a cause to work for that (which) shall not be shattered by his death."[267]

FINDING MORE MEANING AND PURPOSE

Frankl explained that there is no one road to meaning and purpose. Each person finds it in his or her own unique way, and on his or her own timetable. Page 330 lists some possible approaches. As an exercise, check an item if it seems like it might be of interest to you, either now or at some future time. Ask yourself as you go, "What do I really want from life?" A balance among all three areas is characteristic of many of the most fully-developed and satisfied people.

CHAPTER 43

Spiritual and Religious Growth

Never shall I forget those moments that murdered my God
And my soul, and turned my dreams to dust.

—Elie Wiesel

Of course, the sovereign cure for worry is religious faith.

*—William James, psychologist,
professor of philosophy at Harvard*

It has been frequently observed that trauma can shake one's religious faith or lead to its rebirth. Sometimes both occur following trauma. As healing occurs, survivors might discover the potential for greater religious faith, perhaps becoming more receptive to spiritual development after returning from "the valley of death."[268]

Freud called religion the "universal neurosis." The famous modern-day psychologist Albert Ellis thinks that religion creates irrational thinking.[269] However, the research presents a different picture.

Scientific polling among Americans reveals that the proportion of Americans who believe in God has remained remarkably constant between 1944 and 1986, around 95 percent.[270] However, in predicting health outcomes, one's religious commitment is more important than the beliefs one professes.

Religious commitment means putting belief into practice/action. It measures not affiliation or denomination but taps the depth of one's faith. Typically, it is operationalized in the research as attendance at church/synagogue/mosque/temple, prayer, and reading sacred works. It also includes a relationship with God, making beliefs an important part of one's life, and connection with others in the religious community. In reviewing the studies published in recent years, psychiatric epidemiologist David Larson concluded that "The impact of religious commitment on physical and mental health has been demonstrated to be overwhelmingly positive."[271] The religiously committed are more satisfied with life and marriage, are mentally and physically healthier, live longer, are less stressed, and are less likely to commit suicide or abuse drugs.

In reviewing the literature, Gartner et al. observed: "The preponderance of evidence suggests that religion is associated with mental health benefits. Furthermore, the best religious predictors of mental health are not religious questionnaire responses (religious attitudes), but real-life religious behavior (such as frequency of church attendance). Behavior predicts behavior."[272]

WHY IS RELIGIOUS COMMITMENT BENEFICIAL?

We might surmise why religious commitment is associated with positive health outcomes. The following are possible reasons:

- *Heightened self-esteem.* Self-esteem is fostered by knowing that one matters and is loved. As one said, "I take comfort in knowing that I am a child of a loving God, with worth and potential." In one study, high self-esteem was associated with loving images of God.[273] An older person might see himself as more than just an aging body, thereby buffering the stress of aging.

- *Greater meaning and purpose.* Sometimes under the stress of living, it is easy for us to lose sight of the meaning and purpose that steadies us and sees us through the difficult times. One woman said, "I don't see the world purely in terms of pleasure and needs; religion helps define who I am and how I fit into the world." And considering his own mortality, a father wrote:[274]

> Help me
> To weave
> The threads of my life
> Into a tapestry that will
> Keep my children warm
> When I die.

Viktor Frankl acknowledged the relationship between psychological and spiritual health, and that the latter included a religious component. He noted that "If there is a meaning in life at all, then there must be a meaning in suffering (and in dying)."[275]

- *Peace of conscience from living a moral life.* Among the world's religions there is agreement on those moral values that lift humanity and promote happiness: fidelity, honesty, respect, fairness, forgiveness, and schooling of the appetites. Settling upon and living these values fosters a sense of inner security. Said one medical professional, "It is relaxing to know you are living a good life." Religious communities can support us in this difficult process. And when we stumble, religion provides a way toward personal forgiveness and reconciliation.

- *Overcoming aloneness.* Said a friend since youth, one of the most quietly saintlike people I know, "It is comforting to know someone is looking down on me lovingly and generously and compassionately, who's trying to help me out." When asked if they were afraid, survivors of a California earthquake said: "I wasn't afraid—I knew God would take care of us."; "I just trusted God. What else can you do?"

- *Eternal perspective.* Seeing things from the eternal view, momentary stressors assume a smaller significance. Said one teenager, "I know I can't mess things up too bad. So the weight of the world is not on my shoulders." Cardiologist George Sheehan said that religion gives one the sense that there "is no final defeat."[276] Rather, there is hope beyond the present, even the grave. As Harvard's Benson says, there are "realities that the senses cannot detect."[277]

  When we don't realize all the goals we impatiently expect, we can take solace in the comforting words that "all these things will be added" eventually if we seek first the godly life. So we need not feel the pressure of rushing to obtain all things immediately. And a woman gained a perspective on her difficult challenges in life. "I understand trials as homework to grow from, not punishment."

- *Reduced death anxiety.* For many, death anxiety is significant. One might assume that dying is an awful experience. Religion can help one face death with greater peace.[278] Dr. Claire Weekes writes that religious beliefs in the afterlife are an "inborn comfort."[279] Consider:

- Dr. Weekes explains that most do not find dying disagreeable: "I speak as a doctor. I have rarely attended a person actually dying who realized that he or she was dying. A few do, but very few. Nature blunts the edge off her sword; even during the years before our death nature helps us." As with birth, we will be the star performer, but we will likely be unaware of the drama. And for those who are aware, the famous physician William Hunter said, "If I had strength enough to hold a pen, I would write how easy and pleasant a thing it is to die."[280]

- Some find going a relief as the tasks of living become more difficult.

- Some consider reunion with God and loved ones with anticipation and curiosity.

- Dreading death takes away the joy of living. We can accept death, but enjoy the precious moments of life as well. In fact, death denial takes energy. Releasing this energy allows us to focus more fully on life. If you fear for the loved ones who survive you, prepare them as best as you can, which is all you can do. Then don't fear. They might be hardier than you assume. They will grieve. If they know that grieving is permissible, they will eventually move beyond the grief. If judgment is fearful, take action. Focus on what you can do now and do it, which is all you can do.

- Some people find a belief in the afterlife comforting in the death of loved ones. One Mother Against Drunk Driving dreamed that her deceased daughter returned, assured her that she was all right, and told her to keep doing what she was doing. The mother took great comfort in this dream, which seemed to affirm her belief in an afterlife.[281]

- *Religion teaches us to share control; to accept loss of control with greater peace.* As one married couple explained, "God will give us ultimate answers, but not here on earth. Religion teaches you how to have faith and not understand everything. This is a good thing." Generally, an active coping style that seeks control favors health. However, there are inevitably areas of life that we can't control. Trusting that God will ensure that all things work out for our eventual good helps us to accept those things. As Byrd and Chamberlain observe, the Western approach to willpower places total reliance on the self. Religion shares control with God.[282] Dr. Martin Luther King, Jr., said, "My obligation is to do the right thing. The rest is in God's hands." A mother whose daughter was killed in a drunk driving crash cried to God, "How big do you think these shoulders are?" Realizing she can share control, she now says, "I give to God what I can't deal with now."[283]

- *Reduced hostility.* Hostility is associated with earlier death from a variety of causes. The world religions teach the principles of charity and forgiveness as antidotes. Interestingly, compassionate behavior increases as people become involved in religious communities.[284]

- *Religious communities support the growth of religious commitment.* While the religious community provides social support, the benefits are more complex.
  - Others who are striving to live the spiritual life can share insights, affirm values, inspire, encourage, and remind us to rise above the weaknesses of human nature. A father opined that his religious community afforded common goals and ideas. "I feel like I am not standing alone in my beliefs, morality, and devotion to a higher being." Said a mother of two, "We need to reach out to people who respect our beliefs in order to define and clarify what we believe. I don't think I'd have a very close relationship with God without sharing with others."

    A teenager put it this way: "Church is a time to be friendly with people of all ages. I feel more secure with God, a part of God's family. Church makes my relationship with God stronger—it helps me think of God more; it's like having another friend."
  - Religious communities can often be a learning lab for values. Sometimes the most difficult people to love are those who worship beside us, and vice versa.

- *Social support.* I don't know Ivan. I've only heard his name spoken with reverence for the way this quiet, elderly gentleman donated his time to help a dear relative cope in time of illness. Sometimes neighbors in religious communities bring meals, health care, or physical labor in times of need. Sometimes rituals, like funerals, help us share the burden of grief. Sometimes the religious community helps us rejoice. And people with severe psychiatric disorders are just as likely to seek help from clergy as from mental health professionals.[285] One interesting study found that religious content improved the effectiveness of psychotherapy for the depressed, even if the therapist was not religious.[286]

- *The Sabbath, whether it be observed on Friday, Saturday, or Sunday, provides a respite from the cares of the world.*

- *Most religions promote family solidarity which buffers stress.*

IMPLICATIONS/CAUTIONS

Certain precautions might help prevent disappointment. As William James noted, "the fruits of religion . . . are, like all human products, liable to corruption by excess."[287] Some members of any institution will be corrupt. Religion does not guarantee that people won't be prejudiced, judgmental, or immoral. It only appears to reduce the likelihood of such attributes or blunt their sharpness.

Religion does not guarantee that life will be problem-free, as Job's account reminds us, although it might help us to bear up a bit better.

Guilt can be a good thing if it causes us to change destructive behavior. Thereafter it serves little purpose and is best released.

Religion does not deal in the realm of scientific proof, which is why heated debates rarely change minds. I have heard people say, "Don't you know it's a sin to worry? Have greater faith." I think that a more wholesome way to look at it is that it is human to worry, although it is not usually in our best interest to do so. Instead of feeling guilty for worrying, just think, "Faith is like a seed. It probably won't flourish overnight." Then relax and cultivate it patiently.

Finally, Harvard psychology professor Gordon Allport stated that the intrinsically religious person lives according to her personal beliefs regardless of outside social pressure or consequences. For the externally religious person, religion is a means to social acceptance and personal safety. He reasoned that only intrinsic orientation facilitated mental health. Research has found that the intrinsically oriented are indeed mentally healthier, showing less anxiety, more openness to emotions, greater self-esteem, and a greater sense of control.[288]

CHAPTER 44

Happiness, Pleasure, and Humor

What is human life's chief concern? . . . It is happiness.
How to gain, how to keep, how to recover happiness, is in
fact for most men at all times the secret motive of all they
do, and of all they are willing to endure.

—*William James*

As people recover from PTSD, the happiness that once appeared irrevocably taken begins to return. The capacity for pleasure and the ability to laugh begin to resurface. Thus, happiness, pleasure, and humor are signs that healing is taking place. They also help us to enjoy life and protect against distress. This chapter explores approaches to facilitating these positive aspects of life.

HAPPINESS

The happier people are, the less distressed they feel. It is fitting, therefore, to begin with the topic of happiness. Two researchers have devoted considerable effort to summarizing the burgeoning research on this topic. They are psychologists David Myers and Michael Fordyce.[289]

According to Myers, most people are quite resilient and happy. Happiness levels remain consistently high across different levels of age, gender, race, education, or place of residence. Once people rise above the misery levels, wealth and health don't predict happiness either. Even those who are handicapped on average bounce back to previous levels after a period of adjustment. So if these outward circumstances do not predict happiness, what does?

The following factors correlate with happiness. Notice that many of these factors are the same as those which help treat or prevent PTSD, and that most are things we can do something about:

- *Self-esteem and peace of mind.*

- *Religious commitment.*

- *Healthy habits* (such as regular exercise, sufficient sleep, wise eating).

- *Rewarding social interaction.* Happy people are more involved with friends, family, and organizations. They reach out and invest themselves to form high-quality, supportive relationships. They are more outgoing and sociable.

- *Active involvement in life.* Frankl observed that happiness ensues from actively pursuing meaning. Happy people are more likely to immerse themselves in things they find meaningful and/or satisfying (family, work, pleasant activities, avocations). They seem to be energized by this activity and don't sit around passively waiting for life to happen to them. Enjoyable activities can be planned; many are spontaneous and inexpensive.

- *Mastery and control.*
  - An active coping style, committed to problem solving and not passive or helpless, shows initiative.
  - Control over time, organized, deliberately planning, moving/progressing toward meaningful goals, nonprocrastinating, efficient, having both long-term and short-term plans.
  - Goals are somewhat modest, compared to the unhappy. But they are realistic and achievable, thus providing more satisfaction. The unhappy tend to overcompensate for their feeling of inadequacy by shooting for grandiose goals, and derive less satisfaction because they are achieved less often. Happy people don't seem to need success as badly as the unhappy. For them, success ensues from what they love to do; it is not directly pursued.
  - Present-oriented. Happy people have cultivated mindfulness, or the ability to become absorbed in and enjoy the present moment. This is considerably easier when one has made reasonable plans for the future; when one experiences the peace of preparation.

- *Optimism.* Optimism is not the naive expectation that everything will turn out rosy. Rather, it is the attitude that no matter what happens, I can find *something* to enjoy; it is the choice to be happy despite obstacles. This is in direct opposition to the pessimistic distortions of overgeneralizing and fortune telling. The happy person:

- anticipates pleasure
- expects something good to happen; some things will probably go well
- reasons that whatever happens will be for the best
- looks to the bright side
- believes that he plays an important role in shaping his own future
- considers how things could be worse and then how to salvage the most possible
- realizes that failure does not equal a character flaw or the end of the world; overcomes failure with new strengths
- has a fighting spirit. The person with this mindset does not make a career of suffering. She won't be defeated, but anticipates problems and is determined to make the best of things.

- *Lower need for success.* Like people with self-esteem, happy people don't seem driven by the need for success in order to prove themselves. Rather, they commit first to happiness, the great energizing motivator; success then follows. Fordyce counsels to do what you love, and productivity and success will follow. He says, "Success may not lead to happiness, but happiness leads to success."[290] He observes that people complete the sentence stem, "I'll be happy when . . . ," with answers like "I am successful, wealthy, married, etc." Happy people tend to answer with, "I am happy now."

- *Internal attitudes that include absence of blame, bitterness, and helplessness.*

Correlations between factors do not necessarily prove causality. However, Fordyce reasoned that acting like happy people would increase happiness, and thereby reduce anxiety, depression, and stress. This assumption has been borne out by measuring happiness and mental health before and after people completed his happiness course. The tasks and skills include:

1. *Get involved.*

2. *Socialize more* (say hello, ask people how they are doing, listen).

3. *Organize and plan.* Have a plan for reaching achievable, meaningful goals—then enjoy reaching them. The future is no more enjoyable than

the present moment. So enjoy the process of throwing yourself into life, mindful of the joy that is experienced in each moment.

4. *Stop worrying.* Do what you can to combat fears *now.* In addition, try writing down your worries for a twenty-five-minute worry period each day—facts and feelings—at the same time and place each day. Then, instead of worrying during the day, tell yourself that you will postpone your worries until your designated worry period. This approach has been found to very effectively reduce worries.

5. *Develop optimism* (e.g., try saying for each bad outcome, "Well, at least . . ." Thus, after you don't get the promotion you'd wanted, you might say, "Well, at least I won't be away from home as much.")

6. *Cultivate a healthy personality.* Be yourself, be expressive, and spontaneous. With self-esteem, this is easier.

PLEASANT ACTIVITIES SCHEDULING*

We tend to feel balanced when we're doing both needed and pleasant activities. Under periods of great stress and pressure, however, we might give up pleasant activities. We can lose balance, falling into the habit of doing only what is needed. If we do this long enough, sadly, we might even forget what used to give us pleasure or assume that it won't be fun anymore. Doing pleasant activities reverses this cycle. As we do things that are pleasant, we begin to feel happier. We feel more active, interested, and encouraged—and less distressed. Maintaining reasonable levels of pleasant activities also helps to prevent drops in mood.

The exercise that follows will both help you to discover (or rediscover) what is pleasant for you and to make a plan to do some of these things.

STEP 1: The "Pleasant Events Schedule" on the next page lists a wide range of activities. In Column 1, check those activities which you enjoyed in the past. Then rate from 1 to 10 how pleasant each checked item was. A score of 1 reflects little pleasure, and 10 reflects great pleasure. This rating goes in Column 1 also, beside each check mark. For example, if you moderately enjoyed being with happy people, but didn't enjoy being with friends/relatives, your first 2 items would look like this:

√ (5) _____ 1. Being with happy people

_____ _____ 2. Being with friends/relatives

---

*The "Pleasant Events Schedule" and the instructions for using it are adapted with permission from Lewinsohn, P., R. Munoz, M. Youngren, and A. Zeiss. 1986. Control Your Depression. New York: Prentice Hall. Copyright © 1986 by Peter M. Lewinsohn. Not to be produced without written permission from Dr. Lewinsohn.

PLEASANT EVENTS SCHEDULE

I. **Social Interactions.** These events occur with others. They tend to make us feel accepted, appreciated, liked, understood, etc.*

COL. I   COL. 2

COL. I	COL. 2		
_____	_____	1.	Being with happy people
_____	_____	2.	Being with friends/relatives
_____	_____	3.	Thinking about people I like
_____	_____	4.	Planning an activity with people I care about
_____	_____	5.	Meeting someone new of the same sex
_____	_____	6.	Meeting someone new of the opposite sex
_____	_____	7.	Going to a club, tavern, bar, etc.
_____	_____	8.	Being at celebrations (birthdays, weddings, baptisms, parties, family get-togethers, etc.)
_____	_____	9.	Meeting a friend for lunch or a drink
_____	_____	10.	Talking openly and honestly (e.g., about your hopes, fears, what interests you, what makes you laugh, what saddens you)
_____	_____	11.	Expressing true affection (verbal or physical)
_____	_____	12.	Showing interest in others
_____	_____	13.	Noticing successes and strengths in family and friends
_____	_____	14.	Dating, courting (this one is for married people, too)
_____	_____	15.	Having a lively conversation
_____	_____	16.	Inviting friends over
_____	_____	17.	Stopping in to visit friends
_____	_____	18.	Calling up someone I enjoy
_____	_____	19.	Apologizing
_____	_____	20.	Smiling at people
_____	_____	21.	Calmly talking over problems with people I live with
_____	_____	22.	Giving compliments, back pats, or praise
_____	_____	23.	Teasing/bantering
_____	_____	24.	Amusing people or making them laugh
_____	_____	25.	Playing with children
_____	_____	26.	Others: _____

*You might feel that an activity belongs in another group. The grouping is not important.

II. Activities that make us feel capable, loving, useful, strong, or adequate.

_____ _____ 1. Starting a challenging job or doing it well

_____ _____ 2. Learning something new (e.g., fixing leaks, new hobby, new language)

_____ _____ 3. Helping someone (counseling, advising, listening)

_____ _____ 4. Contributing to religious, charitable, or other groups

_____ _____ 5. Driving skillfully

_____ _____ 6. Expressing myself clearly (out loud or in writing)

_____ _____ 7. Repairing something (sewing, fixing a car or bike, etc.)

_____ _____ 8. Solving a problem or puzzle

_____ _____ 9. Exercising

_____ _____ 10. Thinking

_____ _____ 11. Going to a meeting (convention, business, civic)

_____ _____ 12. Visiting the ill, homebound, or troubled

_____ _____ 13. Telling a child a story

_____ _____ 14. Writing a card, note, or letter

_____ _____ 15. Improving my appearance (e.g., seeking medical or dental help, improving my diet, going to a barber or beautician)

_____ _____ 16. Planning/budgeting time

_____ _____ 17. Discussing political issues

_____ _____ 18. Doing volunteer work, community service, etc.

_____ _____ 19. Planning a budget

_____ _____ 20. Protesting injustice, protecting someone, stopping fraud or abuse

_____ _____ 21. Being honest, moral, etc.

_____ _____ 22. Correcting mistakes

_____ _____ 23. Organizing a party

_____ _____ 24. Others: _____

III. Intrinsically Pleasant Activities

_____ _____ 1. Laughing

_____ _____ 2. Relaxing, having peace and quiet

_____ _____ 3. Having a good meal

_____ _____ 4. A hobby (e.g., cooking, fishing, woodworking, photography, acting, gardening, collecting things)

_____ _____ 5. Listening to good music

_____ _____ 6. Seeing beautiful scenery

_____ _____ 7. Going to bed early, sleeping soundly, and awakening early

_____ _____ 8. Wearing attractive clothes

_____ _____ 9. Wearing comfortable clothes

_____	_____	10.	Going to a concert, opera, ballet, or play
_____	_____	11.	Playing sports (e.g., tennis, softball, racquetball, golf, horseshoes, frisbee)
_____	_____	12.	Trips or vacations
_____	_____	13.	Shopping/buying something I like for myself
_____	_____	14.	Being outdoors (e.g., beach, country, mountains, kicking leaves, walking in the sand, floating in lakes)
_____	_____	15.	Doing artwork (e.g., painting, sculpture, drawing)
_____	_____	16.	Reading sacred works
_____	_____	17.	Beautifying my home (redecorating, cleaning, yardwork, etc.)
_____	_____	18.	Going to a sports event
_____	_____	19.	Reading (novels, poems, plays, newspapers, etc.)
_____	_____	20.	Going to a lecture
_____	_____	21.	Going for a drive
_____	_____	22.	Sitting in the sun
_____	_____	23.	Visiting a museum
_____	_____	24.	Playing or singing music
_____	_____	25.	Boating
_____	_____	26.	Pleasing my family, friends, employer
_____	_____	27.	Thinking about something good in the future
_____	_____	28.	Watching TV
_____	_____	29.	Camping, hunting
_____	_____	30.	Grooming myself (e.g., bathing, combing hair, shaving)
_____	_____	31.	Writing in my diary/journal
_____	_____	32.	Taking a bike ride, hiking, or walking
_____	_____	33.	Being with animals
_____	_____	34.	Watching people
_____	_____	35.	Taking a nap
_____	_____	36.	Listening to nature sounds
_____	_____	37.	Getting or giving a backrub
_____	_____	38.	Watching a storm, clouds, the sky, etc.
_____	_____	39.	Having spare time
_____	_____	40.	Daydreaming
_____	_____	41.	Feeling the presence of the Deity in my life; praying, worshiping, etc.
_____	_____	42.	Smelling a flower
_____	_____	43.	Talking about old times or special interests
_____	_____	44.	Going to auctions, garage sales, etc.
_____	_____	45.	Traveling
_____	_____	46.	Others: _____

STEP 2: In Column 2, check if you've done the event in the last thirty days.

STEP 3: Circle the number of events that you'd probably enjoy (when you're feeling good, on a good day).

STEP 4: Notice if there are many items you've enjoyed in the past that you are not doing very often (compare the first and second columns).

STEP 5: Using the completed Pleasant Events Schedule for ideas, make a list of the twenty-five activities that you feel you'd enjoy most.

STEP 6: Make a written plan to do more pleasant activities. Start with the simplest activities and the ones you are most likely to enjoy. When depressed or anxious, it is common to find that your old favorite activities are now the most difficult to enjoy, particularly if you tried them before when you were very upset and failed to enjoy them. You might say, "I can't even enjoy my favorite activity," making you feel even more stressed. These events will become pleasant again. For now, start with other, simple activities. Gradually try your old favorites as your mood lifts. Do as many pleasant events as you reasonably can. We suggest doing at least one each day, perhaps more on weekends. *Write* your plan on a calendar, and carry out this written plan for at least two weeks. Each time you do an activity, rate it on a 1 to 5 scale for pleasure (5 being highly enjoyable). This tests the idea that *nothing* is enjoyable. Later, you can replace less enjoyable activities with others.

Certain blocks (such as negative thoughts, guilt, or a feeling that "I don't deserve pleasure") can interfere with your enjoyment. You know how to deal with distortions. If you feel guilty about the past or feel that you should be doing something "constructive," remind yourself that prolonged guilt serves no one, and that work becomes more efficient after a period of recreation.

Some Tips for Pleasant Event Scheduling

- *Tune into the physical world.* Pay less attention to your thoughts. Feel the wind, or the soap suds as you wash the car. See and hear. This is living in the present.

- *Before doing an event, set yourself up to enjoy it.* Identify three things you will enjoy about it. Say, "I will enjoy _____ (the sunshine, the breeze, talking with brother Bill, etc.). Relax and imagine yourself enjoying each aspect of the event as you repeat each statement.

- *Ask yourself, "What will I do to make the activity enjoyable?"* Sometimes the answer is to just relax and enjoy it, without trying to control it.

- *If you are concerned that you might not enjoy some activity that you'd like to attempt, try breaking it up into steps.* Think small, so you can be satisfied in reaching your goal. For example, start by only cleaning the house for ten minutes, then stop. Then reward yourself with a "Good job!" pat on the back.

- *Check your schedule for balance.* Can you spread out the "need to's" to make room for some "want to's"?

- *Time is limited, so use it wisely.* You needn't do activities you don't like just because they're convenient.

Happiness Meditation

There is a very beautiful meditation practice. After having completed the skills up to this point, you are ready to enjoy it. The Vietnamese monk Thich Nhat Hanh, who was nominated for the Nobel Peace Prize, explains that joy, peace, and serenity can be found in simple moments—eating, walking, breathing, driving—if we are living in the present and receptive to its pleasures. He suggests this simple meditation exercise.[291] Simply recite these four lines silently as you breathe in and out:

> Breathing in, I calm my body.
>
> Breathing out, I smile.
>
> Dwelling in the present moment,
>
> I know this is a wonderful moment!

He teaches that breathing is a joyful, soothing experience. Smiling relaxes the many muscles of the face and signals mastery of your body. Practice many times throughout the day, in various situations. Relax your body as you breathe in, as if drinking a glass of cool lemonade on a hot day. Smile as you breathe out and enjoy the subtle shift in mood.

Loving Kindness Meditation

Jack Cornfield teaches a beautiful way to meditate for fifteen to twenty minutes during the day.[292] Sit in a relaxed way. Let your heart be soft and your mind free of preoccupations. Recite inwardly these phrases:

> May I be filled with loving kindness.
>
> May I be well.

May I be peaceful and at ease.

May I be happy.

As you repeat these phrases silently, you might think of times when you were surrounded with love. Be patient and allow kind feelings to develop over time. When you feel that you have developed and experienced a sense of loving kindness, then expand this meditation to include others. First, select loved ones (May he be filled with loving kindness, etc.). Then expand this meditation to include others, even those you might not feel kindly toward. You can also use this meditation in traffic jams or other stressful situations.

HUMOR

A combat veteran relates:[293]

> I was standing at the counter of our neighborhood dry cleaner, which had been recently bought by a Lebanese family. Suddenly a truck backfired nearby with two loud bangs.
>
> I instinctively hit the floor, face down. Embarrassed, I got to my knees and peered over the counter, only to see the owner also in a prone position.
>
> "Saigon '68," I said. We both laughed when she stood up and replied, "Beirut '79."

By now the benefits of humor are well documented. Humor connects us to other humans, as we share a laugh over life's absurd moments. Like love, humor warmly surrounds and soothes pain, making it more bearable. When we can laugh at our problems, we gain distance, perspective, and a sense of mastery. Humor says, "Things might not be so great right now, but that's okay. I might not be perfect, but I'm a darn sight better than I look." A humor break can recharge creative batteries. In addition, laughter results in numerous beneficial effects on the body: relief from pain, cardiovascular conditioning, improved breathing, muscle relaxation, and improved immune system functioning.

Several cautions apply to humor, however—no kidding.

1. *The overuse of humor can be a form of avoidance, which can prevent one from processing pain.*

2. *Sarcasm or "put-down" humor is a thinly disguised form of hostility, and is rarely appropriate.* Humor, like sex, works best when surrounded by love.

3. *Making light of someone's pain can seem insensitive and can undermine trust.* When in doubt, check it out. You might say, "I was just being humorous there. Was that all right?" Humor may require that a certain degree of healing has taken place. It may be premature to try to get someone to laugh at intense pain. Likewise, it may be premature to expect yourself to laugh too soon.

4. *Humor is not a panacea, nor a substitute for therapy.* Humor can, however, support the healing process if it is suited to you.

Given these precautions, these principles might help to incorporate more humor into our lives.

1. *Be willing to "play the fool" at times.* This openness undermines the rigid need to be perfect, which, of course, no one is. Laughing at ourselves says, in effect, "Isn't it funny that a person of my caliber has such funny quirks." This is really practice in self-acceptance.

2. *Just be willing to play.* If we plan to have lightly structured time, light moments might spring up unexpectedly. Thus, planning a day at the zoo or time for stories with a child creates a place for humor to bubble up.

3. *Humor does not require that one be a joke teller or loud laugher.* A sense of humor includes simply appreciating a good joke. Humor can also mean simply noticing life's incongruities with a light heart.

4. *Humor is not an all-or-none skill.* A sense of humor is standard issue, and each person has the capacity to develop it over time.

5. *Don't be discouraged if not many things seem funny to you.* Trauma can bury anyone's sense of humor—it is hard to laugh when one is emotionally numb. Instead, simply allow time for healing. With time you'll probably become open to humor at your own pace and in your own way.

Think of humor as a skill or a hobby that becomes more enjoyable with time. You might create a humor file of things that make you laugh, or a humor bulletin board. You might also take some time to reflect on this. Have you ever been in a place where you laughed when humor "wasn't appropriate?"[294] For some reason, I think of musical solos in church services that were not intended to be funny. About fifteen minutes spent on this exercise might return some surprising, pleasurable dividends.

CHAPTER 45

Relapse Prevention

> A lapse is often part of a larger pattern of recovery and
> (some people) may have to cope with a future lapse in
> order to continue on (their) way.
>
> —*Dr. Francis Abueg and colleagues*[295]

Life is not linear. It is comprised of ups and downs. It would be nice if once we were headed on a good course at a good pace no slips, setbacks, or falls were to occur. However, as you move ahead you will undoubtedly have periods where some PTSD symptoms return. Such troubling periods are normal in PTSD and do not invalidate your recovery work or detract from your gains. They can actually be useful opportunities to overlearn previously encountered coping skills and/or to process unresolved memory material. This chapter deals with anticipating and preventing symptoms and situations before they occur. We'll also explore how to prevent the return of some symptoms from evolving into a full-blown relapse. Relapse prevention is a wonderful way to put your skills together and continue to practice them.

Relapse prevention consists of six parts:

1. Understand the dynamics of "failure."
2. Identify and anticipate high-risk situations or cues.
3. Develop a sound coping plan.
4. Rehearse the plan.
5. Try out the plan in real life.
6. Evaluate and make improvements if needed.

We'll now look at these six parts in turn.

UNDERSTAND THE DYNAMICS OF "FAILURE"

Let's say that your PTSD symptoms have greatly lessened. For several months you are noticeably less troubled by the past. Then you encounter a setback. Perhaps you encounter a feared situation. Maybe it's a place that reminds you of the traumatic event. Maybe it is a social situation that stirs up old feelings of not fitting in. You notice the return of intrusive thoughts and arousal. Perhaps you have a nightmare. Although these experiences are normal and to be expected, symptoms can be lessened or worsened, depending upon our actions and reactions. So let's understand how setbacks occur and how viewing them as failure can worsen symptoms.

Some setbacks are simply a part of the normal recovery process. Other setbacks are set up. That is, sometimes we do things along the way that will influence an outcome. For example, we are more prone to setbacks when we have not taken care of our health, practiced our coping skills, anticipated difficult challenges, or monitored our self-talk. Sometimes stressful situations pile up and set us up for more intense stress reactions. Let's say you've gotten less sleep lately because you have many things to do. During the day you feel tired and let some of your needed chores slip. Your car has been acting up but you don't bother to get it checked out. You like to spend time with your family, but you don't take the time to plan that enjoyable evening, and when that evening comes you just feel too busy. Instead you return home from work after the family is in bed, and watch TV to unwind until quite late. You oversleep the next day, and find that your car won't start. You are quite late for work, and fall behind on an all-important project. At the end of the week, you blow up at your spouse and go to the company party angry. And then the symptoms hit. You feel out of touch and distant from your colleagues like you don't fit in. Your anger and frustration begin to mount. You think "Why bother?" as you start to think about drowning your troubles with alcohol. Here managing time better, budgeting time for sleep, recreation, and chores, might have prevented stress from building to the breaking point.

The way you think about setbacks, or lapses, is also very important. You might think of the return of symptoms as failure, which might remind you of past failures. What kind of things go through your head when you fail at something? This exercise might shed light on what failure means to you:[296]

> Relax. I'm going to ask you to close your eyes if you feel comfortable. Otherwise just look down at the floor and breathe regularly and deeply. I want you to see yourself as a young child. You may be five years old, ten years old; you may be a teenager. At the count of three I'd like you to see yourself facing an important

task or challenge. Unfortunately, it's a task that you are unable to do or complete. At the count of three (again, if you are comfortable close your eyes): one, two, three. Good. See yourself facing this challenge. Where are you? What do you look like? Who is around, if anyone? Let the action unfold and notice your physical and emotional reaction. What does your face look like? How did it feel? Hold onto these impressions, remember them. What happens later? See the details as best you can. Good. Now let go of the image and return to regular relaxed breathing. I'll count backward from twenty to one. You will become more and more alert as I count. Twenty, nineteen, eighteen . . .

What do you learn about why failure might be uncomfortable for you now? Perhaps you learned to associate failure with rejection, abandonment, or punishment.

Failure can be so painful that people try to explain it in a way that makes sense. Often the explanations are so negative that the fear of future failure becomes excessive. When failure recurs, the negative thoughts return with a vengeance, and the fear is reinforced. We will now learn how to stop the cycle of negativity as early as possible. This approach, described by Abueg and colleagues, has been found to reverse depression and pessimism. When you experience failure, Abueg continues:

1. Immediately: *Stop, look, and listen.* Take a minute if you can to step out of the flow of events and try to get as rational a view as possible. Look for your own cognitive distortions as they are developing.

2. *Keep as calm as you can* so you can function in the situation.

3. After the crisis is past: *Think of the situation as external, specific, and changeable. External* means that we focus on the event, and do not condemn ourselves at the core. *Specific* means that we keep what is happening in the here-and-now. We do not assume that what is happening is a reflection of life in general. *Changeable* means that things can improve. The opposite of external, specific, and changeable is *internal, global,* and *unchangeable*.

   The pessimistic way to think of a setback is:

Internal	It's me. I am so incompetent. I have no willpower.
Global	I do this all the time.
Unchangeable	This failure is proof that I can't change.

   This way of explaining failure leads to further distress. It might set one up to find solace from the pain in drink or drugs. At any rate, it will likely depress one's mood and undermine the motivation to keep trying to improve. In short, it sets you up to fail in the future by creating the expectation of failure. Notice the difference when one looks at a setback more optimistically:

External	This is a difficult situation. I was tired and overworked.
Specific	This isn't the way I always act.
Changeable	This isn't a signpost for the rest of my life. In a few days I'll probably be back in balance again. This is more changeable than I now think. This is a chance to learn a better coping style.

Rather than focusing on judging the self, focus on the situation and what you did and what you would do in the future. For example, you might think, "I made the mistake of getting out of balance. In the future, I'll do better at being rested so that I can be more efficient during the day." Blaming and judging are eliminated, so one feels motivated to improve.

4. *Keep setbacks from getting worse by looking at other self-talk.* Many reactions get worse by self-defeating reactions such as shame, self-disgust, impatience, or discouragement. These emotions maintain arousal. They are preceded by negative self-talk. So learn constructive vs. destructive reactions.

- *Cognitive dissonance.* This refers to the gap between seeing yourself as totally recovered and present reality. Filling the gap with negative self-talk, such as "I should be better by now," creates frustration. Instead, you could think, "It's too bad that symptoms return sometimes. But this is normal—not a catastrophe. They'll pass."

- *Replace the word* failure. Failure has a self-defeating all-or-nothing quality to it. Instead of failure, think of a return of symptoms as a setback, lapse, temporary detour, opportunity, normal and expected challenge, falling short of the ideal, a wake-up call for needed attention.

- *Stand your ground and renew your commitment to recover.* Don't give in to "What's the use?" (fortune telling) or "I've blown it" (all-or-nothing). Remind yourself that setbacks are normal. Remember the benefits of recovering.

IDENTIFY AND ANTICIPATE HIGH-RISK SITUATIONS (CUES)

The most effective copers have been found to anticipate stressful times so that they can be better prepared for them. They form an action plan rather than avoiding thinking about stressful times or constantly worrying without making a plan. In order to make an action plan, we first identify high-risk situations, or cues. As you look ahead, what situations are likely to be challenging for you? Consider a variety of possible triggers, the return of PTSD symptoms, and new situations.

- places
- things
- people
- symptoms (e.g., nightmares)
- funerals
- significant dates, such as the anniversary of the trauma, when a deceased child would have graduated, when you reach the age of a parent who died, a wedding that a deceased loved one doesn't attend, the birth of a child without the loved one being present, holidays without loved ones, Veterans Day
- fatigue, illness, hormone swings
- stressful times with negative emotions (Consider what increases the urge to drink. What situations contribute to depression, anxiety, anger, guilt, loneliness, or stress—such as financial problems, crime, work overload, or medical exams?)
- interpersonal conflict
- social situations: can't open up and express yourself, no confidence, feelings of hostility or intolerance, afraid of meeting people, feeling isolated from people, being reminded that you can't forget problems and relax, fear of being boring, fear of intrusive thoughts, fear of rejection, tension, nervousness about having sex
- overconfidence: on top of the world; telling yourself that nothing can go wrong, you're permanently fixed and don't need to practice your skills or anticipate difficult situations
- other triggers

Not all arousal, of course, is bad. It is comforting to realize that some arousal over new lifestyle choices is excitement or normal curiosity and concern. Try to distinguish the various forms of arousal.

To increase awareness of high-risk situations, list in the first column of Table 45.1 the high-risk situations that you thought of. In the second column, indicate the likelihood of encountering the situations as a percentage. In the third column, indicate your expected reactions. Emotional reactions might be anger, sadness, or fear. Physical reactions might be difficulty breathing or tension. Behaviors might include leaving the situation early, or using food for sedation. In the fourth column, see if you can connect the high-risk situation to a past trauma. It helps to understand this connection, but then separate present fearful situations from past trauma. You might decide that the high-risk situation is just a new feared situation. If you think there is a connection to the past but the connection is not clear, just continue. (This might be a fruitful area to explore with your counselor.) The fifth column is a percentage rating of how much distress you anticipate. This helps to view the situation in the gray areas, the middle ground—and avoid extreme predictions. The last column indicates how much distress you actually experience, and will be completed after you make a coping plan and try it out. It can be motivating to find that distress was less than predicted.

Table 45.1
HIGH-RISK SITUATION RECORD

High-Risk Situation	Likelihood of Encountering (%)	Expected Reactions (emotional, physical, behavioral)	Connection to Past Trauma	Anticipated Distress (%)	Actual Distress (%)

DEVELOP A SOUND COPING PLAN

There is a certain amount of peace in preparation. The next step is to make a coping plan for each high-risk situation. The plan is made well in advance, perhaps two months before the high-risk situation occurs, to permit time to practice and gain confidence. The plan involves multiple elements or tools which will be used at the same time. For each situation, we consider the coping strategies that are available to us. Table 45.2 lists coping strategies that are usually adaptive versus those that are not.

Note that selective avoidance might be a wise coping approach at times. For example, it is wise to steer clear of people with tendencies to batter or abuse in selecting intimate partners. The characteristics of potential batterers are well-documented (tendency to control and isolate, jealousy, insecurity, criticism, anger, etc.). Discuss these with your therapist, and don't expect "love" to change this kind of person. (Love does not expect to change someone but accepts others as they are.) You might wish to avoid social situations that you find uninteresting, but ask yourself if you are depriving yourself of a potentially pleasant opportunity.

For each high-risk situation, write out a specific plan. Consider all the things you need to do to cope effectively. What would you do to cope? What will you do to ensure that a setback does not become a full-blown relapse? Who would you contact for help? What do you need to tell yourself? What would you do first? In what order would all these things occur?

Part of the coping plan involves preplanned, self-instructional statements.[297] Imagine confronting a difficult situation. Imagine eliminating unproductive thoughts, such as "Here we go again" (fortune-telling, all-or-nothing) and "I'll never be okay" (fortune-telling). Instead, you have a battery of thoughts planned for before, during, and after the situation (see Table 45.3).

One way to plan for high-risk situations is to break the feared down situation into parts. Make a written total hierarchy of the feared situation. Think of the situation as one pearl in a string of life pearls. Think of pleasant things that will occur after you encounter the feared situation. Think of pleasant events preceding the feared situation. Then break down the feared situation into chronological steps. Decide what is needed for each part of the feared situation. Anticipate unproductive thoughts and figure out replacement thoughts at each step.[298]

Also, make a plan for immediate recovery, should a setback be encountered. Review the skills in this book, and identify those that will help you return to

Table 45.2
COPING OPTIONS

Usually Unproductive	Usually Productive
Hostility (judging, revenge, acting out anger)	Empathize, compassion, remain calm enough to be effective, anger control techniques.
Withdraw, freeze, avoid, give up, do nothing, be passive, wait to be rescued, be helpless	Gather facts, make plan, problem solve, take rational action, ask for help, replace trigger with something constructive (e.g., read pleasant book instead of watching news), learn needed skills.
Isolate yourself, suffer alone	Make connections with mental health professionals, support groups, or individuals.
Allow abusive treatment	Assert, negotiate, compromise.
Placate	Acknowledge feelings constructively.
Deny problems	Acknowledge problems, but don't stew.
Sedation, escape	Take responsibility for coping; healthy distractions, relaxation, talk it over.
Make excuses	Acknowledge external factors, improve behavior.
Take total blame	Acknowledge all influences; accept rational responsibility with self-acceptance.
Cynicism, fatalism, pessimism	Laughter, soft humor, optimism.
Constant worry	Confine worry to twenty-five-minute daily worry period. Worry in writing, with an eye toward solutions. Then do something else that's distracting/ pleasant.
Despair	See how far you've come, replace distortions (e.g., Is this symptom actually occurring all the time, or is it actually less severe or frequent than it was?). Normalize the symptoms.

balance after the setback. Write these down. The plan might include a booster session with your therapist.

REHEARSE THE PLAN

This is an opportunity to put everything together and practice your plan, much like an actress or athlete would rehearse in relatively low-stress situations. Re-

Table 45.3
PREPLANNED, SELF-INSTRUCTIONAL STATEMENTS

Before	• Realistically, what are the odds that something bad will happen?
	• I've been through this before. I know what to expect.
	• I'm prepared. I know what to do. Just stay calm and think what you need to do.
	• Things might go well. If not, that's okay. I'll do my best and see what happens.
	• A good job is okay—no need for perfection.
	• Some upset is to be expected. It's normal. It will pass.
	• Be gentle. Relax into the symptoms.
	• I have better coping skills now.
	• I'm capable.
	• Challenges to grow are just a part of life.
During	• No need to be too upset.
	• Just use arousal as a cue to cope.
	• This is just a moment. It will pass. I can handle this. I can ride this out.
	• It will end soon. I'm doing fine.
	• I am capable. I can figure out ways to calm myself down.
	• Just relax and breathe calmly.
	• I've survived all sorts of things—I'll survive this.
	• This is inconvenient, not the end of the world.
	• These are just harmless memories. No need to take them too seriously or pay attention to them now.
After	• I did pretty well. Maybe not perfectly, but all in all pretty well.
	• Next time will probably be easier now.
	• *Some* symptoms do not mean total relapse.
	• It's normal to have upset. That's life. I know how to restore balance.
	• I just had a bad day. It's silly to expect perfect peace. I'll feel better again.
	• A setback means I made some progress.
	• What have I learned to help me cope in the future?

hearsing can be done in image or in role play.

In imagery, you imagine yourself encountering the feared situation and coping successfully. Abueg and colleagues instruct the individual as follows:

1. *Take two to three minutes to recall all your coping actions—all the elements of your coping plan.*

2. *Begin to get comfortable in your chair, and slowly close your eyes.* Allow yourself to begin to feel relaxed and comfortable. Take a deep breath, hold

it, and then release it, noticing yourself getting rid of tension and becoming more relaxed. Good. (Do a relaxation technique here.)

Now, imagine a black screen in front of your eyes. You can't see a thing, just a dark black screen in front of your eyes. Just a deep black screen like you're looking out into deep space. As you look at the blackness, you begin to see your high-risk scene. Look around the scene and notice what you see, the colors, shapes, things in the room or on the ground. Notice what sounds you hear and listen to the sounds. Notice what other people look like and what they're doing. Now, visualize yourself coping positively and effectively. Good. Now I'd like you to turn your attention back to this room and become aware of your surroundings here. When you're ready, open your eyes and return your focus to the present.

3. *Discuss.* How well did the coping routine work? Which parts seemed effective and not so effective? At what points did you notice strong emotions? What are the lessons learned? How would the imagined situation compare with the real situation?

4. *Practice a daily five-minute visualization of positive coping.* You can change the high-risk situation from day to day if you like.

This form of imagery is called mastery imagery, because you imagine yourself mastering the situation. Some people find it more realistic to first imagine yourself being distressed, but then rebounding and coping well.[299]

TRY OUT THE PLAN IN REAL LIFE

When sufficiently confident, implement your plan with a scientist's eye. Without judging yourself, just see how well your plan works and how well you coped.

EVALUATE AND MAKE IMPROVEMENTS IF NEEDED

If the plan worked well, or even partially, give yourself credit for making and executing it. If the plan needs improvements, identify what they would be and practice them.

CHAPTER 46

Summing Up

Having worked your way through this book, you are now familiar with an array of skills that can help you lessen your PTSD symptoms and cope with stress throughout life. Like most other skills, you will probably need to practice them to keep sharp. It will not be unusual to need to return to this book to review certain principles and skills.

Try to keep your life in balance. Remember to do things that keep you physically fit, nourished, and rested. It is also important to include pleasurable and satisfying activities in your life. Be kind to yourself when you are less than perfect, or when things don't go as smoothly as you'd like. And finally, remember that help is available when you need or want it (see Appendix 10 for a variety of resources).

To summarize and reinforce what you have learned, please flip back through the pages of this book and list those ideas and skills that you most want to remember. Complete the following:

I. The ideas that have had the most meaning to me are . . .

2. The skills that I most wish to return to and use again are . . .

3. What do I need right now? Are there skills that I would like to spend more time with? (If so, make a plan and take the time to do so.)

I close with my earnest wishes for your healing, recovery, and growth.

Appendices

The History of PTSD*

It is instructive to review the history or PTSD, and understand that people have experienced this and coped with it throughout history.

1900 B.C.	Egyptian physicians first report hysterical reactions.
8th century B.C.	Homer's *The Odyssey* describes the "travails of Odysseus," a veteran of Trojan Wars, including flashbacks and survivor's guilt.
490 B.C.	Herodotus writes of a soldier going blind after witnessing the death of a comrade next to him.
1597	Shakespeare vividly describes war sequelae (Lady Percy in *King Henry IV*).
1600	Samuel Pepys describes symptoms in survivors of the great fire of London.
1879	Rigler coins term *compensation neurosis*.
1880s	Pierre Janet studies and treats traumatic stress; eventually describes "hysterical and dissociative symptoms, inability to integrate memories, biphasic nature" of suppression and intrusion, and other symptoms often resulting from abuse.
1899	Helmut Oppenheim coins term *traumatic neurosis*.
1890s	Freud believes patients; develops seduction theory, which relates symptoms to traumatic sexual experience. Unfortunately,

---

*The interested reader will find an excellent historical overview in Figley, C. R., foreword in J. P. Wilson and B. Raphael, eds., *International Handbook of Traumatic Stress Syndromes* (New York: Plenum, 1993): xvii–xx, from which this is primarily adapted. Quotations are his.

	within a few years, he recants in favor of the theory that patients' accounts are just fantasized sexual desires.
WWI	The term *shell shock* describes symptoms believed to be caused by artillery barrages.
WWII	The terms *battle fatigue, combat exhaustion, and traumatic neurosis* describe symptoms thought to be caused primarily by the stress of combat.
	Gen. George Patton slaps soldier nervously incapable of combat.
1980	PTSD becomes a diagnostic category in DSM III.
1985	Society for Traumatic Stress Studies formed (*Journal of Traumatic Stress*).
1980s	False Memory Foundation urges caution in some cases since memories can change over time.
1991	Dr. George Everly coins the term *psychotraumatology* to describe the study of traumatic experience and the prevention and treatment of symptoms.
Present	Thousands specialize worldwide in psychotraumatology.

APPENDIX 2

Assessing Abuse

Some people are uncertain whether or not what happened to them was abuse. The following questions from Cruz and Essen might help.[300]

1. *Sexual Abuse.* Has anyone ever fondled you; touched, held, or kissed you inappropriately; forced you to look at or touch another person's private parts; forced you into a prone position; forced you to listen to off-color stories or look at pornography; forced you to go nude, touch, or masturbate yourself; raped you; required you to share a bed after toddlerhood; given enemas when unnecessary? Were you threatened or told to keep such actions secret? Did the other person's actions cause you to feel frightened, ashamed, or cause other negative reactions?

2. *Physical Abuse.* How were you disciplined? Were you hit, slapped, spanked? Where? Did it cause marks? Were you kicked, pinched, shoved, punched, bitten, scratched, choked, thrown? Did it cause broken bones? Were you restrained? Were your arms twisted? Were you forced to eat or drink bad food, or forced to eat or drink large quantities? Did your caretakers minimize or deny abuse? Were you hit with an object or threatened with a weapon?

3. *Emotional Abuse.* Were you frequently called names, put down, insulted, ridiculed, ignored, rejected, humiliated, teased, threatened with harm or abandonment, bullied, isolated, told you were no good or wrong? Did your caretakers demand all your attention? Did they fail to protect you from emotional attacks by others? Did others force you to depend on them and forbid you to form friendships with others?

Cruz and Essen suggest that old photographs might help you to assess abuse, revealing what you were like before, during, and after. Photographs might help one to see the impact of abuse at different stages of life. Photographs can also help you to rediscover disowned parts of yourself. What do you notice regarding your face, body, expression, and physical sensations? What did you like? What were you proud of? What were your beliefs about self, others, and the world—compared to now? What meaning does the photo have for you now? What do you learn about yourself and others? Sometimes a photo helps break denial (e.g., a man insisted that his childhood was idyllic, yet the picture tells a different story). Draw comparisons: What differences between the three phases do you notice—remember sights, sounds, smells, or tactile sensations? What feelings did you have then that you no longer have? Do you have any physiological reactions to those feelings? What feelings are still evident today? Are you able to soothe yourself? Keep a picture of your pretrauma self, in a special frame, as a reminder of feelings you can again experience—such as love, acceptance, respect, and joy.

The Brain and Memory

Neuroscientists are beginning to understand how the brain processes memories. The limbic system is the emotional center of the brain. The amygdala, part of the emotional center, begins processing emotional memories. It sends memories that are fragmented, emotional, and irrational to the hippocampus for integration.

Sitting next to the amygdala, the hippocampus performs critical roles of memory integration. The hippocampus helps:

- connect aspects of a single memory to each other

- connect a single memory to other memories

- locate a memory in time and space, permitting one to recall a memory in the context of one's life history (i.e., the memory is filed in an organized way alongside other memories)

- give memories "narrative coherence" by sending them to the prefrontal cortex for interpretation. A certain area of the left frontal cortex, Broca's area, generates names for emotions and verbally integrates memories. This gives a memory logic and understanding and allows it to make sense. This process allows strong emotions to settle so that the memory can be stored in long-term memory. We say that the hippocampus is emotionally cool—it permits us to recall memories without being overwhelmed by uncontrolled emotions.

The locus ceruleus is the brain's alarm or stress center. Located in the brain stem near the limbic system, it communicates directly with the amygdala and hippocampus. In response to fear, the locus ceruleus fires, sending alarm messages throughout the brain and starting a cascade of changes in chemical messengers, or neurotransmitters, throughout the brain. Once sensitized, the locus ceruleus reacts to smaller stressors as if they were recurrences of the original trauma.

Traumatic memories seem to be processed and stored differently than normal memories. The hippocampus becomes smaller in traumatized individuals and appears to become less functional during subsequent stressful periods. Broca's area shuts off and other prefrontal areas become less active. At the same time, the amygdala seems to become more active under stress or when reliving traumatic memories. Charged negative emotions seem to be "stuck" in the right hemisphere, split from the more logical left hemisphere. This accounts for the speechless terror of PTSD. As a result, trauma material remains fragmented, emotionally charged, nonverbal, and unstable. Now relatively harmless triggers can cause trauma memories or memory fragments to flood one's awareness. The material is emotionally distressing and does not make sense. It cannot be put away as just one memory in a file of memories. Rather, it seems as if the trauma memory is the only memory on file. Because the memory cannot be expressed verbally, it is often expressed as physical symptoms.

References

Everly, G. S. Jr., and J. M. Lating, eds. *Psychotraumatology: Key Papers and Core Concepts in Post-Traumatic Stress.* New York: Plenum, 1995.

van der Kolk, B. A., A. C. McFarlane, and L. Weisaeth, eds. *Traumatic Stress: The Effects of Overwhelming Experience on Mind, Body, and Society.* New York: Guilford, 1996.

van der Kolk, B. A., and J. Saporta. "Biological Response to Psychic Trauma," in J. P. Wilson and B. Raphael, eds. *International Handbook of Traumatic Stress Syndromes.* New York: Plenum, 1993, 25–34.

Psychiatric Disorders

These disorders might result in response to trauma. They usually develop by early adulthood. However, there are other factors that can contribute and not all victims of trauma develop these disorders.

ANTISOCIAL PERSONALITY DISORDER (sociopathy/psychopathy)

Think of Adolf Hitler or Saddam Hussein and you will have an image of this disorder. Brutally abused as children, they became indifferent to the suffering or well-being of others. This disorder is defined as extreme disregard for, and violation of, the rights of others. It is marked by aggression to people or animals, destruction of property, deceit, manipulation or bullying, stealing or other criminal behavior, inability to keep a job or remain in relationships, anger, revenge, irresponsibility (failing to pay child support or debts), lack of compassion or remorse, and cockiness. The victim might become the victimizer, thinking, "I should do what I can get away with—push before I'm pushed; It's okay to lie; I'm entitled to what I want; I count, you don't."[301] This disorder prevents the bonding that would otherwise help heal.

BORDERLINE PERSONALITY DISORDER

Think of a woman who was abused and abandoned in childhood. As an adult, she clings desperately to relationships, yet fears she will be abandoned. This personality disorder is characterized by extreme instability in relationships, mood, and self-image. It is seen frequently in people who come from homes marked by abuse (especially incest), abandonment, conflict, or neglect. Interestingly, 70 percent of people diagnosed with dissociative identity disorder (DID) also share a diagnosis of borderline personality disorder, suggesting common roots.[302] Its diagnostic features include:

- Poor self-esteem that might lift when the person is in an intense relationship, but falls with any threat of rejection or abandonment.

- A profound need to be in an intense relationship, coupled with a feeling of impending rejection. They make unreasonable demands on lovers/caregivers, idealizing them when they are sufficiently devoted, and demonizing them when they show insufficient attention (either the loved one is a devil or an angel). They rage at perceived slights (such as being kept waiting), which seem to confirm their lack of worth. They can become very angry and sarcastic when caregivers or lovers are not attentive enough.

- Rejection or being alone may lead to impulsive, self-destructive behavior: self-mutilating, suicide, gambling, binge eating, drug abuse, or unsafe sex.

- Plagued by feelings of emptiness, boredom, inability to be alone, and neediness.

The psychological underpinnings—low self-esteem, fear of being unloved (a symptom of low self-esteem), and fear of being alone with dissociated material—all suggest antidotes to the disorder.

NARCISSISTIC PERSONALITY DISORDER

An air of superiority and the need for admiring attention suggests an underlying lack of self-love. Their self-absorption does not permit empathy or love for others. Instead, the narcissist will exploit others in order to succeed. Narcissism may be viewed as compensation for uncertain self-worth and self-protection from vulnerability.[303]

DISSOCIATIVE IDENTITY DISORDER

Although not a personality disorder, this condition affects the personality. According to the International Society for the Study of Dissociation, a person with DID is a single person who experiences having separate parts of the mind that function with some autonomy. The patient is not a collection of separate people sharing the same body. The terms *personality* and *alter* (short for alternate personality) refer to dissociated parts of the mind that alternately influence behavior. Some clinicians prefer terms such as *disaggregate self state, part of the mind*, or *part of the self*.

Whenever possible, treatment should move the patient toward a sense of integrated functioning and connectedness among the different alternate personalities. Individual psychotherapy generally involves two to three sessions per week, over a period of three to five years (or more in complex cases). Treatment modalities include psychodynamic, modified cognitive-behavioral, and hypnosis—most commonly for calming, soothing, containment, and ego strengthening. While some believe that hypnotic techniques are useful in memory retrieval, others believe that hypnotically facilitated memory processing increases the patient's chances of mislabeling fantasy as real memory and increases the patient's level of belief in "retrieved" imagery that may actually be fantasized. Therapists, therefore, should minimize the use of leading questions that may in some cases alter the details of what is recalled in hypnosis. Group psychotherapy is not a viable primary treatment modality and may prove destabilizing for some people with DID. However, carefully structured, time-limited groups can be a useful adjunct to promote a sense that survivors are not alone in coping with their symptoms.

References

The descriptions are adapted from the American Psychiatric Association, 1994: *DSM IV*.

Dissociative identity disorder treatment guidelines are adapted from *Guidelines for Treating Dissociative Identity Disorder (Multiple Personality Disorder) in Adults*, 1997. Copyright ©1994, 1997. International Society for the Study of Dissociation, 4700 West Lake Avenue, Glenview, IL 60025–1485.

Scott, M. J. and S. G. Stradling. *Counseling for Post-Traumatic Stress Disorder.* 1992. London: Sage.

Braun, B. G. 1993. "Multiple Personality Disorder and Post-traumatic Stress Disorder," in J. P. Wilson and B. Raphael, eds. *International Handbook of Traumatic Stress Syndromes*. New York: Plenum, 1993, 35–47.

Parson, E. R. 1993. "Post-traumatic Narcissism: Healing Traumatic Alterations in the Self Through Curvilinear Group Psychotherapy," in J. P. Wilson and B. Raphael, eds., 821–40.

APPENDIX 5

72-Hour Emergency Preparedness

An emergency kit that will sustain you for several days can provide a tremendous sense of security for a variety of emergencies: natural disasters, the need to flee an abuser, or civil unrest. As much as possible, store items in a single container (e.g., a suitcase, duffel, backpack) in a safe and accessible place. This inventory list can be kept with the container.

ITEM	ON HAND (√)	PURCHASE (√)
sleeping bag and pad		
light tent		
clothing (coat, change of clothes)		
underwear		
socks		
gloves		
hat		
footwear		
whistle		
money: credit cards, $20 plus coins for phone calls		
important papers (notarized copies) driver's license, car title birth certificate		

will

insurance

important phone numbers & addresses

assets (locations, amounts)

military discharge, passport

food: ready-to eat meals, tuna,
    peanut butter, etc.

candles and flares

waterproof matches

blanket

poncho

flashlight (rechargeable, batteries)

can opener

pocket knife

toilet articles—soap, toothbrush, floss,
    toilet paper, towelettes, etc.

pencil, pen, paper

sunscreen

insect repellent

first aid

    tweezers

    aspirin

    adhesive tape

    gauze bandage

    medications

canteen with water and additional water

sewing kit

entertainment—reading, games, etc.

Other items to take (not stored with container) and their location:

Time Management

**One hour spent in effective planning saves
three to four hours in execution.**

Many time-management approaches simply train people to be *efficient* workers. However, the larger goal is to manage time with wisdom, enjoyment, and balance. The driven person, for example, might be very efficient at using time to accomplish tasks, but not allow time for activities that promote balanced health. This person might be rich in achievements but impoverished in joy and health.

"Burnout" refers to the exhaustion resulting from demand overload, particularly when the demands yield little joy. There are several antidotes to burnout. One (a short-term solution) is to take a vacation that is long enough to restore sanity. A second antidote is to develop and use a plan that balances work, love, and play. The "want to's" are just as essential to overall well-being as the "need to's" because the former promote growth, satisfaction, joy, and emotional well-being. This is not to diminish the importance of "need to's." There is nothing wrong with well-defined career goals that promote prosperity. This strategy, however, will challenge you to also meet your essential emotional, physical, and spiritual needs, so that you are more likely to achieve your professional goals without burning out and losing the "joie de vivre." Get some sheets of paper, and be prepared to write.

STEP 1: **Life Goals.** Finish the following sentence stems. Write as quickly as you can. Do not worry about whether what you write is doable or makes sense. Just write quickly.

- My personal definition of success is . . . (Try to think beyond the material. Those whose central goals are solely financial tend to have poorer mental health.)

- If I were to live more fully functioning and happily I would be more . . . and less . . . (For this one, indicate personal traits.)

- My life overall would be just about ideal/complete if I were to . . . (Imagine you were taking a video of yourself. What would you see yourself doing?)

- My retirement goals are . . .

- My goals for ten years from now are . . .

- My goals for five years from now are . . .

- My goals for one year from now are . . .

- If someone looking into a crystal ball were to tell me that I had only six months to live, I would do the following:

STEP 2: **Balance Check.** You have just made a substantial list of goals that are important to you. Now you'll check your goals for balance. Goals typically fall under one or more of the following categories:

1. *Physical health* (weight, fitness, rest, eating, medical care)

2. *Personal* (character/spiritual development, personality traits, emotional health, possessions you'd like to acquire)

3. *Relationships* (family, friends, groups)

4. *Recreation* (entertainment, hobbies, travel)

5. *Professional* (career or educational)

Beside each response to the sentence stems in Step 1, place a 1, 2, 3, 4 and/or a 5 according to the five categories above. When you finish this step, pause. What do you notice? Are your goals balanced? Make any desired adjustments.

STEP 3: **Backward Planning.** There is peace in preparation, in having a sound written plan to refer to during times of distraction and distress. In this step, translate your general life goals to more specific goals that are achievable. Start by making a five-year goal sheet as follows:

FIVE-YEAR GOALS

for Period _____ 20 __ to _____ 20 __
[month/year]   [month/year]

Goals	What I'll Do to Reach Goals	Starting Date	How I'll Know I Reached Goal	How I Did (evaluate at end of period)

Considering all your life goals, list several goals under each of the five categories listed at Step 2. Try to make each goal as specific and measurable as possible. For example, instead of the vague physical health goal of "improve appearance," you might write "lose one inch off waistline." Instead of "improve personal relationships," you might write, "spend fifteen minutes of uninterrupted time with my son each day." In the second column, list specific steps that will enable you to reach each goal. For example, a way to lose one inch from the waistline might be to walk thirty minutes six days per week. In the third column, specify when you will begin to work on each goal. In the fourth column, describe how you will measure/observe the successful achievement of each goal (e.g., achieve waist measurement of 30 inches). The last column is completed after the five-year time period.

Continue the backward planning process by completing a one-year goal sheet next. Make a separate sheet for your goals for the next year, following the same procedures as for the five-year goal sheet.

STEP 4: **Monthly Planning.** Next, complete a monthly calendar for the upcoming month. What will you do each day to bring you closer to your one and five year goals? Anticipate and record here major events coming up during the month such as medical or professional appointments, work tasks, and recreational dates. You might wish to make or buy a monthly planner to continue planning for each month.

STEP 5: **Weekly Planning.** Plan a typical week, using a form such as this:

TYPICAL WEEKLY WORK AND RECREATION SCHEDULE

Hours	Sunday	Monday	Tuesday	Wednesday	Thursday	Friday	Saturday
6–7 A.M.							
7–8							
8–9							
etc.							

It is wise to start by blocking out some of the essentials such as sleep, eating, and exercise, and daily sanity breaks) before you block out other demands (commuting, work, meetings). Remember, recovery is a marathon. You'll run farther and accomplish more if you are conditioned, rested, and nourished. You'll probably want to include perhaps an hour of time beforehand to plan the week.

Pause here for a moment. Have you allowed time each day for emotional, spiritual, and physical nourishment? If not, you will probably not give your best to self, others, or your tasks. Is ample time allocated to accomplish your monthly goals? If overloading is evident, what would happen if you softened expectations or spread out the less essential goals? Remember, you can do almost anything you choose to do, but you can't do everything, and you can't do it all at once. Do what you can, and then release worry as much as you can.

STEP 6: **Daily "To Do" List.** Keep a single list of things you choose to do for the upcoming day, by priority. Do the highest-priority items first. Try to make a list with reasonable expectations, allowing sufficient time to accomplish each item. If you don't get to all the items, place the unfinished items on tomorrow's "to do" list, again listed by priorities. You might wish to make a "to do" list at least an hour or two before bedtime, and review it at the start of the next day. It is also suggested that you keep all your planning sheets together, perhaps in a single notebook, with your daily "to do" list first, where you can refer to it often.

Rape and Sexual Assault Facts and Myths*

Rape refers to criminal sexual assault committed by a man against a woman. The legal definition of *criminal sexual assault* is: "any genital, anal, or oral penetration, by a part of the accused's body or by an object, using force or without the victim's consent." Lack of consent includes the inability to give consent due to being underage or due to impaired mental function caused by alcohol and/or drugs, sleep, or unconsciousness.

The American Medical Association has compiled common myths believed by rape victims. These myths can lead to inappropriate guilt:

1. *A woman who truly resists can't be raped. If she didn't fight back she must have wanted it.* Some women are too afraid of physical harm to fight back. Particularly in acquaintance rape, the woman is often too shocked to believe that someone whom she knows and trusts would rape her. She is not mobilized to hurt the other person and hopes that he will come to his senses and stop.

2. *A woman who gets drunk deserves to be raped.* Getting drunk may reflect poor judgment, but does not justify being assaulted.

3. *A woman who goes to a man's room after a party deserves it.* Consenting to go to someone's room to "see my new salt-water fish collection," or for any other reason, does not equate to consent to have sex.

*Source: American Medical Association. 1995. *Strategies for the Treatment and Prevention of Sexual Assault*. Chicago, Ill.: American Medical Association. Copyright ©1995 by the AMA.

4. *Agreeing to some degree of sexual intimacy means she wants intercourse.* Consenting to some physical closeness is not the same as consenting to intercourse.

5. *A woman must want it if it has happened before and she allows it to happen again.* People who have been abused before often feel helpless to protect themselves. A condition called *learned helplessness* develops that probably includes biologically based changes.

6. *Women really want to be raped.* There is a difference between intimacy and rape.

7. *Since women aren't physically hurt by rape, they'll get over it.* Emotional wounds are often more debilitating than physical ones, and usually last longer.

8. *If the woman is not a virgin, it is not a big deal.* Any sexual assault can severely traumatize and impede interpersonal and intimate relationships for a very long time. Even prostitutes can be traumatized, although they rarely report it because they are seldom taken seriously.

9. *Sexual assault is only perpetrated by strange men against women.* Rape is just one type of sexual assault. Sexual assault can also be committed by women against men. Most sexual assault is committed by acquaintances, not strangers.

Other myths:

- *If the woman had an orgasm, she wanted to be raped.* Orgasm is a physiological response that can happen when the genital area is stimulated. This can happen without wanting it to happen. An orgasm does not mean that the victim wanted to be raped, or enjoyed it.

- *Something about the victim caused the rape.* Rape is a criminal act. The perpetrator is responsible for it, not the victim.

Medication Facts and Guidelines

> I've never seen anyone cured of PTSD with a pill.
>
> —*Dr. George Everly*

Psychotropic medication is sometimes used to lessen certain symptoms of PTSD. All have side-effects of varying degrees, and none reduce all symptoms. None seem to work well in reducing guilt, grief, interpersonal difficulties, or moral outrage. However, medications can reduce intrusions (nightmares, recollections, flashbacks) and physical arousal (insomnia, irritability, startle reactivity). They can be useful when symptoms are so severe that therapy cannot proceed. The medications that are sometimes tried are:

Antidepressants. These may especially lessen symptoms of both depression and anxiety, as well as chronic pain with little risk of dependence.

- Newer antidepressants (the serotonergic drugs such as Prozac, Paxil, Luvox, Zoloft) have fewer side-effects than older antidepressants and are currently thought to be the first line of treatment for chronic PTSD. They might also help to reduce numbing and avoidance.

- Tricyclics. Imiprimine (Tofranil) and amitriptyline (Elavil) are the most studied.

- MAO inhibitors. Phenelzine (Nardil) has been studied the most. Extreme side-effects occur if dietary restrictions are not followed.

Mood stabilizers may help to reduce arousal, mood swings, rage, violent impulses, hallucinations, and/or delusions. These include:

- Lithium (Eskalith)
- Antikindling agents, such as carbamazepine (Tegretol) and sodium valproate (Depakote)

Clonidine (Catapres, an alpha-2 agonist) and propranolol (Inderal, a beta-blocker) help reduce arousal, intrusions, and angry outbursts without risk of abuse or addiction.

Opioid antagonists block opiates, which result in numbing and stress-induced analgesia. Naltrexone may reduce self-mutilation.

Benzodiazepines (anti-anxiety drugs or minor tranquilizers) can quickly lessen symptoms of anxiety but their use is quite controversial. They can be quite addictive and discontinuing their use can be difficult. Rebound anxiety can follow discontinuation, especially when discontinuation is too abrupt. The use of benzodiazepines can induce depressive symptoms, which should be monitored. The benzodiazepines include:

- Diazepam (Valium)
- Alprazolam (Xanax)
- Clonazepam (Klonopin; has somewhat less-distressing withdrawal symptoms)
- Lorazepam (Ativan)

Buspirone (Buspar), which is not a benzodiazepine, also helps reduce arousal and causes less dependence and withdrawal symptoms.

Antipsychotics or neuroleptics such as Clozaril and Thorazine reduce psychotic thoughts such as hallucinations. These are not usually used unless antidepressants or other drugs are not working because hallucinatory flashbacks in PTSD are consistent with dissociation, not psychosis.

SPECIAL CONSIDERATIONS:

Several points are important to keep in mind when taking medication:

- Medications have side effects (such as dry mouth, constipation, dizziness, sleepiness, nervousness). These are generally mild and tend to lessen with treatment.

- It takes awhile for antidepressants and other medications to work. During the first few weeks you may experience side effects, but little relief from PTSD symptoms. Therefore, your doctor may ask you to stick with a medication for six to twelve weeks. If no improvement is then noticed, your doctor may try a different medication or combination of medications. Careful adjustment of dosage and monitoring for side effects require that you work closely with your doctor.

- Maintenance periods might last a year or longer, or until recovery is stabilized.

- Before taking any medication, give your doctor a complete history of all drugs you use, including alcohol, marijuana, caffeine, and cocaine. Even one drink a day can interfere with the effects of antidepressant medication. Some drugs can trigger anxiety symptoms. Some can react with anti-anxiety drugs, causing severe side-effects.

- It is important to consult a physician who is familiar both with diagnosing PTSD and with properly prescribing medication. As a rule, a psychiatrist (or a team with one) is preferable to a family physician in prescribing drugs for PTSD. A psychiatrist is usually more experienced in recognizing symptoms of mental disturbance and is usually more knowledgeable about the medications used. If you wish reassurance that a medication is properly prescribed, consult a current edition of *Drug Facts and Comparisons* or *Physicians Desk Reference* (check your library or a medical school library), or get a second opinion.

- After prolonged use, do not stop taking medication all at once. Abrupt withdrawal of medication might cause confusion, nausea, sleep disruption, or relapse. The likelihood of keeping symptoms manageable is greatest if you have learned sound coping skills and if discontinuation is tapered over the course of several weeks or months. However, the return of symptoms is the rule after discontinuation. Discuss *any* changes in medication with your doctor. And do not miss doses.

- Be sure you completely understand instructions for taking your medications. Prescriptions can be confusing. If you are confused at all, ask your doctor to help you. Reasonable questions to ask are:

  "What is the name of the drug, and what is it supposed to do?"

"How and when do I take it, and when do I stop taking it?"
"What are the side-effects, and what should I do if they occur?"
"Is this drug addictive?"
"How long does it take to be effective?"
"What food, drink, drugs, or activities should I avoid while taking it?"
"What should I do if I forget to take a dose?"
"Is there any written information about the drug?"

- Ask your pharmacist for information. They can often give you information about side effects, medications, foods to avoid, etc.

- Some antidepressants (Prozac and other serotonin enhancers) do not work well if there is inadequate intake of protein, so make sure you are eating balanced meals.

Victim, Survivor, Thriver

Although the terms *victim* and *survivor* are often used interchangeably, the terms *victim, survivor,* and *thriver* often reflect attitudinal distinctions as follows.

VICTIM	SURVIVOR	THRIVER
helpless	satisfying sense of having gotten through intact or mostly in-tact	committed to move forward
out of control		planning for the future
angry		active
hoping to be rescued	beginning to feel strong	self-determined
perception of lacking choices	perception that one has re-sources and choices	feels joy day to day
self-pity		achieving mastery
passive	recognition of one's potential to change and grow	self-esteem; sees self as more than a victim—a valuable person
payoffs (secondary gains) per-suade person to remain in victim role	living one day at a time; coping from day to day; present life is primary focus	reaching out to others; finding meaning and purpose
identity as a victim		
in pain, numb	beginning to take control	ennobled by the experience; has grown from the trauma
defeated	beginning to "thaw out" or heal	
avoidance of feelings	living moderately well	living well
"I'm still in the trauma"	suffering begins to lessen	can endure remaining PTSD symptoms with relative com-fort or acceptance
controlled by memories	neutral about life—not de-pressed, but not happy	
controlled by depression, anxi-ety, hatred, bitterness, re-venge, physical complaints	realization that one is outside of the trauma; one has gotten through it	guilt has been resolved
has not yet learned from the experience, likely to repeat trauma, victimization	extricated self from abuse (ei-ther in actuality or at least one has mentally triumphed over it)	generally satisfied with life
shame, self-dislike		perception that one has moved beyond the trauma
self-destructive, addictions		

VICTIM	SURVIVOR	THRIVER
hiding	confronting trauma	acquiring peace, happiness, renewal, commitment to life, optimism despite scars, empowerment
feeling fragile, vulnerable, defenseless	beginning to integrate	
	guilt beginning to be resolved	
sense of no future, preoccupation with the past	committed to healing, trusting, and restoring boundaries	committed to physical health
discouraged, immobilized	influenced, but not controlled, by past	committed to loving again
	mostly back to normal	feeling strong, compassionate—able to connect with others who are suffering and imperfect without a need to hide
		resilient, renewed
		has learned coping skills that did not exist before the trauma
		sense of humor
		"beginner's mind"—openness to possibilities
		finds ordinary life interesting—does not need "adrenaline fix"

Resources

REFERRALS: FINDING MENTAL HEALTH PROFESSIONALS

In addition to the following resources, check with police, rape crisis hotlines, women's shelters, and crisis /sexual assault centers for referrals.

Sidran Foundation, 2328 West Joppa Road, Suite 15, Lutherville, MD 21093 (410) 825-8888. Free referrals to psychotherapists specializing in PTSD.

International Society for Traumatic Stress Studies, 60 Revere Drive, Suite 500, Northbrook, IL 60062; (847) 480-9028. Provides resource list for services and information.

American Professional Society on the Abuse of Children (APSAC), 407 South Dearborn, Suite 1300, Chicago, IL 60605; (312) 554-0166. Refers children and adults through state chapters.

Childhelp USA, 15757 North 78 Street, Scottsdale, AZ 85260; 1-800-422-4453. In addition to referrals to therapists, crisis centers, and child protective services, hotline also provides crisis counseling for children, troubled parents, and adult survivors. Free literature on child abuse, parenting, and recovery.

TIR Association, 13 North West Barry Road, Suite 214, Kansas City, MO 64155-2728; (816) 468-4945. Referrals to clinicians offering traumatic incident reduction (TIR).

EMDR Institute, P.O. Box 51010, Pacific Grove, CA 93950; (831) 372-3900 ext. 16; 1-800-780-3637. Referrals for clinicians trained in eye movement desensitization and reprocessing.

American Art Therapy Association, 1202 Allanson Road, Mundelein, IL 60060 (847) 949-6064. Referrals for registered art therapists through local chapters.

American Dance Therapy Association, 2000 Century Plaza, Suite 108, 10632; Little Patuxent Parkway, Columbia, MD 21044 (410) 997-4040. Referrals for registered dance therapists. Co-located with National Coalition of Arts Therapies Association.

American Music Therapy Association, 8455 Colesville Road, Suite 1000, Silver Spring, MD 20910-3392; (301) 589-3300. Registered music therapists.

Association for Play Therapy, 5130 East Clinton Way, Fresno, CA 93727; (209) 253-2278. Referrals to registered play therapists.

National Association for Drama Therapy, 15245 Shady Grove Road, Suite 130, Rockville, MD 20850; (301) 258-9210. Referrals to registered drama therapists who have training in drama and psychotherapy.

Association for Poetry Therapy, P.O. Box 551, Port Washington, NY 11050; (516) 944-9791. Maintains registry of registered poetry therapists who use the language arts in therapy.

Anxiety Disorders Association of America, 11900 Parklawn Drive, Suite 100, Rockville, MD 20852-2624; (301) 231-9350. Provides members with a list of professionals who specialize in the treatment of anxiety disorders. Also provides information on self-help and support groups in your area. Has a catalog of available brochures, books, and audiocassettes. Newsletter. Annual national conference.

National Mental Health Association, 1021 Prince Street, Alexandria, VA 22314-2971; (703) 684-7722 or 1-800-969-NMHA. Provides list of affiliate mental health organizations in your area who can provide resources and information about self-help groups, treatment professionals, and community clinics.

Center for Mental Health Services, 5600 Fishers Lane, Room 13-103, Rockville, MD 20857; 1-800-789-2647. Refers to local community mental health centers and family service agencies, both of which provide mental health services on a sliding fee scale. Also supplies information about mental health agencies, support groups, and clearinghouses.

American Psychiatric Association, 1400 K Street, N.W., Washington, DC 20005; (202) 682-6220. Call or write the Public Affairs office for referrals to psychiatrists in your area. (An on-call psychiatrist from the Washington Psychiatric Foundation answers your questions 9:00 A.M. to 5:00 P.M. weekdays at (202) 371-1522.

American Psychological Association, 750 First Street, N.E., Washington, DC 20002; (202) 336-5500 or 5800 or 1-800-374-2721. Call or write for referrals to psychologists in your area.

Association for Advancement of Behavior Therapy, 305 Seventh Avenue, Suite 16A, New York, NY 10001; (212) 647-1890. Provides a membership listing, including specialty areas, of mental health professionals focusing in behavior therapy and cognitive behavior therapy in your state, along with a complimentary brochure, "Guidelines for Choosing a Behavior Therapist."

American Academy of Child and Adolescent Psychiatry, 3615 Wisconsin Avenue, N.W., Washington, DC 20016; (202) 966-7300; 1-800-333-7636. Call or write for referral information about child and adolescent psychiatrists in your area.

National Board for Certified Counselors, 3 Terrace Way, Suite D, Greensboro, NC 27403; (336) 547-0607). Referrals for certified clinical mental health counselors.

National Association of Social Workers, 750 First Street, N.E., Suite 700, Washington, DC 20002-4241; (202) 408-8600 or 1-800-638-8799. Referrals to qualified clinical social workers in your area.

Family Service America, 11700 West Lake Park Drive, Milwaukee, WI 53224; 1-800-221-2681. Referrals to family/social service agencies which accept payments on a sliding scale.

American Association for Marriage and Family Therapy, 1133 Fifteenth Street, N.W., Suite 300, ATTN: Referrals, Washington, DC 20005; (202) 452-0109. Marriage and family therapists.

American Association of Pastoral Counselors, 9504A Lee Highway, Fairfax, VA 22031; (703) 385-6967. Many who seek help in times of need turn first to a clergy person. This association provides referrals to certified pastoral counselors who consider both spiritual and psychological needs.

American Nurses' Association, 600 Maryland Avenue, S.W., Suite 100W, Washington, DC 20024-2571; (202) 554-4444 or 1-800-284-2378, and ask for your state's nurses' association for referrals to psychiatric nurses.

SURVIVOR AND SUPPORT GROUPS

In addition to the following, check your local newspaper, white pages, library, police, hospitals, mental health professional, or mental health agency listings.

American Self-Help Clearinghouse, St. Clares-Riverside Medical Center, 25 Pocono Road, Denville, NJ 07834; (973) 625-3037 or 1-800-367-6274 in New Jersey only. Directs caller to diverse self-help groups. Inexpensive sourcebook lists national and model self-help groups, guidelines for forming self-help groups, and other clearinghouses.

National Self-Help Clearinghouse, 25 West 43rd Street, Room 620, New York, NY 10036; (212) 354-8525. Directs callers to self-help and support groups. Also trains facilitators.

National Helpline 1-800-662-HELP. Referrals to diverse self-help and support groups.

National Mental Health Consumers' Self-Help Clearinghouse, 1211 Chestnut Street, Philadelphia, PA 19107; 1-800-553-4539. Technical assistance for self-help groups plus help in locating self-help groups. Also furnishes inexpensive informational packets.

Below is a sampling of self-help/support groups whose numbers may be obtained from the above clearinghouses/helplines. Many are based on the Alcoholics Anonymous Twelve-step model.

Alcoholics Anonymous

Adult Children of Alcoholics

Al-Anon Family Groups and **Alateen**. For those whose lives have been affected by the drinking of a family member.

Incest Survivors Anonymous

Survivors of Incest Anonymous. Also provides a hotline and bimonthly bulletins.

Narcotics Anonymous. Support groups for users.

Nar-A-Non. Support groups for families of users of illegal drugs.

Overeaters Anonymous

Gamblers Anonymous

Sex Addicts Anonymous

Debtor's Anonymous

Cocaine Anonymous

Parents Anonymous. For parents who batter and wish to learn effective parenting. Professionally facilitated and peer-led. Not a Twelve-step program.

Theos (They Help Each Other Spiritually). Helps widowed persons move successfully through the grieving process. Non-denominational.

The Compassionate Friends. Information and referrals to support groups for bereaved parents, siblings, and grandparents who grieve the death of a child.

Widowed Persons Service, American Association of Retired Persons. Referrals for widows and widowers to information, services, and support programs.

Parents of Murdered Children. Support groups for anyone who has lost someone to homicide. Also court accompaniment, antiviolence advocacy, questions related to unsolved cases of suicide/homicide, training for support groups, and sensitivity to violence.

Survivors of Suicide. For families and friends of suicide victims.

SIDS Alliance (sudden infant death syndrome).

Parents United International and **Adults Molested as Children**. For sexually abused victims of all ages, offenders, and support persons (spouses, parents, etc.).

Society of Military Widows

National Amputation Foundation

National Burn Victim Foundation

National Head Injury Foundation

Prostitutes Anonymous

National Council on Sexual Addiction and Compulsivity (NCSAC), 1090 Northchase Parkway, Suite 200 South, Marietta, GA 30067; (770) 989-9754. Helps individuals find a Twelve-step program for sexual addiction, and counselors with interest in treating this condition.

National Council on Alcoholism and Drug Dependence, 12 West 21st Street, New York, NY 10010; (212) 206-6770 or 1-800-622-2255. Referrals to self-help groups and low-cost treatment facilities.

Pregnancy and Infant Loss Center, 1421 East Wayzata Boulevard, Suite 30, Wayzata, MN 55391; (612) 473-9372. Grief support for miscarriage, stillbirth, and infant death. Resources and education. Referrals to support groups.

National SHARE Office, St. Joseph Health Center, 300 First Capitol Drive, St. Charles, MO 63301; (314) 947-6164 or 1-800-821-6819. Support for families who have suffered perinatal loss.

AGENCIES/ORGANIZATIONS/VICTIMS' SERVICES

Check the telephone directory for violence shelters, counseling and support groups, hotlines, legal services, welfare, etc., under: crises intervention, domestic abuse information and treatment centers, social services, human services, shelters, women's organizations, or family services.

International Critical Incident Stress Foundation, 10176 Baltimore National Pike, Suite 201, Ellicott City, MD 21042; (410) 750-9600. Develops and disseminates crisis intervention, stress education, and recovery programs for all those affected by work-related stress, disasters, and other traumatic events. Annual conference and newsletter. Known for developing critical incident stress debriefing.

Sidran Foundation, 2328 West Joppa Road, Suite 15, Lutherville, MD 21093; (410) 825-8888. National nonprofit organization devoted to education and information in support of survivors of traumatic experiences. Publishes books on PTSD and DID. Computerized information database of educational resources, therapists, organizations, conferences, training, and treatment facilities.

National Domestic Violence Hotline. (512) 453-8117 or 1-800-799-SAFE or TTY 1-800-787-3224. Twenty-four-hour hotline with multilingual and deaf capabilities. Serves victims and concerned family and friends. Helps victims with issues of safety, shelter, counseling, and legal advice. Also helps batterers get help. Printed information.

National Organization for Victims Assistance (NOVA), 1757 Park Road, N.W., Washington, DC 20010; (202) 232-6682 or 1-800-TRY-NOVA. Support and advocacy for crime victims. Referrals to victim assistance programs (battered women's programs, support groups, rape crisis centers, legal and medical advice, etc.). Crisis Response Team Project formed to deal with community crisis. Training and education for helpers.

National Victim Center, 2111 Wilson Boulevard, Suite 300, Arlington, VA 22201; 1-800-FYI-CALL. Referrals to victims of any violent crime (sexual abuse, domestic violence, stalking, hate crimes, etc.) to shelters, support groups, and legal advocacy programs. Also information bulletins on these topics.

Crime

- All states have a crime victims compensation program for violent crimes (including domestic violence) that are reported within specified periods. Benefits usually apply to medical and certain legal expenses, counseling, lost income, funerals, and shelter. Assistance programs advise victims of rights, help victims through the legal system, and help them secure protection. If local authorities do not direct you, call the Office for Victims of Crime, Washington, D.C. The OVC Resource Center/Clearinghouse 1-800-627-6872 refers callers to the appropriate state or other helpful agencies. The clearinghouse also offers a wide range of printed and audio-visual information, most of which is free.

- Contact police, social service agencies, or the local bar association or legal aid society to find victim-assistance centers which provide information about legal, financial, and psychological help. Sometimes pro bono (free) legal assistance is available.

- The state department of social services or state worker compensation board will discuss worker compensation for victims of violence on the job.

- Contact the Social Security Administration to apply for disability benefits if you are disabled due to crime.

Mothers Against Drunk Driving (MADD), 511 East John Carpenter Freeway, Suite 700, Irving, TX 95062; 1-800-GET-MADD. Victim-to-victim support services include support groups, diverse publications (crash victim, mourning, legal issues, etc.), court accompaniment, help with navigating the criminal justice system, and training.

Rape, Abuse and Incest National Network (RAINN), 252 Tenth Street, N.E., Washington, DC 20002. Calling 1-800-656-HOPE (ext. 1) will automatically connect a victim of sexual assault to the nearest sexual assault center. These centers provide confidential twenty-four-hour crisis hotlines for free advice and support. Also free or sliding scale private counseling and/or groups treatment.

National Committee to Prevent Child Abuse, P.O. Box 2866, Chicago, IL 60690; (312) 663-3520 or 1-800-835-2671 or 1-800-CHILDREN. Extensive printed material. Healthy Families America is a home-visiting service for parents which teaches parenting skills, links parents to resources, and provides a helping hand.

National Clearinghouse for Child Abuse and Neglect Information, P.O. Box 1182, Washington, DC 20013-1182; (703) 385-7565 or 1-800-394-3366. Information of all aspects of child mistreatment for the public and professionals. Referrals to services.

American Foundation for Suicide Prevention, 120 Wall Street, 22nd Floor, New York, NY 10005; 1-888-333-AFSP. Survivors of suicide support groups. Also referral to crisis hotlines. Free materials on coping.

Group Project for Holocaust Survivors and Their Children, 345 East 80th Street, New York, NY 10021; (212) 737-8524. Referrals, training for therapists and others working with all types of trauma survivors. Literature and bibliographies may be purchased. Counseling and intergenerational community meetings. Dr. Y. Danieli, Director.

Post-Abortion Stress

- Open Arms, P.O. Box 9292, Colorado Springs, CO 80932; (719) 573-5790. Christian support groups. Newsletter and phone support.

- Institute for Pregnancy Loss, 111 Bow Street, Portsmouth, NH 03801-3819; (603) 778-1450. Vincent M. Rue, Director. Counseling, research, and consulting organization providing compassionate information regarding traumatic pregnancy losses (induced and spontaneous abortion, stillbirth, and adoption).

- National Office of Post-Abortion Reconciliation and Healing, P.O. Box 07477, Milwaukee, WI 53207; 1-800-5WE CARE. Support services directory, audio-visual materials, annual conference. Directs Project Rachel, a Catholic counseling project which is for people of all faiths.

Gift From Within, R.R.1 Box 5158, Camden, ME 04843; (207) 236-8506 or 1-800-888-5236. Educational material. Roster of survivors for peer support by telephone and letters.

National Mental Health Services Knowledge Exchange Network, P.O. Box 42490, Washington, DC 20015; 1-800-789-2647. Provides information on disaster and emergency assistance via publications, videos, website, electronic bulletin board, and telephone services. Referrals to mental health associations, clearinghouses, advocacy organizations.

National Institute of Mental Health, Anxiety Disorders Education Program,

Room 7-99, 5600 Fishers Lane, Rockville, MD 20857; 1-888-8-ANXIETY. Free publications about PTSD and other anxiety disorders.

Grief Recovery Helpline 1-800-445-4808. Trained grief counselors handle calls from 9 A.M. to 5 P.M., Pacific time.

Outward Bound, National Headquarters, Route 9D, R2 Box 280, Garrison, NY 10524-9757; (914) 424-4000. A range of challenging wilderness environments coupled with emotional support to inspire self-respect and care for others, community, and environment. Since 1941.

Martial Arts for Peace Association, P.O. Box 816, Middlebury, VT 05753; (802) 388-0922 or 1-800-848-6021. Helps children learn how to avoid violence and stand up to abusers in nonviolent ways. Beautiful publications.

MILITARY/VETERANS SERVICES

Veterans Affairs Facilities. The Department of Veterans Affairs (DVA) is the acknowledged expert in treating war-related trauma. DVA offers various treatment options:

- Outpatient clinics, mental health clinics, day hospitals, and day treatment centers provide a full range of services including individual psychotherapy and medication, group and/or family therapy. Located at DVA medical centers or independent sites.

- Over two hundred vet centers provide individual, family, and group counseling services. Veterans who are not close to a vet center may receive a referral to non-DVA providers. Also provides assistance with employment or benefits.

- Inpatient treatments upon admission to DVA hospitals include:
  - general psychiatry units
  - specialized inpatient PTSD units (currently there are several PTSD/substance use projects)

For compensation, educational, housing, medical, job training, or other benefits for PTSD, call or write your local DVA facility (e.g., vet center, regional office). If unable to locate one, call **Department of Veteran's Affairs**, 1120 Vermont Avenue, Washington, DC 20420; 1-800-827-1000.

National Center for PTSD, Department of Veteran Affairs, VA Medical Center, White River Junction, Vermont 05009; (802) 296-5132. Referrals and information, including the *PTSD Research Quarterly*. PILOTS Website provides PTSD research material for vets or anyone else (http://www.dartmouth.edu/dms/ptsd/).

Veterans of the Vietnam War, National Headquarters, 760 Jumper Road, Wilkes-Barre, PA 18702; (717) 825-7215. Volunteer organization. Refers veterans to rehabilitation services. Information newsletter.

Vietnam Veterans of America, 1224 M Street, N.W., Washington, DC 20005; (202) 628-2700 or 1-800-882-1316. Congressionally chartered. Helps veterans and families. Referrals to all services (legal, medical, vet centers, etc.).

Military Family Resource Center, 4040 North Fairfax Drive, Room 420, Arlington, VA 22203; (703) 696-9053. Extensive information on child/spouse abuse and deployment stress. Referrals to family centers for family members.

Ripcord Report, Chuck Hawkins, editor, 13140 Lakehill Drive., Nokesville, VA 20181; (703) 791-5005. Newsletter for Vietnam veterans in Ripcord or 101st Airborne Division.

Disabled American Veterans, 807 Maine Avenue, S.W., Washington, DC 20024; (202) 554-3501. Free assistance in gaining benefits and referrals to mostly VA rehabilitation services.

Also American Legion, Veteran's Outreach Program, and veterans associations for Jewish, blinded, disabled, and paralyzed veterans are all headquartered in Washington, D.C.

BOOKS

Cohen, B. M., M. Barnes, and A. B. Rankin. 1995. *Managing Traumatic Stress Through Art*. Lutherville, Md.: Sidran. An excellent, practical workbook for survivors.

Frankl, V. 1959. *Man's Search for Meaning*. Boston: Beacon. The classic work on discovering meaning in one's life out of suffering. Written by the Holocaust survivor who founded logotherapy.

Geisel, Theodor. 1990. *Oh, the Places You'll Go*. New York: Random House. Part of the Dr. Seuss series; a clever, humorous treatise on human growth and fallibility. Written for kids. Or is it?

Hanh, T. N. 1991. *Peace Is Every Step: The Path of Mindfulness in Everyday Life*.

New York: Bantam. Nominated for the Nobel Peace Prize by Dr. Martin Luther King, Jr., this peaceful monk describes many practical ways to cultivate inner peace, joy, serenity, and balance. Useful while you are healing or after. Highly recommended.

Hendrix, H. H. 1988. *Getting the Love You Want: A Guide for Couples.* New York: Harper Perrenial. Helps couples to understand the deeper issues underlying conflict and turn that conflict into growth. Many practical skills.

Kushner, H. S. 1981. *When Bad Things Happen to Good People.* New York: Avon. A compassionate treatise on suffering that happens to good people, and how to cope with it.

Markman, H., S. Stanley, and S. L. Blumberg. 1994. *Fighting for Your Marriage: Positive Steps for Preventing Divorce and Preserving a Lasting Love.* San Francisco: Jossey-Bass. Research at the University of Denver found that the program described increased marital satisfaction and decreased divorce. This practical and down-to-earth guide shows how to discuss difficult issues safely and clearly, manage and resolve conflict, and enhance fun and intimacy.

Pennebaker, J. W. 1997. *Opening Up: The Healing Power of Expressing Emotion.* New York: Guilford. Explains why verbalizing grief and upsetting events from the past reduces distress.

Schiraldi, G. 1990. *Hope and Help for Depression: A Practical Guide.* Detailed instructions for diverse self-managed approaches. Also explains professional treatments and how to find them. ("The bottom line: Highly recommended!"—*American Journal of Health Promotion.*) Available by mail: Send $12.00 (plus S/H) to Chevron Publishing Corporation, 5018 Dorsey Hall Drive, Suite 104, Ellicott City, MD 21042; (410) 740-0065 or Fax: (410) 740-9213 prepaid or purchase order.

————. 1996. *Facts to Relax By: A Guide to Relaxation and Stress Reduction.* Detailed instructions for five relaxation exercises plus exercise and nutrition guidelines, assertiveness, time management, changing stressful attitudes, and other ways to reduce stress. Available by mail: Send $5.95 to: Utah Valley Regional Medical Center, Education Department, 1034 North 500 West, Provo, UT 84603. (Also available from Chevron Publishing, below.)

————. 1997. *Conquer Anxiety, Worry and Nervous Fatigue: A Guide to Greater Peace.* Step-by-step instructions for recognizing, reducing, and preventing anxiety and its troubling symptoms. From hyperventilation to worrisome thought patterns. Extensive resource list. Also explains how to find professional help if it is needed. ("Dr. Schiraldi has brought together information from a variety of mental health disciplines, translated them into language that is easily understood, and sprinkled it all with the wisdom of some of the greatest minds known to man. A great job."—Robert J. Hedaya, MD, Biopsychiatrist.) Send $19.00 (plus S/H) to Chevron Publishing Corporation, 5018 Dorsey Hall Drive, Suite 104, Ellicott City, MD 21042; (410) 740-0065 or Fax: (410) 740-9213 prepaid or purchase order.

————. 1999. *Building Self-Esteem: A 125-Day Program*. A clear, effective guide to understanding and improving self-esteem. Based upon the Stress and the Healthy Mind course, University of Maryland. Sound principles. Many practical skills with complete instructions. Available by mail: Send $16.00 (plus S/H) to Chevron Publishing Corporation, 5018 Dorsey Hall Drive, Suite 104, Ellicott City, MD 21042; (410) 740-0065 or Fax: (410) 740-9213 prepaid or purchase order.

Shapiro, F., and M. S. Forrest. 1997. *EMDR: The Breakthrough Therapy for Overcoming Anxiety, Stress, and Trauma*. New York: Basic. Shows individuals how EMDR has been used to effect healing.

Hazelden Educational Materials, Box 176, Pleasant Valley Road, Center City, MN 55012; 1-800-328-9000 for free catalog on wide range of books and audiovisual materials on all areas of substance abuse.

Compassion Books, 477 Hannah Branch Road, Burnsville, NC 28714; (704) 675-9670. Catalog for books and videos on dying, grief, loss, and trauma for all ages.

Trauma Recovery Publications, 3302 College Drive., Columbus, GA 31907; (706) 563-9893. Distributes materials with a spiritual perspective, such as *Rainbows for Recovery*—tender Christian meditations for survivors of trauma.

RESOURCES FOR PROFESSIONALS

James, B. 1989. *Treating Traumatized Children: New Insights & Creative Interventions*. Lexington, Mass.: Lexington. A brilliant compilation of practical approaches, most of which are applicable to adults.

Meichenbaum, D. 1994. *A Clinical Handbook/Practical Therapist Manual for Assessing and Treating Adults with Post-Traumatic Stress Disorder (PTSD)*. Contact

Dr. Meichenbaum at University of Waterloo, Department of Psychology, Waterloo, Ontario, Canada N2L3G1; (519) 885-1211, ext. 2551. Price: $50.

Shapiro, F. 1995. *Eye Movement Desensitization and Reprocessing: Basic Principles, Protocols, and Procedures*. New York: Guilford. EMDR appears to have potential as a component of comprehensive treatment program for anxiety disorders. EMDR was originally developed to treat PTSD. A thorough, well-written book.

Wilson, J. P. and B. Raphael, eds. 1993. *International Handbook of Traumatic Stress Syndromes*. New York: Plenum. Comprehensive research on a broad range of PTSD aspects.

The International Society for Traumatic Stress Studies, 60 Revere Drive, Suite 500, Northbrook, IL 60062; (847) 480-9028. Shares research, clinical strategies, theoretical, and policy concerns. *Journal of Traumatic Stress*, quarterly newsletter. Annual meeting. Members include many survivors.

The International Society for the Study of Dissociation, 60 Revere Drive, Suite 500, Northbrook, IL 60062; (847) 480-0899. Sponsors conferences; publishes a dissociation journal and *ISSD News*.

Association of Traumatic Stress Specialists, 7338 Broad River Road, Irmo, SC 29063; (803) 781-0017. Certifies trauma counselors and other helpers. Training conferences and newsletter.

Glossary

Anxiety—Worry plus physical and emotional arousal.

Anxiety Disorder—A mental illness characterized by persistent and/or excessive anxiety. In addition to PTSD, anxiety disorders include generalized anxiety disorder, obsessive-compulsive disorder, panic disorder, and phobias. PTSD is the only anxiety disorder which includes a stressful event as one of its diagnostic criteria.

Cognitive Restructuring—A systematic process of modifying habitual, disturbing thoughts which race through one's mind so quickly that they are hardly noticed let alone tested for reasonableness. This is a major skill for the treatment of anxiety, depression, and other distressing conditions. Also called cognitive reframing.

Counting Method—A treatment strategy whereby a survivor silently and briefly recalls a disturbing memory, linking that memory to the soothing sound of the therapist's voice as they count to 100. In this way, a greater feeling of control over the memory is established. The experience is then processed verbally to facilitate processing of the memory.

Dissociation—A mental process whereby one attempts to escape distressing memories or situations. One's mind might appear to separate from distressing bodily experience. Or the mind might separate traumatic memories from the main body of consciousness. These "dissociated memories" are stored in a fragmented way and often intrude into awareness in distressing ways.

Dissociative Identity Disorder (formerly **Multiple Personality Disorder**)—Forming at least two personality states, at least one of which contains unacceptable memory material. Healing and recovery involve integrating the diverse personality states into one.

Expressive Art Therapies—Treatment strategies which make use of painting, sculpture, drawing, dance, music, literature, drama, etc., to help survivors process trauma material and facilitate healing.

Eye Movement Desensitization and Reprocessing (EMDR)—A treatment approach that is thought to accelerate the processing of traumatic memories. The client holds a disturbing aspect of the memory in their mind while moving the eyes rapidly back and forth (or performing a similar repetitive action). The negative thoughts, emotions, and sensations are integrated, neutralized, and fused with more positive thought(s).

Flashbacks—The perception that one is somehow reliving the traumatic event; flashbacks can include any or all sensations, emotions, and/or behaviors.

Foreshortened Future—The sense that a normal or pleasant future will not exist as the survivor seems to focus on the injury caused by the traumatic event and the likelihood that unpleasant outcomes will recur.

Healing—The process of becoming whole again; uniting pieces of self that have been shattered by trauma.

Hyperventilation (overbreathing)—The rapid expiration of carbon dioxide, usually occurring with rapid, shallow "chest" breathing (or sometimes deep breathing). The resulting drop in the level of blood CO_2 leads to a host of symptoms of anxiety. This condition may be caused by stress-induced tension, lung or airway disorders, certain postures or speech stylistics, constrictive clothes, or other causes. Treatment of this condition often helps to reduce anxiety symptoms.

Hypervigilance—The extreme caution survivors take to protect against further harm, or the fearful anticipation of real or recalled threats.

Hypnosis—A state of deep relaxation and heightened concentration where one is more open to helpful suggestions.

Memory Work/Processing—Recalling and exploring aspects of traumatic memories so that memory fragments can be connected to each other, neutralized emotionally, and stored in long-term memory much like other memories.

Numbing—A shutdown of emotions or memory in order to protect survivors from distressing feelings.

Post-Traumatic Stress Disorder—The understandable response to an overwhelmingly stressful event(s). The symptoms of the resulting emotional wounding include re-experiencing the event(s) in distressing ways, emotional and physical arousal, and attempts to distance oneself from reminders of the event(s).

Prolonged Exposure—A method of inviting all aspects of a traumatic memory fully into awareness in a controlled way in a safe setting, until one feels mastery over the feared memory.

Recovery—A return to the former state of functioning.

Rewind Technique—Similar to visual-kinesthetic dissociation, this treatment strategy enables survivors to view traumatic events in imagery forwards and backwards, connecting memories to the safe time preceding the traumatic event and, sometimes, to a time following the event when the survivor was assured of surviving.

Stress—Originally, the response of the body to a threat. In the anxiety disorders, the stress response becomes exaggerated, too easily triggered, and/or chronic. Because the mind and body are connected, physical arousal is accompanied by emotional arousal and sometimes behavioral changes.

Subjective Units of Distress (SUDs)—A rating of discomfort ranging, for example, from 0 (none) to 10 (severe). Quantifying discomfort facilitates client-therapist communication. Changes in SUD ratings can indicate how effectively a treatment strategy is working.

Systematic Relaxation—Forms of relaxation that are structured and practiced regularly, such as meditation, progressive muscle relaxation, and autogenic training. These practices tend to reduce physical and emotional arousal, and can be an important part of a survivor's coping and recovery.

Thought Field Therapy—A process by which survivors briefly recall a traumatic event, then neutralize the memory through a series of tapping movements, sometimes combined with various activities.

Traumatic Death Circumstance—One which involves "suddenness and lack of anticipation; violence, mutilation, and destruction; preventability and/or randomness; loss of a child; multiple death"; or a brush with death following a "significant threat to survival or a massive and/or shocking confrontation with the death and mutilation of others" (Rando's foreword to C. R. Figley, B. E. Bride, and N. Mazza, eds., *Death and Trauma: The Traumatology of Grieving* [Washington, D.C.: Taylor and Francis, 1997]). Recovery from such circumstances might be especially challenging and require professional help.

Traumatic Incident Reduction—A treatment strategy whereby the survivor views a traumatic memory in imagery, then verbally describes the event in a condition of safety. The "videotape" is then rewound and the memory is viewed and described again. With successive repetitions the client often notices that negative emotions diminish and positive insights and emotions rise.

Trigger—A cue that reminds one of a traumatic event and elicits distressing intrusions.

Endnotes

1. G. R. Schiraldi, *Conquer Anxiety, Worry, and Nervous Fatigue: A Guide to Greater Peace* (Ellicott City, Md.: Chevron, 1997), from the foreword.

2. R. Figley, ed., *Trauma and Its Wake: The Study and Treatment of Post-traumatic Stress Disorder* (New York: Brunner/Mazel, 1985).

3. PTSD patients have higher scores than psychiatric or normal controls on all MMPI scales. The MMPI is a widely used inventory of psychological disturbance. (P. A. Saigh, "History, Current Nosology, and Epidemiology," in P. A. Saigh, *Post-traumatic Stress Disorder: A Bipolar Approach to Assessment and Treatment* [Boston: Allyn and Bacon, 1992], 1–27.) Especially noteworthy is that PTSD patients are higher in anxiety, depression and hostility. (J. C. Jones and D. H. Barlow, "A New Model of Post-traumatic Stress Disorder: Implications for the Future," in Saigh, *Post-traumatic Stress Disorder*, 147–65.)

4. M. J. Scott and S. G. Stradling, *Counseling for Post-Traumatic Stress Disorder* (London: Sage, 1992), 28.

5. As Schopenhauer observed, "Suffering which falls to our lot in the course of nature, or by chance, or fate, does not seem so painful as suffering which is inflicted on us by the arbitrary will of another." (Quoted by M. A. Simpson, "Bitter Waters: Effects on Children of the Stresses of Unrest and Oppression," in J. P. Wilson and B. Raphael, eds., *International Handbook of Traumatic Stress Syndromes* [New York: Plenum, 1993], 613.)

6. Some experts think that emotional abuse alone is not sufficient to cause PTSD, but it must occur in combination with other forms of abuse.

7. This example was described by M. Crocq, J. Macher, J. Barros-Beck, S. J. Rosenberg, and F. Duval, "Posttraumatic Stress Disorder in World War II Prisoners of War from Alsace-Lorraine Who Survived Captivity in the USSR," in Wilson and Raphael, *International Handbook*, 253–61.

8. K. C. Peterson, M. F. Prout, and R. A. Schwarz. *Post-Traumatic Stress Disorder: A Clinician's Guide*, New York: Plenum, 1991.

9. Ibid.

10. Dr. George S. Everly, Jr. (Second World Congress on Stress, Trauma and Coping in the Emergency Services Professions, International Critical Incident Stress Foundation, Baltimore, Md., April 1993).

11. Saigh, *Post-traumatic Stress Disorder*.

12. For example, catecholamines and thyroxin are elevated, while cortisol, which may be depleted, is lowered.

13. For example, the constant "partyer" may be denying that wounding has occurred.

14. H. Krystal, "Beyond the DSM-III-R: Therapeutic Considerations in Posttraumatic Stress Disorder," in Wilson and Raphael, *International Handbook*, 848.

15. J. G. Allen, *Coping with Trauma: A Guide to Self-Understanding*, (Washington, D.C.: American Psychiatric Press, 1995); R. B. Flannery, Jr., *Post-Traumatic Stress Disorder: The Victim's Guide to Healing and Recovery* (New York: Crossroad, 1992).

16. Krystal, "Beyond the DSM-III-R."

17. Example provided by C. R. Hartman and A. W. Burgess, "Treatment of Victims of Rape Trauma," in Wilson and Raphael, *International Handbook*, 507–16.

18. The olfactory nerves are proximate to the amygdala and hippocampal areas of the brain.

19. B. A. van der Kolk and J. Saporta, "Biological Response to Psychic Trauma," in Wilson and Raphael, *International Handbook*, 25–34.

20. The amygdala is the part of the brain that arouses state-dependent memories.

21. M. Keane, J. A. Fairbank, J. M. Caddell, R. T. Zimering, and M. E. Bender, "A Behavioral Approach to Assessing and Treating Post-Traumatic Stress Disorder in Vietnam Veterans," in Figley, *Trauma and Its Wake*, 257–94.

22. Flannery, *Victim's Guide*.

23. A similar case was reported in T. M. Keane et al., "A Behavioral Approach."

24. R. Janoff-Bulman, "The Aftermath of Victimization: Rebuilding Shattered Assumptions," in Figley, *Trauma and Its Wake*, 15–35; S. Epstein, "The Self-Concept, the Traumatic Neurosis, and the Structure of Personality," in D. Ozer, J. M. Healy, Jr., and R. A. J. Stewart, eds., *Perspectives on Personality*, vol. 3 (Greenwich, Conn.: JAI, 1991); R. M. Scurfield, "War-Related Trauma: An Integrative Experiential, Cognitive, and Spiritual Approach," in M. B. Williams and J. F. Sommer, Jr., eds., *Handbook of Post-Traumatic Therapy* (Westport, Conn.: Greenwood Press, 1994), 179–204; J. D. Lindy, "Focal Psychoanalytic Psychotherapy of Posttraumatic Stress Disorder," in Wilson and Raphael, *International Handbook*, 803–9; M. Crocq, J. Macher, J. Barros-Beck, S. J. Rosenberg, and F. Duval, "Posttraumatic Stress Disorder in World War II Prisoners of War from Alsace-Lorraine Who Survived Captivity in the USSR," in Wilson and Raphael, *International Handbook*, 253–61.

25. Peterson et al., *A Clinician's Guide*, 36.

26. Ibid; Flannery, *Victim's Guide*; J. T. R. Davidson et al., "Posttraumatic Stress Disorder in the Community: An Epidemiological Study," *Psychological Medicine* 2 (1991): 713–21.

27. Indeed, Op den Veld and colleagues feel that exhaustion should be a diagnostic criterion for PTSD. (W. Op den Veld et al., "Posttraumatic Stress Disorder in Dutch Resistance Veterans from WWII," in Wilson and Raphael, *International Handbook*, 219–30.)

28. Dr. R. Bruce Lydiard, Medical Director and Director of Psychopharmocology Unit, Anxiety Disorders Research, Medical University of South Carolina, explains the relationship between anxiety and the gut. Some parts of the brain regulate both anxiety states and gut

function. For example, locus ceruleus activation inhibits the stomach and small intestine, while increasing motility contractions in the lower colon and rectum. This explains why antianxiety drugs help irritable bowel syndrome. Stimulating the gut in turn activates the locus ceruleus. Unlike other cells outside the brain, the enteric nervous system, the "little brain," shows properties of the brain. "Gut hormones," such as cholecystokinin and vaso-active intestinal peptide, are also found in the brain. Gut sensors lead to the brain, which in turn regulates acid secetion, contractions, and hormone secretions. It is common to find a history of sexual and physical assault in irritable bowel syndrome patients. (ADAA *Reporter* 7, no. 3 [fall 1996]: 1–25.)

29. K. A. Lee, G. E. Vaillant, W. C. Torrey, and G. H. Elder, "A 50-year Prospective Study of the Psychological Sequelae of World War II Combat," *American Journal of Psychiatry* 152, no. 4 (1995): 141–48.

30. B. G. Braun, "Multiple Personality Disorder and Posttraumatic Stress Disorder," in Wilson and Raphael, *International Handbook*, 35–47.

31. L. R. Daniels and R. M. Scurfield, "War-Related PTSD: Chemical Addictions and Non-chemical Habituating Behaviors," in Williams and Sommer, *Handbook*, 205–18.

32. A. Matsakis, *Post-Traumatic Stress Disorder: A Complete Treatment Guide* (Oakland, Calif.: New Harbinger, 1994), 93–95. Dr. Matsakis has cogently explained a number of the reasons underlying self-mutilation, from which the discussion below is primarily adapted.

33. van der Kolk and Saporta, "Biological Response."

34. Friedman points out that Vietnam vets show higher pain thresholds after watching the movie *Platoon,* due to sudden increases in opioid levels (M. J. Friedman, "Psychobiological and Pharmacological Approaches to Treatment," in Wilson and Raphael, *International Handbook*, 785–94). van der Kolk uses the term "addiction to trauma," which might also help explain repetition compulsion and risk-taking behavior.

35. Krystal, "Beyond the DSM-III-R."

36. M. A.Simpson, "Bitter Waters."

37. Flannery, *Victim's Guide*.

38. Flannery estimates that half of bulimics are victims of past abuse.

39. Neurological changes may interfere with the victim's ability to recognize danger, read and interpret facial expressions, and so forth.

40. J. G. Allen provides these cogent insights and the term "shred of affection" (Allen, *Coping with Trauma*, 158).

41. A discussion of alexithymia in PTSD may be found in Krystal, "Beyond the DSM-III-R." See also N. Milgram, "War-related Trauma and Victimization: Principles of Traumatic Stress Prevention in Israel," in Wilson and Raphael, *International Handbook*, 811–20; and J. P. Wilson, "The Need for an Integrative Theory of Post-Traumatic Stress Disorder," in Williams and Sommer, *Handbook,* 3–18.

42. Some people exhibit PTSD symptoms in response to so-called stressors of normal living (e.g., divorce, being fired, business loss, chronic illness, death from natural causes). This response is usually characterized as an adjustment disorder, rather than PTSD, although sometimes the distinction is blurry.

43. N. Breslau , G. C. Davis, and P. Andreski, "Traumatic Events and Post Traumatic Stress Disorder in an Urban Population of Young Adults," *Archives of General Psychiatry* 48 (1991): 216–22.

44. Some argue that expected events can also be traumatic, such as repeated incest. However, at least the first occurrence is usually not expected, nor completely prepared for.

45. D. W. Foy, S. S. Osato, B. M. Houskamp, and D. A. Neumann, "Etiology of Post Traumatic Stress Disorder," in Saigh, *Post-traumatic Stress Disorder,* 28–49.

46. F. Flach, "The Resilience Hypothesis and Posttraumatic Stress Disorder," in M. E.Wolf and A. D. Mosnaim, eds., *Post-traumatic Stress Disorder: Etiology, Phenomenology, and Treatment* (Washington, D.C.): American Psychiatric Press, l990) 36–45. Cited in Allen, *Coping with Trauma,* 187. See also J. N. Lam and F. K. Grossman, "Resilience and Adult Adaptation in Women with and without Self-reported Histories of Childhood Sexual Abuse," *Journal of Traumatic Stress* 10, no. 2 (1997): 175–96.

47. L. L. Harkness, "Transgenerational Transmission of War-related Trauma," in Wilson and Raphael, *International Handbook,* 635–43.

48. A. A. Feinstein, "Prospective Study of Victims of Physical Trauma," in Wilson and Raphael, *International Handbook,* 157–64. See review by A. Y. Shalev, "Stress versus Traumatic Stress: From Acute Homeostatic Reactions to Chronic Psychopathology," in B. A. van der Kolk, A. C. McFarlane, and L. Weisaeth, eds., *Traumatic Stress: The Effects of Overwhelming Experience on Mind, Body, and Society* (New York: Guilford, 1996), 77–101. Also see J. D. Bremner and E. Brett, "Trauma-related Dissociative States and Long-term Psychopathology in Post-traumatic Stress Disorder," *Journal of Traumatic Stress* 10, no. 1 (1997): 37–49.

49. Troops returned from the Gulf War to nationally televised victory parades; our troops who served in Vietnam received no such welcoming ritual. Dr. Jim Reese, of the International Critical Incident Stress Foundation, relates that he got off the plane in San Francisco following his tour in Vietnam. He was emaciated and exhausted. The customs inspector said, "You don't have any contraband, do you? Welcome home, son." One wishes for such support for all survivors.

50. M. J. Horowitz, "Stress-Response Syndromes: A Review of Posttraumatic Stress and Adjustment Disorders," in Wilson and Raphael, *International Handbook,* 49–60.

51. This oft-stated estimate is somewhat misleading. Children, particularly those who are traumatized prior to personality integration (i.e., eight to ten years of age) fare much worse. About half of WWII survivors (armed forces and concentration camp survivors) have been found to suffer PTSD forty years after the war. This estimate generally applies to adults experiencing criminal assault, rape, natural disasters, and other events of relatively limited duration.

52. Long-term studies are instructive: 84 percent of Dutch resistance fighters had PTSD at some time after WWII, 55 percent had it more than forty years after the war, and many got worse after retirement (Op den Veld et al., "Dutch Resistance Veterans").

53. Figley, *Trauma and Its Wake.*

54. Wilson, "Need for an Integrative Theory."

55. S. Berglas, "Why Did This Happen to Me?" *Psychology Today* (February 1985), 44–48.

56. This term is used by R. P. Kluft, "Multiple Personality Disorder," in A. Tasman and S. Goldfinge, eds., *Review of Psychiatry* (Washington, D.C.: American Psychiatric Press, 1991), 375–84.

57. J. H. Albeck, "Intergenerational Consequences of Trauma: Reframing Traps in Treatment Theory—A Second-Generation Perspective," in Williams and Sommer, *Handbook*, 106–25.

58. Foy et al., "Etiology."

59. M. A. Donaldson, and R. Gardner, Jr., "Diagnosis and Treatment of Traumatic Stress among Women After Childhood Incest," in Figley, *Trauma and Its Wake*, 356–77.

60. Matsakis, "Dual, Triple and Quadruple Trauma Couples: Dynamics and Treatment Issues," in Williams and Sommer, *Handbook*, 78–105.

61. Op den Veld et al., "Dutch Resistance Veterans."

62. See, for example, J. J. Sherman, "Effects of Psychotherapeutic Treatments for PTSD: A Meta-Analysis of Controlled Clinical Trials," *Journal of Traumatic Stress* 11, no. 3 (1998): 413–35. This study indicates that cognitive-behavioral therapies substantially reduce symptoms of PTSD, anxiety, and depression by the end of treatment, and these effects are maintained at follow-up three to twelve months later.

63. Allen, *Coping with Trauma*. van der Kolk concurs that dissociation may cause distortions (B. A. van der Kolk, "Trauma and Memory," in van der Kolk et al., *Traumatic Stress*, 279–302). Everstine and Everstine echo the fact that extreme emotions interfere with the hippocampus's ability to store memories accurately in time (D. S. Everstine and L. Everstine, L., *The Trauma Response: Treatment for Emotional Injury* [New York: Norton, 1993]).

64. D. Meichenbaum, *A Clinical Handbook/Practical Therapist Manual for Assessing and Treating Adults with Post-Traumatic Stress Disorder* (Waterloo, Ontario: Institute Press, 1994), 14.

65. Adapted from Cambridge Hospital Victims of Violence program resolution criteria by psychologist Mary Harvey. In M. P. Koss, "Date Rape," *Harvard Mental Health Letter* 9, no. 3 (September 1992): 6.

66. Cited in Allen, *Coping with Trauma*, 213.

67. B. James, *Treating Traumatized Children: New Insights and Creative Interventions* (Lexington, Mass.: Lexington, 1989), 58.

68. A well-written book on boundaries from a Biblical perspective is H. Cloud and J. Townsend, *Boundaries: When to Say Yes, When to Say No, to take Control of Your Life* (Grand Rapids, Mich.: Zondervan Publishing, 1992.) I am grateful for the ideas it suggests as regards PTSD.

69. *From Peace Is Every Step* by Thich Nhat Hanh. Copyright © 1991 by Thich Nhat Hanh. Used by permission of Bantam Books, a division of Random House, Inc., 51–56.

70. Everstine and Everstine, *Trauma Response*.

71. Items 3, 4, and 6 are adapted from Scurfield, "War-Related Trauma."

72. Adapted with permission from F. Shapiro, *Eye Movement Desensitization and Reprocessing: Basic Principles, Protocols, and Procedures* (New York: Guilford, 1995).

73. Consider soldiers in combat. They drink to bond and deaden the pain. The bonding is superficial and the anesthesia soon wears off. They deny danger and put on a brave, self-sufficient front. The thrilling violence of combat provides a temporary distraction from emotional pain, which must be deadened to survive. The trauma survivor might repeat retraumatizing behaviors for their temporary gains.

74. This quote is suggested by K. Olness and D. P. Kohen, *Hypnosis and Hypnotherapy with Children*, 3d ed. (New York: Guilford, 1996).

75. Shapiro presents a cogent discussion of secondary gains, from which these examples and questions are adapted. See Shapiro, *Eye Movement*.

76. Flannery, *Victim's Guide*, 159.

77. Matsakis, *Complete Treatment Guide*, 224.

78. F. Ochberg, "Posttraumatic Therapy," in Wilson and Raphael, *International Handbook*, 773–84.

79. L. A. Pearlman and I. L. McCann, "Integrating Structured and Unstructured Approaches to Taking a Trauma History," in Williams and Sommer, *Handbook*, 42.

80. An excellent overview of assessment issues may be found in B. T. Litz and F. W. Weathers, "The Diagnosis and Assessment of Post-Traumatic Stress Disorder in Adults," in Williams and Sommer, *Handbook*, 19–37.

81. This list is slightly adapted and reprinted with permission from Matsakis, *Complete Treatment Guide*. Copyright © 1994 Aphrodite Matsakis.

82. F. R. Abueg and J. A. Fairbank, "Behavioral Treatment of PTSD and Co-occurring Substance Abuse," in Saigh, *Post-traumatic Stress Disorder*, 111–46; K. S. Calhoun and P. A. Resick, "Post-Traumatic Stress Disorder," in D. H. Barlow, ed., *Clinical Handbook of Psychological Disorders: A Step-by-Step Treatment Manual* (New York: Guilford, 1993), 48–98.

83. Survivors can be damaged by groups that are poorly managed; thus caution is advised. Esther Giller, Executive Director, Sidran Foundation, adds that group members often dump trauma material into a group in a graphic and triggering manner, causing other group members to react problematically. Flashbacks are contagious. Therefore, she suggests these ground rules: Members should not describe traumatic events graphically, nor should they compare war stories to see which is more horrible. The focus of communication should be on the present, and leaders should vigilantly monitor members for grounding versus dissociation.

84. In some cases, the even more sensitive TRH stimulation test might be used. PTSD might cause elevated levels of blood thyroxine, with a normal TRH stimulation test. M. J. Friedman, "Biological and Pharmacological Aspects of the Treatment of PTSD," in Williams and Sommer, *Handbook*, 496–509.

85. Get as much calcium as you can from foods, especially dairy products. Most of your calcium requirements will be met if you follow the USDA Food Guide Pyramid. Send a $1.00 check, payable to Superintendent of Documents, to: Consumer Information Center, Department 159-Y, Pueblo, Colorado 81009. Calcium supplements, such as calcium carbonate, can supply the remaining needs.

86. D. R. Catherall, *Back from the Brink: A Family Guide to Overcoming Traumatic Stress* (New York: Bantam, 1992), 160.

87. C. Weekes, *More Help for Your Nerves.* (New York: Bantam, 1984), 23.

88. Ibid., 27.

89. Some clinicians also train panic disorder patients to distract from their symptoms when they need to function (e.g., when driving). This can be done, for example, by sensing colors around you, noticing sounds in the environment, feeling the floor supporting you, counting backward, and so forth, until the symptoms subside. This counters the tendency to catastrophize about the symptoms and helps the person instead focus on functioning.

90. C. Patel, cited in B. H. Timmons and R. Ley, eds., *Behavioral and Psychological Approaches to Breathing Disorder* (New York: Plenum, 1994), ix. British chest physician Claude Lum calls hyperventilation the "great mimic."

91. Perhaps 10 percent of patients visiting general internists complain of signs and symptoms associated with hyperventilation, according to G. J. Magarian, "Hyperventilation Syndromes: Infrequently Recognized Common Expressions of Anxiety and Stress," *Medicine* 61 (1982): 219–36. Hyperventilation appears to be seen in a majority of those with anxiety disorders. In 60 percent of patients with anxiety neurosis or anxiety hysteria at Lahey Clinic, hyperventilation was a significant cause of symptoms (W. I. Tucker, "Hyperventilation and Differential Diagnosis," *Medical Clinics of North America* 47 [1963]: 491–97). Also, 50 to 60 percent of phobics seen in the Department of Clinical Psychology, University of Amsterdam, showed signs of hyperventilation syndrome. (H. Van Dis, "Hyperventilation in Phobic Patients," in C. D. Spielberger and I. G. Sarason, eds., *Stress and Anxiety*, Vol. 5 [New York: Hemisphere, 1978]). Prevalence ranges from 10 to25 percent of the population. It accounts for 60 percent of ambulance calls (R. Fried, *The Breath Connection* [New York: Plenum, 1990]).

92. Technically, "overbreathing" means that you expel carbon dioxide faster than the rate required by the metabolic demand for oxygen (i.e., faster than the cells are using oxygen). It is like smoke clearing the chimney faster than the fire is burning (Dr. Ronald Ley, personal communication, 22 January 1996).

93. Dr. Richard Gevirtz uses the metaphor of a milk wagon that brings milk to the house but can't drop it off at the door. In the same way, blood cannot release oxygen that it delivers to the cells when the blood becomes alkaline.

94. For example, calcium and phosphorous enter muscles and/or nerves, making them more active.

95. Barelli explains that breathing during sleep is unilateral, shifting from one nostril to another, and causing the body to turn during sleep, preventing various symptoms. Impaired nasal functioning may disturb sleep. A good overview of nasopulmonary problems is provided by P. A. Barelli, "Nasopulmonary Physiology," in Timmons and Ley, *Breathing Disorders*, 47–57.

96. Rosenman and Friedman observed this in Type As, as reported by D. Boadella, "Styles of Breathing in Reichian Therapy," in Timmons and Ley, *Breathing Disorders*, 233–42.

97. To restore the acid-base balance, the kidney excretes bicarbonate, an important biochemical buffer. The next episode of hyperventilation will then induce rapid changes in pH and ionic balance.

98. L. C. Lum., "The Syndrome of Habitual Chronic Hyperventilation," in O. Hill, ed., *Modern Trends in Psychosomatic Medicine*, 3 vols. (London: Butterworth, 1976), 196–230.

99. Magarian, "Hyperventilation Syndromes."

100. A capnograph compares the resting end-tidal PCO_2 with levels following the provocation test. This test is sometimes the only way to be certain that one is hyperventilating. Capnographs are found in research settings and some clinics.

101. For this reason, some psychotherapists use this test as a cognitive-behavioral strategy. Others avoid this, however, fearing that the provocation test might trigger adverse cardiovascular symptoms (angina, arrhythmias, spasms of coronary arteries, etc.). If cardiovascular disorders are suspected, it is essential that this test be conducted under proper medical supervision.

102. P. G. F. Nixon and L. J. Freeman, "The 'Think Test': A Further Technique to Elicit Hyperventilation," *Journal of the Royal Society of Medicine* 81 (1988): 277–79.

103. This section incorporates the ideas of E. A. Holloway, "The Role of the Physiotherapist in the Treatment of Hyperventilation," in Timmons and Ley, *Breathing Disorders*, 157–75. The writings of Barlow and Ross have also been helpful.

104. Explains Dr. Michael Johnson, Anxiety Disorders Clinic, Medical School, University of South Carolina: "My own experience is that the addition of mental counting to the breathing practice helps the individual stay focused and has the added benefit of distracting him/her from other worries. I will have people count at the end of their inhalation and think 'relax' at the end of their exhalation. The idea of pausing (slightly) at the end of inhalation and at the end of exhalation is very useful in helping people to slow their breathing rate" (personal communication, 1 November 1995).

105. J. H. Weiss "Behavioral Management of Asthma," in Timmons and Ley, *Breathing Disorders*, 205–19.

106. H. Benson, *Beyond the Relaxation Response* (New York: Berkley, 1984).

107. A richer, more complete discussion of meditation may be found in S. Rinpoche, *The Tibetan Book of Living and Dying* (San Francisco: Harper, 1993).

108. Weekes, *More Help*.

109. Later in the course of treatment, you might abandon the method of meditation altogether, and simply contemplate quietly what arises. At times, you'll access your true nature, which had once perhaps been covered by the trauma. At other times you will view with a wise, kind mind what is needed and/or how to heal. At other times, you might contemplate satisfying directions for the course of your life.

110. "Visitor From the Future" by Ron Klein is adapted and reprinted with permission. Copyright © 1989–1991 by Ron Klein, American Hypnosis Training Academy, Inc. The exercise is adapted from the original work of Steve Andreas, Richard Bandler, and Neurolinguistic Programming, Division of Training and Research. The client's role is to

stop if there is discomfort in doing this exercise, and to tell the therapist if images on the screen are difficult to "hold on to." More mundane images may be practiced if this occurs.

111. At any time during this procedure, if the client feels overwhelmed by negative feelings or "pulled into" the earlier experience, either the client or the therapist may interrupt the procedure to restore a sense of safety, security, and separateness from the earlier experience. The procedure may be started again when the client feels ready.

112. R. DiGiuseppe, "Developing the Therapeutic Alliance with Angry Clients," in H. Kassinove, ed. *Anger Disorders: Definition, Diagnosis and Treatment* (Washington, D.C.: Taylor and Francis, 1995), 131–49.

113. This technique was developed by Dr. Larry D. Smyth, Sheppard and Enoch Pratt Hospital, as a useful modification of Dr. Francine Shapiro's Eye Movement Desensitization and Reprocessing. Detailed instructions may be found in L. D. Smyth, *Treating Anxiety Disorders with a Cognitive-Behavioral Exposure Based Approach and the Eye-Movement Technique: Video and Viewer's Guide* (Havre de Grace, Md.: RTR Publishing, 1996). Copyright © 1996 by Larry Smyth, Ph.D., from which this chapter is adapted with permission.

114. I am grateful to Dr. Bethany Brand, Trauma Disorders Unit, Sheppard Pratt Hospital, for articulating these approaches. B. Brand and N. N. Funk, *The Basics of Treating Dissociative Patients*, Maryland Psychological Association/MPAF Annual Convention, 6 June 1997.

115. For flashbacks occurring in therapy, the therapist says loudly, "_____ (say name), I know you are having a flashback. You are here now. Come toward my voice. 1. Coming closer. 2. Almost here. 3. Here now." When the therapist detects the first signs of dissociation, she might ask, "I wonder where you went just now."

116. This technique is adapted primarily from Shapiro, *Eye Movement*.

117. Williams suggests that the safe place might be the place where one went in imagination during abuse. M. B. Williams, "Establishing Safety in Survivors of Severe Sexual Abuse," in Williams and Sommer, *Handbook*, 162–78. Some people find it helpful to look through magazines to find a soothing place to use, then hang up this picture as a reminder of safety.

118. Dr. Brand suggests bringing the frightened child to a safe place during sexual relations.

119. The freezing and dirty laundry strategies are adapted with permission from undated handout, "Containment Techniques," courtesy of Dr. Bethany Brand.

120. M. B. Williams, "Interventions with Child Victims of Trauma in the School Setting," in Williams and Sommer, *Handbook*, 69–77.

121. R. M. Scurfield, "Treatment of Posttraumatic Stress Disorder among Vietnam Veterans," in Wilson and Raphael, *International Handbook*, 879–88.

122. Beverly James uses the metaphor of a photograph album of an event with children. B. James, "Long-Term Treatment for Children with Severe Trauma History," in Williams and Sommer, *Handbook*, 52–68.

123. T. Beck, G. Emery, and R. L. Greenberg, *Anxiety Disorders and Phobias* (New York: Basic Books, 1985).

124. Emery uses this term in Beck et al., *Anxiety Disorders and Phobias*, 206.

125. Your concern probably indicates that you will not be violent. If it truly seems likely that you might hurt someone, discuss this completely and immediately with your therapist. Or call a crisis hotline, such as Parents United.

126. The exception to the rule rebuttal was suggested by G. S. Everly, Jr. "Short-Term Psychotherapy of Acute Adult Onset Post-Traumatic Stress: The Role of Weltanschauung." *Stress Medicine* 10 (1994): 191–96.

127. G. S. Everly, Jr. and J. T. Mitchell, Third World Conference on Stress, Trauma and Coping, Baltimore, Md., April 1995.

128. Dr. Aaron Beck originated the process of questioning to uncover the core beliefs. David Burns popularized the technique in *Feeling Good* (New York: New American Library, 1980), calling it "the downward arrow technique."

129. Act iv, scene 3, line 208.

130. Confronting the trauma is not the same as confronting an abuser, which is often counterproductive.

131. W. Zeigarnik, "Aber das behalten von erledigten und unerledigten handlungen," *Psychologische Forschung*, 1927; K. Lewin, *A Dynamic Theory of Personality* (New York: McGraw-Hill, 1935). Both cited in J. W. Pennebaker, *Opening Up: The Healing Power of Expressing Emotion* (New York: Guilford, 1997).

132. J. Murray, A. D. Lamnin, and C. S. Carver, "Emotional Expression in Written Essays and Psychotherapy, " *Journal of Social and Clinical Psychology* 8 (1989): 414–29. Emotional expression plus cognitive reappraisal was superior to simple affective discharge.

133. Dr. Judith Herman of Harvard asserts that retelling should involve all the senses—sights, smells, feelings, thoughts, bodily sensations (racing heart, tension, weakness in the legs, etc.), and the meaning of the event to the survivor and important people in his/her life-to facilitate the association of memory fragments. J. Herman, *Trauma and Recovery* (New York: Basic Books, 1997).

134. Donnelly, and E. J. Murray, "Cognitive and Emotional Changes in Written Essays and Therapy Interviews," *Journal of Social and Clinical Psychology* 10 (1991): 334–50. See also D. L. Segal and E. J. Murray, "Emotional Processing in Cognitive Therapy and Vocal Expression of Feeling," *Journal of Social and Clinical Psychology* 13 (1994): 189–206. Also, E. J. Murray and D. L. Segal, "Emotional Processing in Vocal and Written Expression of Feelings About Traumatic Experiences," *Journal of Traumatic Stress* 7 (1994): 391–405.

135. Dr. A. Dean Byrd offers this helpful point: "Dealing with the past is useful insofar as there are intrusions into the present. Bringing the past forward often provides more benefits than taking the person back into the past" (personal communication, 23 January 1996).

136. B. Bettelheim, afterword to C. Vegh, *I Didn't Say Goodbye*, R. Schwartz, trans. (New York: E. P. Dutton, 1984), 166.

137. James, "Children with Severe Trauma History."

138. Matsakis, *Complete Treatment Guide*, 230.

139. State-dependent memories are dissociated memories that are only recalled when the individual is feeling an emotion similar to that associated with the original event.

140. Quoted in van der Kolk, et al., *Traumatic Stress*, 551.

141. van der Kolk and Saporta, "Biological Response," 30.

142. R. Figley, *Helping Traumatized Families* (San Francisco: Jossey-Bass, 1989).

143. Reprinted with permission from Scurfield, "War-Related Trauma."

144. This personal experience was related by Jim Reese of the Critical Incident Stress Foundation.

145. Matsakis, *I Can't Get Over It: A Handbook for Trauma Survivors* (Oakland, Calif.: New Harbinger, 1992).

146. Everstine and Everstine, *Trauma Response*.

147. Donaldson and Gardner, "Women after Childhood Incest."

148. Matsakis, *Complete Treatment Guide*, 181.

149. M. A. Simpson, "Traumatic Stress and the Bruising of the Soul: The Effects of Torture and Coercive Interrogation," in Wilson and Raphael, *International Handbook*, 667–84.

150. Ibid.

151. L. D. Smyth, *Clinician's Manual for the Cognitive-Behavioral Treatment of Post Traumatic Stress Disorder* (Havre de Grace, Md.: RTR Publishing, 1994), 77.

152. Janoff-Bulman, "Aftermath of Victimization."

153. Rinpoche, *Tibetan Book*.

154. This contemplation is adapted from the Tibetan phowa practice, which is beautifully and completely described in Rinpoche, *Tibetan Book*.

155. A variation is to approach the presence and feel embraced by that loving being.

156. This is equivalent to the rewind technique presented in the next chapter.

157. In slightly modified form this is called visual-kinesthetic (VK) dissociation. The dissociation refers to seeing yourself separated from the trauma. The term *visual-kinesthetic* refers to seeing yourself moving away from and then into the film, experiencing all sensations.

158. D. C. Muss, "A New Technique for Treating Post-Traumatic Stress Disorder," *British Journal of Clinical Psychology* 30 (1991): 91–92.

159. D. C. Muss, *The Trauma Trap* (London: Doubleday, 1991), 132.

160. This chapter is summarized with permission primarily from Shapiro, *Eye Movement*. Copyright © 1995 by Francine Shapiro; also F. Shapiro and M. S. Forrest, EMDR: *The Breakthrough Therapy for Overcoming Anxiety, Stress and Trauma* (New York: Basic Books, 1997). Copyright © 1997 by Francine Shapiro.

161. For example, a meta-analysis of sixty-one studies found EMDR produced effects similar to those produced by conventional behavioral and cognitive-behavioral therapy for PTSD (M. L. Van Etten and S. Taylor, "Comparative Efficacy of Treatments for Posttraumatic Stress Disorder: A Meta-analysis," *Clinical Psychology and Psychotherapy* 5 (1998): 126–44.

162. van der Kolk, et al., "A General Approach to Treatment of Posttraumatic Stress Disorder," in van der Kolk et al., *Traumatic Stress*, 435. Figley has called EMDR one of the most significant developments in psychotherapy (C. Figley, "Adult Traumatization." The National Conference on Loss and Transition: Finding Hope in Broken Places. 14–16 May 1997).

163. The combination of elements in EMDR from the major psychological modalities can be effective even without eye movements. If eye movements are inappropriate (e.g., the client has visual problems or a child cannot follow the fingers), other forms of rhythmical stimulation can also be effective. Various clinicians have effectively used alternating hand taps, tones, or finger snaps. The clients can tap their own legs with their fingers. A handheld instrument can also provide alternating pulses of varying length or rate.

164. Throughout the desensitization process, the clinician interactively determines the next focus of attention and does unblocking procedures as needed.

165. A technique whereby the client is flooded with intense memories and sensations of the traumatic experience until the arousal runs its course and the client realizes that the memories are no longer able to control him. This approach can be quite upsetting for the unprepared client. Some feel that the Counting Method can also be upsetting if the exposure is too intense. If in doubt, discuss this with your therapist.

166. From D. Barrett, ed., *Trauma and Dreams* (Cambridge, Mass.: Harvard University Press, 1996), 3. Copyright © 1996 by the President and Fellows of Harvard College. Reprinted by permission of Harvard University Press, in which book Canetti's quotation also appears.

167. Compiled from Barrett, *Trauma and Dreams*.

168. L. Zadra, "Recurrent Dreams: Their Relation to Life Events," in Barrett, *Trauma and Dreams*, 231–47.

169. J. A. Lipovsky, "Assessment and Treatment of Post-Traumatic Stress Disorder in Child Survivors of Sexual Assault," in D. W. Foy, ed., *Treating PTSD: Cognitive-Behavioral Strategiesm* (New York: Guilford, 1992).

170. J. King and J. R. Sheehan, "The Use of Dreams with Incest Survivors," in Barrett, *Trauma and Dreams*, 62.

171. Some people can be verbally logical, yet still quite distressed. Healing images can be more profoundly emotionally soothing. It is thought that the images in the right hemisphere are more closely linked to the limbic system, or emotional center of the brain.

172. A number of great teachers have influenced the development of this exercise, including the skilled psychologist Arnold Lazarus, who taught time tripping at the First Annual Eastern Regional Conference in Advances in Cognitive Therapies: Helping People Change, Washington, D.C., 21–23 October 1988. The dialogue is a Gestalt technique for finishing uncompleted business. Dr. A. Dean Byrd has provided invaluable instruction in touching the past with love.

173. Adapted and reprinted with permission of the publisher, Health Communications, Inc., Deerfield Beach, Florida, from John Bradshaw, *Healing the Shame That Binds You* (Deerfield Beach, Fl.: Health Communications, Inc., 1988). The corrective experience was adapted from what first appeared in P. Levin, *Cycles of Power* (Deerfield Beach, Fl.: Health Communications, Inc., 1988).

174. The Menninger Clinic, *Imagery and Grief Work: Healing the Memory* (Topeka, Kans.: The Menninger Clinic, 1989).

175. One Vietnam vet said, "This is what our country meant to give us, and would have if the politics had been different then. I'm pretending this parade is for me, too."

176. Catherall, *Back from the Brink*.

177. From J. P. Wilson, "Treating the Vietnam Veteran," in F. M. Ochberg, ed., *Post-Traumatic Therapy and Victims of Violence* (New York: Brunner/Mazel, 1988), 254–77; B. Colodzin, *How to Survive Trauma: A Program for War Veterans and Survivors of Rape, Assault, Abuse or Environmental Disaster* (Barrytown, N.Y.: Station Hill, 1993).

178. G. C. Wilson, "Vietnam Revisited: Veterans Go Back to Battlefields to Lay Their Nightmares to Rest," *Washington Post Health Journal* (6 February 1990): 12–15.

179. A memorial to Jane Austen, Winchester Cathedral, reads, "Their grief is in proportion to their affection; they know their loss to be irreparable, but in their deepest affliction they are consoled by a firm though humble hope that her charity, devotion, faith and purity have rendered her soul acceptable in the sight of her Redeemer."

180. The grief literature suggests that symptoms of unresolved grief parallel PTSD symptoms. Survivors often increase the use of alcohol, tobacco, or drugs to medicate the pain. Visits to physicians often increase. Anniversaries, meaningful dates, and other triggers can cause grief spasms.

181. For instance, long after a fetal death, a couple realized that they had stopped developing as parents, spouses, and lovers. It was as if they had been frozen in many regards at the time of the trauma. For them it was useful to affirm, "We are parents of a dead child." This permitted them to acknowledge their loss and begin to develop again.

182. Rando discusses the concepts of tangible, intangible, and secondary losses, on which this discussion is based, in T. A. Rando, *Treatment of Complicated Mourning* (Champaign, Ill.: Research Press, 1993).

183. The discussion of uncomplicated and complicated mourning are adapted from Rando, *Complicated Mourning*.

184. "Bereavement and Grief—Part I," excerpted from the March 1987 issue of the *Harvard Mental Health Letter*. Copyright © 1987 by the President and Fellows of Harvard College.

185. Shapiro, *Eye Movement*, suggests this thought.

186. Flannery, *Victim's Guide*.

187. H. S. Kushner, *When Bad Things Happen to Good People* (New York: Avon, 1981).

188. Quoted in R. N. Ostling and M. Levin, "U.S. Judaism's Man of Paradox," *Time* (8 October 1984), 66.

189. A. Whitman, "Secret Joys of Solitude," *Reader's Digest* (April 1983), 128–32.

190. S. Vanauken, *A Severe Mercy* (New York: Bantam, 1977).

191. The suggestion to be responsible for one's suffering does not blame victims or minimize their suffering. Rather, it empowers by providing tools to understand and process suffering.

192. R. A. Schwarz, "Hypnotic Approaches in Treating PTSD: An Ericksonian Framework," in Williams and Sommer, *Handbook*, 401–17.

193. Executive Committee of the American Psychological Association, Division of Psychological Hypnosis.

194. R. A. Schwarz, "Hypnotic Approaches."

195. G. Ambrose, "Hypnosis in the Treatment of Children," *American Journal of Clinical Hypnosis* 11 (1968): 1–5, as described in Olness and Kohen, *Hypnosis with Children.*

196. D. Spring, "Art Therapy as a Visual Dialogue," in Williams and Sommer, *Handbook,* 337–51.

197. A pilot study by Charles Morgan and David Johnson at the National Center for PTSD in West Haven, Connecticut, which appeared in the December 1995 issue of the journal *Art Therapy,* found that drawing pictures of nightmares decreased the frequency and intensity of the nightmares, while writing about the nightmares led to increases. Perhaps drawing more directly discharges imagery aspects of memory, which are stored in the right brain.

198. Shapiro, *Eye Movement,* suggests reinforcing the positive images with sets of eye movements.

199. G. Roth, *Maps to Ecstasy* (San Rafael, Calif.: New World Library, 1987).

200. R. Milliken, "Dance/Movement Therapy with the Substance Abuser," *The Arts in Psychotherapy* 17 (1990): 309–17.

201. Roth, *Maps to Ecstasy.*

202. R. L. Blake and S. R. Bishop, "The Bonny Method of Guided Imagery and Music (GIM) in the Treatment of Post-Traumatic Stress Disorder (PTSD) with Adults in the Psychiatric Setting," in B. L. Wilson and M. A. Scovel, eds., "Psychiatric Music Therapy (special issue)," *Music Therapy Perspectives* 12, no. 2 (1994): 125–29.

203. Ibid.

204. H. L. Bonny, "Twenty-One Years Later: A GIM Update," in Wilson and Scovel, "Psychiatric Music Therapy," 73.

205. C. S. Off, "Drumming Technique for Assertiveness and Anger Management in the Short-Term Psychiatric Setting for Adult and Adolescent Survivors of Trauma," in Wilson and Scovel, "Psychiatric Music Therapy," 111–16.

206. T. Alston, "Storytelling: A Tool for Vietnam Veterans and Their Families," in D. K. Rhoades, M. R. Leaveck, and J. C. Hudson. *The Legacy of Vietnam Veterans and Their Families: Papers from the 1994 National Symposium* (Washington, D.C.: Agent Orange Class Assistance Program, 1995), 384–95, quote 385. Reprinted with permission.

207. J. Campbell, *The Hero with a Thousand Faces,* 3d ed. (New York: Meridian, 1975); J. Campbell, and W. Moyers, *The Power of Myth,* edited by B. S. Flowers (New York: Doubleday, 1988).

208. J. Ruth Gendler, "Fear," in *The Book of Qualities* (New York: HarperCollins Publishers, Inc., 1987).

209. With gratitude for information provided by the National Association for Drama Therapy.

210. Create Therapy Institute, 4905 Del Ray Avenue, Suite 301, Bethesda, MD 20814 ([301] 652–7183). Dr. Miller and cofounder Rebecca Milliken can often provide referrals to expressive art therapists around the country. Sand-tray example is excerpted from the in-

stitute newsletter, 1, no. 2 (August 1997): 4. Appreciation also to art therapist Dr. Eliana Gil of Rockville, Md., for assistance with this section.

211. Both examples are from M. I. Lewis and R. N. Butler, "Life-Review Therapy: Putting Memories to Work in Individual and Group Psychotherapy," *Geriatrics* 29, no. 11 (1974): 165–73.

212. See for a review: L. B. Taft and M. F. Nehrke, "Reminiscence, Life Review, and Ego Integrity in Nursing Home Residents," *International Journal of Aging and Human Development* 30, no. 3 (1990): 189–96.

213. Reprinted with slight adaptation with permission from Colodzin, *How to Survive Trauma.* Copyright © 1993 by Olympia Institute.

214. Love for others and love for self are not mutually exclusive. Ideally, the attitude of loving encircles both.

215. J. Gauthier, D. Pellerin, and P. Renaud, "The Enhancement of Self-Esteem: A Comparison of Two Cognitive Strategies," *Cognitive Therapy and Research* 7 (1983): 389–98.

216. Reprinted with permission from J. H. Childers, Jr., "Looking at Yourself Through Loving Eyes," *Elementary School Guidance and Counseling* 23 (1989): 204–9. Copyright © by American Counseling Association. No further reproduction authorized without written permission of the American Counseling Association.

217. Paraphrased from Hanh, *Peace Is Every Step*, 59.

218. The word resentment derives from words meaning "to feel again" and suggests indignation for a past offense.

219. This is itself a very complex issue. Some people's hearts are softened by compassion, by those who refuse to retaliate and instead express forgiveness and hope for the offender. For example, on *The Donahue Show*, Reginald Denny expressed compassion for the offender who severely injured him in the Los Angeles riots. He said, "It doesn't mean I'm not angry. But I truly love him." The offender's mother said that Denny was the first person to soften her son's anger. On the other hand, some hardened individuals repeatedly inflict severe suffering on others, despite repeated jailings. Perhaps stricter discipline rather than leniency is called for in such cases.

220. Quoted by Mary Grunte in D. Hales, "Three Words That Heal," *McCall's* (June 1994).

221. Dr. Judith Herman explains that mourning is not completed until we give up the hope of getting even. Revenge does not compensate for or change the harm that was done. Acts of revenge make the victim feel as bad as the offender, and waiting for compensation from the offender (e.g., an apology, acknowledgment of wrongdoing, public humiliation, or shame) holds the victim hostage to the offender's whim. Herman suggests instead that the survivor think in terms of holding the offender accountable for the crime. The survivor joins with society in bringing the offender to justice, not as a personal vendetta, but for the safety of self and the community. Even if the survivor loses the legal case, she knows she did all she could. See Herman, *Trauma and Recovery.*

222. Drs. Robert Enright and Suzanne Freedman found that incest survivors who attended forgiveness workshops had far less anxiety and depression than those who did not (*Psychology Today* [July/August 1996]: 12).

223. D. Hope, "The Healing Paradox of Forgiveness," *Psychotherapy* 24, no. 2 (1987): 240–44.

224. Related in *Fight For Your Life*, dir. M. Mears and J. Distel-Schwartz, The Fight for Your Life Co., videocassette. The Fight for Your Life Co., c/o Varied Directions, Camden, Maine, 1-800-888-5236.

225. 2 Chron. 20:15.

226. S. Trout, *To See Differently* (Washington, D.C.: Three Roses, 1990), 31.

227. Scott and Stradling, *Counseling*.

228. E. M. Carroll and D. W. Foy, "Assessment and Treatment of Combat-Related Post-Traumatic Stress Disorder in a Medical Center Setting," in Foy, *Treating PTSD*, 39–68; E. B. Foa, D. E. Hearst-Ikeda, and C. V. Dancu, *Cognitive Therapy and Prolonged Exposure (CT/PE) Manual* (Philadelphia: Allegheny University of the Health Sciences/Eastern Pennsylvania Psychiatric Institute, 1994); Smyth, *Clinician's Manual*.

229. Prolonged exposure can also be effectively applied to hierarchies for nightmares.

230. M. A. Dutton, "Assessment and Treatment of Post-Traumatic Stress Disorder Among Battered Women," in Foy, *Treating PTSD*, 69–98. Dutton feels that the client often gets sufficient exposure from simply telling the story.

231. Some may be dissociative for up to hours in therapy due to flooding of memories (C. R. Figley, "From Victim to Survivor: Social Responsibility in the Wake of Catastrophe," in Figley, *Trauma and Its Wake*, 398–415). Exacerbations in psychiatric disorders (e.g., depression, suicide, panic attacks) and drug relapse have also been reported (for review, see Meichenbaum, *Clinical Handbook*).

232. See Meichenbaum, *Clinical Handbook*, for review of these stringent criteria.

233. H. S. Resnick and T. Newton, "Assessment and Treatment of Post-Traumatic Stress Disorder in Adult Survivors of Sexual Assault," in Foy, *Treating PTSD*, 99–126.

234. Scott and Stradling, *Counseling*.

235. Scurfield, "Treatment among Vietnam Veterans"; C. M. Stuhlmiller, "Action-Based Therapy for PTSD," in Williams and Sommer, *Handbook*, 386–400.

236. Adapted from Stuhlmiller, "Action-Based Therapy."

237. O. J. Brende, *Trauma Recovery for Victims and Survivors* (Sparta, Ga.: Trauma Recovery, 1994).

238. Quoted by Carol Clurman in *USA Weekend*.

239. R. G. Tedeschi and L. G. Calhoun. "The Posttraumatic Growth Inventory: Measuring the Positive Legacy of Trauma." *Journal of Traumatic Stress* 9, no. 3 (1996): 455–71. Growth was positively correlated with optimism, religiosity, extroversion, openness, agreeableness, and conscientiousness. Spiritual change was correlated with being more optimistic, religious, and extroverted.

240. For example, van der Kolk writes, "In the Grant Study, a 50-year study of Harvard men from the 1940s to the 1990s, the men who developed PTSD after World War II were much more likely to be listed in *Who's Who in America* than their nontraumatized peers" (van der Kolk et al., *Traumatic Stress*, 28. The original study is Lee et al., "A 50-Year Prospective Study").

241. Adapted slightly and reprinted with permission from Scurfield, "Treatment among Vietnam Veterans," 886.

242. Bonding can occur even when the traumatic events are dissimilar. I am reminded of two young women in my class who formed a special friendship. One had survived a recent rape; the other deaths of eleven family members and close friends over a period of months. As they heard each other disclose their suffering, they were drawn by a sense of compassion, respect, and the bond of shared suffering.

243. R. C. Sipprelle, "A Vet Center Experience: Multievent Trauma, Delayed Treatment Type," in Foy, *Treating PTSD*, 13–38, quote 36.

244. I am grateful to Suzanne Kobasa for this concept.

245. Reprinted with the permission of The Free Press, a Division of Simon and Schuster, Inc. from James, *Treating Traumatized Children*, 173–74. Copyright © 1989 by Lexington Books.

246. Z. Harel, B. Kahana, and E. Kahana, "Social Resources and the Mental Health of Aging Nazi Holocaust Survivors and Immigrants," in Wilson and Raphael, *International Handbook*, 241–52.

247. Y. Danieli, "The Treatment and Prevention of Long-term Effects and Intergenerational Transmission of Victimization: A Lesson from Holocaust Survivors and Their Children," in Figley, *Trauma and Its Wake*, 295–313.

248. Adapted with permission from P. L. Sheehan, "Treating Intimacy Issues of Traumatized People," in Williams and Sommer, *Handbook*, 94–105.

249. F. R. Abueg and J. Fairbank, "A Behavioral Treatment of PTSD and Co-occurring Substance Abuse," in Saigh, *Post-traumatic Stress Disorder*, 111–46.

250. E. J. Letourneau, P. A. Schewe, and B. C. Frueh, "Preliminary Evaluation of Sexual Problems in Combat Veterans with PTSD," *Journal of Traumatic Stress* 10 (1997): 125–32.

251. W. I. Miller, *The Anatomy of Disgust* (Cambridge, Mass.: Harvard University Press, 1997).

252. This principle is from Hanh, *Peace Is Every Step*.

253. I am grateful to Allison Grad, whose research assisted in the compilation of this section.

254. Reprinted with the permission of The Free Press, a Division of Simon and Schuster, Inc. from James, *Treating Traumatized Children*, 90–91. Copyright © 1989 by Lexington Books.

255. B. Engel, *Raising Your Sexual Self-Esteem* (New York: Fawcett Columbine, 1995), 242.

256. Ibid., 217. Published by Ballantine Books, a division of Random House, Inc.

257. Y. M. Dolan, *Resolving Sexual Abuse: Solution-Focused Therapy and Ericksonian Hypnosis for Adult Survivors* (New York: Norton, 1991), 176; and Engle, *Sexual Self-Esteem*.

258. B. Rothschild, *An Annotated Trauma Case History: Somatic Trauma Therapy* (Online at http://users.lanminds.com/~eds/article.html, 1995).

259. S. H. Spence, *Psychosexual Therapy: A Cognitive-Behavioral Approach* (London: Chapman and Hall, 1991).

260. The interested reader is referred to L. Wallas, *Stories That Heal: Reparenting Adult Children of Dysfunctional Families Using Hypnotic Stories in Psychotherapy* (New York: Norton, 1991).

261. V. Frankl, *Man's Search for Meaning* (Boston: Beacon, 1959), 110.

262. Scurfield, "Treatment among Vietnam Veterans."

263. I am grateful to Brian Richmond for suggesting this question.

264. Yalom suggests this on page 216 of his *Existential Psychotherapy*.

265. I. Yalom, *Existential Psychotherapy* (New York: Basic Books, 1980), 439.

266. A. Maslow, "Self-actualizing and Beyond," in *The Pleasures of Psychology*, edited by D. Goleman and D. Heller, 299 (New York: New American Library, 1986).

267. W. Durrant, On the Meaning of Life (New York: Ray Long and Richard R. Smith, 1932,) 128–29.

268. Mother Teresa's life is instructive here. Born into wealth, the untimely death of her father (some feel it was a politically motivated murder) plunged her quickly into poverty before she began her odyssey of service and faith.

269. A. Ellis, "Psychotherapy and Atheistic Values: A Response to A. Bergin's 'Psychotherapy and Religious Values,'" *Journal of Consulting and Clinical Psychology* 48 (1980): 635–39.

270. Princeton Religious Research Center, *Religion in America 1992–1993* (Princeton, N.J.: Princeton Religious Research Center, 1993).

271. D. B. Larson and S. S. Larson, *The Forgotten Factor in Physical and Mental Health: What Does the Research Show?* (Rockville, Md.: National Institute for Healthcare Research, 1994), 35. Larson, a psychiatrist and former senior researcher for the National Institutes of Health, is presently president of the National Institute for Healthcare Research. This volume contains the summary of the religious research that follows.

272. J. Gartner, D. B. Larson, and G. Allen, "Religious Commitment and Mental Health: A Review of the Empirical Literature," *Journal of Psychology and Theology* 19, no. 1 (1991): 6–25. Cited in Larson and Larson, *Forgotten Factor*.

273. P. L. Benson and B. P. Spilka, "God-image as a Function of Self-esteem and Locus of Control," in *Current Perspectives in the Psychology of Religion*, edited by H. N. Maloney (Grand Rapids, Mich.: Eerdmans, 1977), 209–24.

274. D. Lowenstein, untitled poem in *Wounded Healers,* edited by R. N. Remen (Bolinas, Calif.: Wounded Healer Press, 1994), 59. Copyright © 1994 by Rachel Naomi Remen, M.D. Used by permission.

275. Frankl, *Man's Search*, 76.

276. Personal communication.

277. Benson, *Relaxation Response*, 10.

278. K. Alvarado, D. Templer, C. Bresler, and S. Thomas-Dobson, "The Relationship of Religious Variables to Death Depression and Death Anxiety," *Journal of Clinical Psychology* 51, no. 2 (1995): 202–4.

279. Weekes, *More Help,* 78. Quote following, 76.

280. Cited in J. Hinton, *Dying* (London: Pelican, 1967).

281. Shared by Karolyn Nunnallee, Mothers Against Drunk Driving.

282. A. D. Byrd and M. D. Chamberlain, *Willpower Is Not Enough* (Salt Lake City, Utah: Deseret, 1995).

283. Shared by Millie Webb, Mothers Against Drunk Driving.

284. Gallup poll analyzed by Robert Wuthnow, Princeton University sociologist, in R. Wuthnow, "Evangelicals, Liberals, and the Perils of Individualism," *Perspectives* (May 1991): 10–13.

285. The National Institute of Mental Health's Epidemiological Catchment Area Survey, cited in Larson and Larson, *The Forgotten Factor*, 11.

286. L. R. Propst, R. Ostrom, P. Watkins, T. Dean, and D. Mashburn, "Comparative Efficacy of Religious and Nonreligious Cognitive-Behavioral Therapy for the Treatment of Clinical Depression in Religious Individuals," *Journal of Consulting and Clinical Psychology* 60, no. 1 (1992): 94–103. I had a very memorable experience with this in a graduate class. I asked my class if anyone wished to demonstrate how cognitive restructuring is used in modifying anger. One volunteered, and chose as the stressor the death of her brother, who had fallen to his death from a building. Her anger centered on his careless supervisors, on her brother for not being careful, and on God for letting the accident happen. It was the latter she chose to work with. Among her self-talk was the idea, "How could a loving God allow such a good twenty-nine-year-old man to die as he did?" As we pondered this question, this idea came to my mind, which I shared, knowing her religious orientation: "How could a loving God allow a perfect thirty-three-year-old man die as He did?" She reported later that that idea helped her dispel her anger in a profound and peaceful way, for the first time in the year since his death. Often, a single question can cause cognitive restructuring at several levels simultaneously, with considerable shifts in the emotional consequences.

287. W. James, *The Varieties of Religious Experience*, (New York: Mentor, 1958), 288.

288. See Larson, *Forgotten Factor*, 88–93.

289. D. G. Myers, *The Pursuit of Happiness: Who is Happy—and Why* (New York: Morrow, 1992). Also, M.W. Fordyce, *Human Happiness: Its Nature and Its Attainment*, 2 vols. (Ft. Myers, Fla.: Cypress Lake Media, n.d.). This, along with videos and course material for the happiness course are available from Dr. Fordyce at Cypress Lake Media, 8192 College Parkway, Ft. Myers, FL 33919 ([813] 482–1660).

290. Fordyce, *Human Happiness*, 171.

291. From Hanh, *Peace Is Every Step*, 10. Copyright © 1991 by Thich Nhat Hanh. Used by permission of Bantam Books, a division of Random House, Inc.

292. J. Cornfield, *Buddha's Little Instruction Book* (New York: Bantam, 1994), 137.

293. George B. Sellarole. Contributed to *Readers Digest* (January 1997).

294. I'm grateful to Brian Richmond for this simple question that caused me such pleasure.

295. I am grateful to Dr. Francis Abueg for the many helpful ideas in this chapter, which are adapted from F. R. Abueg, A. J. Lang, K. D. Drescher, J. I. Ruzek, N. Sullivan, and J. F. Aboudarham, *Trauma Relevant Relapse Prevention Training (TRRPT): A Group Psychotherapy Protocol for PTSD and Alcoholism* (Menlo Park, Calif: National Center for PTSD, 1993). Available from F. R. Abueg at Trauma Resource Consulting, Suite 115, 4966 El Camino Real, Los Altos, CA 94022.

296. From Abueg et al., *TRRPT*.

297. The psychologist Donald Meichenbaum is recognized for developing this approach.

298. Clinicians familiar with EMDR might also process any disturbance that arises at each step. Some disturbance might be new aspects of past trauma, or it might be related to fears of failure, or fears that successful recovery will lead to abandonment by the therapist.

299. EMDR practitioners will use eye movements to reinforce the image of coping successfully and positive feelings, once negative material has been processed and ceases to come up.

300. Reprinted with permission from F. G. Cruz and L. Essen, *Adult Survivors of Childhood Emotional, Physical, and Sexual Abuse: Dynamics and Treatment* (Northvale, N.J.: Jason Aronson, 1994), 125–27. Their ideas are supplemented with those of M. A. Dutton, "Post-Traumatic Therapy with Domestic Violence Survivors," in Williams and Sommer, *Handbook*, 146–61.

301. Scott and Stradling, *Counseling*, 23.

302. Braun, "Multiple Personality Disorder."

303. E. R. Parson, "Posttraumatic Narcissism: Healing Traumatic Alterations in the Self Through Curvilinear Group Psychotherapy," in Wilson and Raphael, *International Handbook*, 821–40.

Bibliography

Abueg, F. R., A. J. Lang, K. D. Drescher, J. I. Ruzek, N. Sullivan, and J. F. Aboudarham. *Trauma Relevant Relapse Prevention Training (TRRPT): A Group Psychotherapy Protocol for PTSD and Alcoholism.* Menlo Park, Calif: National Center for PTSD, 1993.

Allen, J. G. *Coping with Trauma: A Guide to Self-Understanding.* Washington, D.C.: American Psychiatric Press, 1995.

Alvarado, K., D. Templer, C. Bresler, and S. Thomas-Dobson. "The Relationship of Religious Variables to Death Depression and Death Anxiety." *Journal of Clinical Psychology* 51, no. 2 (1995): 202–4.

American Psychiatric Association. *Diagnostic and Statistical Manual of Mental Disorders.* 4th ed. Washington, D.C.: American Psychiatric Association, 1994.

Barlow, D. H., and M. Craske. *Mastery of Your Anxiety and Panic.* Albany, N.Y.: Graywind, 1989.

Barlow, D. H., ed. *Clinical Handbook of Psychological Disorders: A Step-by-Step Treatment Manual.* 2d ed. New York: Guilford, 1993.

Barrett, D., ed. *Trauma and Dreams.* Cambridge, Mass.: Harvard University Press, 1996.

Beck, A. T., G. Emery, and R. L. Greenberg. *Anxiety Disorders and Phobias.* New York: Basic Books, 1985.

Benson, H. *Beyond the Relaxation Response.* New York: Berkley, 1984.

Benson, P. L., and B. P. Spilka. "God-image as a Function of Self-esteem and Locus of Control." In *Current Perspectives in the Psychology of Religion*, edited by H. N. Maloney, 209–24. Grand Rapids, Mich.: Eerdmans, 1977.

Borkovec, T. D., L. Wilkinson, R. Folensbee, and C. Lerman. "Stimulus Control Applications to the Treatment of Worry." *Behavior Research and Therapy* 21 (1983): 247–51.

Bremner, J. D., and E. Brett. "Trauma-related Dissociative States and Long-term Psychopathology in Post-traumatic Stress Disorder." *Journal of Traumatic Stress* 10, no.1 (1997): 37–49.

Brende, J. O. *Trauma Recovery for Victims and Survivors*. Sparta, Ga.: Trauma Recovery, 1994.

Breslau, N., G. C. Davis, and P. Andreski. "Traumatic Events and Post Traumatic Stress Disorder in an Urban Population of Young Adults." *Archives of General Psychiatry* 48 (1991): 216–22.

Byrd, A. D., and M. D. Chamberlain. *Willpower Is Not Enough*. Salt Lake City, Utah: Deseret, 1995.

Campbell, J. *The Hero with a Thousand Faces*. 3d ed. New York: Meridian, 1975.

Campbell, J., and W. Moyers. *The Power of Myth*. Edited by B. S. Flowers. New York: Doubleday, 1988.

Carnes, P., and J. M. Moriarity. *Sexual Anorexia: Overcoming Sexual Self-Hatred*. Center City, Minn.: Hazelden, 1997.

Catherall, D. R. *Back from the Brink: A Family Guide to Overcoming Traumatic Stress*. New York: Bantam, 1992.

Cloud, H., and J. Townsend. *Boundaries: When to Say Yes, When to Say No, To take Control of Your Life*. Grand Rapids, Mich.: Zondervan Publishing, 1992.

Cohen, B. M., M. Barnes, and A. B. Rankin. *Managing Traumatic Stress Through Art*. Lutherville, Md.: Sidran, 1995.

Coleman, V. D., and P. M. Farris-Dufrene. *Art Therapy and Psychotherapy: Blending Two Therapeutic Approaches*. New York: Taylor and Francis, 1996.

Colodzin, B. *How to Survive Trauma: A Program for War Veterans and Survivors of Rape, Assault, Abuse or Environmental Disaster*. Barrytown, N.Y.: Station Hill, 1993.

Cornfield, J. *Buddha's Little Instruction Book*. New York: Bantam, 1994.

Cruz, F. G., and L. Essen. *Adult Survivors of Childhood Emotional, Physical, and Sexual Abuse: Dynamics and Treatment*. Northvale, N.J.: Jason Aronson, 1994.

Davidson, J. R. T., and E. B. Foa, eds. *Posttraumatic Stress Disorder: DSM-IV and Beyond*. Washington, D.C.: American Psychiatric Press, 1993.

Dolan, Y. M. *Resolving Sexual Abuse: Solution-Focused Therapy and Ericksonian Hypnosis for Adult Survivors*. New York: Norton, 1991.

Durrant, W. *On the Meaning of Life*. New York: Ray Long and Richard R. Smith, 1932.

Engel, B. *Raising Your Sexual Self-Esteem*. New York: Fawcett Columbine, 1995.

Everly, G. S., Jr. "Short-Term Psychotherapy of Acute Adult Onset Post-Traumatic Stress: The Role of Weltanschauung." *Stress Medicine* 10 (1994): 191–96.

Everly, G. S., Jr., and J. M. Lating, eds. *Psychotraumatology: Key Papers and Core Concepts in Post-Traumatic Stress*. New York: Plenum, 1995.

Everstine, D. S., and L. Everstine. *The Trauma Response: Treatment for Emotional Injury*. New York: Norton, 1993.

Figley, C. R., ed. *Trauma and Its Wake: The Study and Treatment of Post-traumatic Stress Disorder*. New York: Brunner/Mazel, 1985.

Figley, C. R. *Helping Traumatized Families*. San Francisco: Jossey-Bass, 1989.

Figley, C. R., B. E. Bride, and N. Mazza, eds. *Death and Trauma: The Traumatology of Grieving*. Washington, D.C.: Taylor and Francis, 1997.

Flannery, R. B., Jr. *Post-Traumatic Stress Disorder: The Victim's Guide to Healing and Recovery*. New York: Crossroad, 1992.

———. *Violence in the Workplace*. New York: Crossroad, 1995.

Foa, E. B., D. E. Hearst-Ikeda, and C. V. Dancu. *Cognitive Therapy and Prolonged Exposure (CT/PE) Manual*. Philadelphia: Allegheny University of the Health Sciences/Eastern Pennsylvania Psychiatric Institute, 1994.

Fontana, A., and R. Rosenheck. "A Causal Model of the Etiology of War-related PTSD." *Journal of Traumatic Stress* 6 (1993): 475–500.

Fordyce, M. W. *Human Happiness: Its Nature and Its Attainment*. 2 vols. Ft. Myers, Fla.: Cypress Lake Media, n.d.

Foy, D. W., ed. *Treating PTSD: Cognitive-Behavioral Strategies*. New York: Guilford, 1992.

Frankl, V. *Man's Search for Meaning*. Boston: Beacon, 1959.

Gauthier, J., D. Pellerin, and P. Renaud. "The Enhancement of Self-Esteem: A Comparison of Two Cognitive Strategies." *Cognitive Therapy and Research* 7 (1983): 389–98.

Gil, E. *The Healing Power of Play: Working with Abused Children*. New York: Guilford, 1991.

Goleman, D., and D. Heller, eds. *The Pleasures of Psychology*. New York: New American Library, 1986.

Green, B. L., and J. Wolfe. "Traumatic Memory Research." *Journal of Traumatic Stress* 8, no. 4 (1995).

Hanh, T. N. *Peace Is Every Step: The Path of Mindfulness in Everday Life*. New York: Bantam, 1991.

Harvey, M. R. "An Ecological View of Psychological Trauma and Trauma Recovery." *Journal of Traumatic Stress* 9, no.1 (1996): 3–23.

Herman, J. *Trauma and Recovery*. New York: Basic, 1997.

Hinton, J. *Dying*. London: Pelican, 1967.

Horowitz, M. J. "Psychological Response to Serious Life Events." In *Human Stress and Cognition*, edited by V. Hamilton and D. M. Warburton. New York: Wiley, 1979.

———. *Stress Response Syndromes*. 2d ed. New York: Jason Aronson, 1986.

Hossack, A. and R. P. Bentall. "Elimination of Posttraumatic Symptomatology by Relaxation and Visual-Kinesthetic Dissociation." *Journal of Traumatic Stress* 9, no.1 (1996): 99–110.

James, B. *Treating Traumatized Children: New Insights and Creative Interventions*. Lexington, Mass.: Lexington, 1989.

James, W. *The Varieties of Religious Experience*. New York: Mentor, 1958.

Kassinove, H., ed. *Anger Disorders: Definition, Diagnosis and Treatment*. Washington, D.C.: Taylor and Francis, 1995.

Kessler, R. C., K. A. McGonagle, S. Zhao, C. B. Nelson, M. Hughes, S. Eshleman, H. Wittchen, and K. S. Kendler. "Lifetime and 12-month Prevalence of DSM-III-R Psychiatric Disorders in the United States." *Archives of General Psychiatry* 51 (1994): 8–19.

Kluft, R. P. "Multiple Personality Disorder." In *Review of Psychiatry*, edited by A. Tasman and S. Goldfinge, 375–84. Washington, D.C.: American Psychiatric Press, 1991.

Kulka, R. A., W. E. Schlenger, J. A. Fairbank, R. L. Hough, B. K. Jordan, C. R. Marmar, and D. S. Weiss. *Trauma and the Vietnam War Generation: Report of Findings from the National Vietnam Veterans Readjustment Study*. New York: Brunner/Mazel, 1990.

Kushner, H. S. *When Bad Things Happen to Good People*. New York: Schocken, 1989.

Larson, D. B., and S. S. Larson. *The Forgotten Factor in Physical and Mental Health: What Does the Research Show?* Rockville, Md.: National Institute for Healthcare Research, 1994.

Lee, K. A., G. E. Vaillant, W. C. Torrey, and G. H. Elder. "A 50-year Prospective Study of the Psychological Sequelae of World War II Combat." *American Journal of Psychiatry* 152, no. 4 (1995): 141–48.

Letourneau, E. J., P. A. Schewe, and B. C. Frueh. "Preliminary Evaluation of Sexual Problems in Combat Veterans with PTSD." *Journal of Traumatic Stress* 10, no.1 (1997): 125–32.

Lewinsohn, P., R. Munoz, M. Youngren, and A. Zeiss. *Control Your Depression.* New York: Prentice Hall, 1986.

Lewis, M. I., and R. N. Butler. "Life-Review Therapy: Putting Memories to Work in Individual and Group Psychotherapy." *Geriatrics* 29, no. 11 (1974): 165–73.

Lowenstein, D. Untitled poem. In *Wounded Healers*, edited by R. N. Remen. Bolinas, Calif.: Wounded Healer Press, 1994.

Marlatt, G. A., and J. R. Gordon, eds. *Relapse Prevention.* New York: Guilford, 1985.

Maslow, A. "Self-actualizing and Beyond." In *The Pleasures of Psychology*, edited by D. Goleman and D. Heller, 299. New York: New American Library, 1986.

Matsakis, A. *I Can't Get Over It: A Handbook for Trauma Survivors.* Oakland, Calif.: New Harbinger, 1992.

———. *Post-Traumatic Stress Disorder: A Complete Treatment Guide.* Oakland, Calif.: New Harbinger, 1994.

Mayo, B. *Jefferson Himself: The Personal Narrative of a Many-Sided American.* Charlottesville,Va.: University Press of Virginia, 1942.

Meichenbaum, D. *A Clinical Handbook/Practical Therapist Manual for Assessing and Treating Adults with Post-Traumatic Stress Disorder.* Waterloo, Ontario: Institute Press, 1994.

Miller, W. I. *The Anatomy of Disgust.* Cambridge, Mass.: Harvard University Press, 1997.

Milliken, R. "Dance/Movement Therapy with the Substance Abuser." *The Arts in Psychotherapy* 17 (1990): 309–17.

Moore, T. *Care of the Soul.* New York: Harper Perennial, 1994.

Mother Teresa. *Total Surrender.* Edited by A. Devananda. Ann Arbor, Mich.: Servant, 1985.

Murray, E. J., A. D. Lamnin, and C. S. Carver. "Emotional Expression in Written Essays and Psychotherapy." *Journal of Social and Clinical Psychology* 8 (1989): 414–29.

Murray, E. J., and D. L. Segal. "Emotional Processing in Vocal and Written Expression of Feelings About Traumatic Experiences." *Journal of Traumatic Stress* 7 (1994): 391–405.

Muss, D. *The Trauma Trap.* London: Doubleday, 1991.

Myers, D. G. *The Pursuit of Happiness: Who is Happy—and Why.* New York: Morrow, 1992.

Olness, K., and D. P. Kohen. *Hypnosis and Hypnotherapy with Children.* 3d ed. New York: Guilford, 1996.

Ozer, D., J. M. Healy, Jr., and R. A. J. Stewart, eds. *Perspectives on Personality.* Vol. 3. Greenwich, Conn.: JAI, 1991.

Pennebaker, J. W. *Opening Up: The Healing Power of Expressing Emotion.* New York: Guilford, 1997.

Peterson, K. C., M. F. Prout, and R. A. Schwarz. *Post-Traumatic Stress Disorder: A Clinician's Guide.* New York: Plenum, 1991.

"Post-Traumatic Stress Disorder—Part II." *The Harvard Mental Health Letter* 13, no. 1 (July 1996): 1–5.

Princeton Religious Research Center. *Religion in America* 1992–1993. Princeton, N.J.: Princeton Religious Research Center, 1993.

Propst, L. R., R. Ostrom, P. Watkins, T. Dean, and D. Mashburn. "Comparative Efficacy of Religious and Nonreligious Cognitive-Behavioral Therapy for the Treatment of Clinical Depression in Religious Individuals." *Journal of Consulting and Clinical Psychology* 60, no. 1 (1992): 94–103.

Reiger, D., W. Narrow, D. Rae, R. W. Manderscheid, B. Z. Locke, and F. K. Goodwin. "The De Facto U.S. Mental and Addictive Disorders Service System: Epidemiologic Catchment Area Prospective 1-year Prevalence Rates of Disorders and Services." *Archives of General Psychiatry* 50 (1993): 85–94.

Rhoades, D. K., M. R. Leaveck, and J. C. Hudson. *The Legacy of Vietnam Veterans and Their Families: Papers from the 1994 National Symposium.* Washington, D.C.: Agent Orange Class Assistance Program, 1995.

Rinpoche, S. *The Tibetan Book of Living and Dying.* San Francisco: Harper, 1993.

Ross, J. *Triumph over Fear: A Book of Help and Hope for People with Anxiety, Panic Attacks, and Phobias.* New York: Bantam, 1994.

Saigh, P. A., ed. *Post-traumatic Stress Disorder: A Behavioral Approach to Assessment and Treatment.* Boston: Allyn and Bacon, 1992.

Schiraldi, G. *Stress Management Strategies.* Dubuque, Iowa: Kendall/Hunt, 1994.

———. *Conquer Anxiety, Worry, and Nervous Fatigue: A Guide to Greater Peace.* Ellicott City, Md.: Chevron, 1997.

———. *Building Self-Esteem: A 125-Day Program.* Ellicott City, Md.: Chevron, 1999.

Scott, M. J., and S. G. Stradling. *Counseling for Post-Traumatic Stress Disorder.* London: Sage, 1992.

Scurfield, R. M. "Treatment of Posttraumatic Stress Disorder among Vietnam Veterans." In *International Handbook of Traumatic Stress Syndromes,* edited by J. P. Wilson and B. Raphael, 879–88. New York: Plenum, 1993.

———. "War-Related Trauma: An Integrative Experiential, Cognitive, and Spiritual Approach." In *Handbok of Post-traumatic Therapy,* edited by M. B.

Williams and J. F. Sommer, Jr., 179–204. Westport, Conn.: Greenwood Press, 1994.

Segal, D. L., and E. J. Murray. "Emotional Processing in Cognitive Therapy and Vocal Expression of Feeling." *Journal of Social and Clinical Psychology* 13 (1994): 189–206.

Shapiro, F. *Eye Movement Desensitization and Reprocessing: Basic Principles, Protocols, and Procedures.* New York: Guilford, 1995.

Simon, S., and S. Simon. *Forgiveness: How to Make Peace with Your Past and Get on with Your Life.* New York: Warner, 1990.

Smyth, L. D. *Clinician's Manual for the Cognitive-Behavioral Treatment of Post Traumatic Stress Disorder.* Havre de Grace, Md.: RTR Publishing, 1994.

——. *Treating Anxiety Disorders with a Cognitive-Behavioral Exposure Based Approach and the Eye-Movement Technique.* Havre de Grace, Md.: RTR Publishing, 1996. Videocassette.

——. *Treating Anxiety Disorders with a Cognitive-Behavioral Exposure Based Approach and the Eye-Movement Technique, Viewer's Guide.* Havre de Grace, Md.: RTR Publishing, 1996.

Solomon, S. D., E. T. Gerrity, and A. M. Muff. "Efficacy of Treatments for Posttraumatic Stress Disorder." *Journal of the American Medical Association* 268, no. 5 (1992): 633–38.

Spence, S. H. *Psychosexual Therapy: A Cognitive-Behavioral Approach.* London: Chapman and Hall, 1991.

Taft, L. B., and M. F. Nehrke. "Reminiscence, Life Review, and Ego Integrity in Nursing Home Residents." *International Journal of Aging and Human Development* 30, no. 3 (1990): 189–96.

Tedeschi, R. G., and L. G. Calhoun. "The Posttraumatic Growth Inventory: Measuring the Positive Legacy of Trauma." *Journal of Traumatic Stress* 9, no. 3 (1996): 455–71.

Timmons, B. H., and R. Ley, eds. *Behavioral and Psychological Approaches to Breathing Disorders.* New York: Plenum, 1994.

Trout, S. *To See Differently.* Washington, D.C.: Three Roses, 1990.

Vanauken, S. *A Severe Mercy.* New York: Bantam, 1977.

van der Kolk, B. A., A. C. McFarlane, and L. Weisaeth, eds. *Traumatic Stress: The Effects of Overwhelming Experience on Mind, Body, and Society.* New York: Guilford, 1996.

Van Dis, H. "Hyperventilation in Phobic Patients." In *Stress and Anxiety*, Vol. 5., edited by C. D. Spielberger and I. G. Sarason. New York: Hemisphere, 1978.

Weekes, C. *More Help for Your Nerves*. New York: Bantam, 1984.

Wells, K. B., G. Goldberg, R. H. Brook, and B. Leake. "Quality of Care for Psychotropic Drug Use in Internal Medicine Group Practices." *Western Journal of Medicine* 145 (1986): 710–14.

Williams, M. B., and J. F. Sommer, Jr., eds. *Handbook of Post-traumatic Therapy*. Westport, Conn.: Greenwood Press, 1994.

Wilson, B. L., and M. A. Scovel, eds. "Psychiatric Music Therapy." *Music Therapy Perspectives* 12, no. 2 (1994).

Wilson, J. P., and B. Raphael, eds. *International Handbook of Traumatic Stress Syndromes*. New York: Plenum, 1993.

Wolf, M. E., and A. D. Mosnaim, eds. *Post-traumatic Stress Disorder: Etiology, Phenomenology, and Treatment*. Washington, D.C.: American Psychiatric Press, 1990.

Yalom, I. *Existential Psychotherapy*. New York: Basic Books, 1980.

Index

About the Author

Glenn R. Schiraldi, Ph.D., has served on the stress management faculties at the Pentagon and the University of Maryland, where he received the Outstanding Teacher Award in the College of Health and Human Performance. He is the author of various articles and books on human mental and physical health, including *Conquer Anxiety, Worry and Nervous Fatigue: A Guide to Greater Peace; Hope and Help for Depression: A Practical Guide; Facts to Relax By: A Guide to Relaxation and Stress Reduction*; and *Building Self-Esteem: A 125-Day Program*. He serves on the Board of Directors of the Depression and Related Affective Disorders Association. He is a graduate of the U.S. Military Academy, West Point, and holds graduate degrees in Health Education from Brigham Young University and the University of Maryland.